Recent Results in Cancer Research 158

Springer
Berlin
Heidelberg
New York
Barcelona
Hong Kong
London
Milan
Paris
Singapore
Tokyo

U. Reinhold W. Tilgen (Eds.)

Minimal Residual Disease in Melanoma

Biology, Detection and Clinical Relevance

With 40 Figures and 45 Tables

Springer

Prof. Dr. med. Uwe Reinhold
Prof. Dr. med. Wolfgang Tilgen

Universitätskliniken des Saarlandes
Haut- und Poliklinik
66421 Homburg/Saar, Germany

ISBN-13:978-3-642-64015-5 e-ISBN-13:978-3-642-59537-0
DOI: 10.1007/978-3-642-59537-0

ISSN 0080-0015

Library of Congress Cataloging-in-Publication Data
Minimal residual disease in melanoma: biology, detection, and clinical relevance / U. Reinhold, W. Tilgen (eds.). p.; cm. – (Recent results in cancer research; 158) Includes bibliographical references and index.
ISBN-13:978-3-642-64015-5 (hardcover: alk. paper) 1. Melanoma. 2. Metastasis. I. Reinhold, Uwe. II. Tilgen W. (Wolfgang), 1944 – III. International Symposium on Minimal Residual Disease in Melanoma (1st: 1999: Homburg, Saarland, Germany) IV. Series. [DNLM: 1. Neoplasm, Residual-diagnosis-Congresses. 2. Melanoma-complications-Congresses. 3. Neoplasm, Metasis-diagnosis-Congresses. 4. Neoplasm, Residual-therapy-Congresses. QZ 202 M6653 2000] RC280.M37 M56 2000 616.99'477-dc21.

Springer-Verlag Berlin Heidelberg New York
a member of BertelsmannSpringer Science+Business Media GmbH

Softcover reprint of the hardcover 1st edition 2001

Production: PRO EDIT GmbH, 69126 Heidelberg, Germany
Typesetting: K+V Fotosatz GmbH, 64743 Beerfelden, Germany

Printed on acid-free paper SPIN 10764787 21/3130göh 5 4 3 2 1 0

Preface

Knowledge about diagnostic procedures in melanoma has increased rapidly within the past few years. Single tumor cells have been identified in normal tissue such as sentinel lymph nodes, as well as in bone marrow, peripheral blood, and other bodily fluids and cells, by molecular technologies. The introduction of polymerase chain reaction-based methods can be regarded as a prototype of this dramatic development towards molecular approaches in new diagnostic procedures. This fact opens up the possibility of clinical use in patients and of influencing treatment strategies. Considerable discrepancies have been described, however, in the success rates of these new techniques for the detection of minimal residual disease in cancer patients. Despite favorable results reported by different groups of investigators, it will take several years to define the clinical and pathophysiological relevance of new diagnostic procedures.

The 1st International Symposium "Minimal Residual Disease in Melanoma: Biology, Detection and Clinical Relevance of Micrometastases", held in September 1999 in Homburg/Saar, Germany, focused on recent developments in this particular area of cancer research. The purpose of the meeting was to stimulate discussion and exchange of new data and ideas by renowned international scientists.

The aim of this volume is to summarize major topics of basic research and clinical investigations presented by invited experts in this fascinating but still controversial field of melanoma research. Despite the fact that especially the basic science of tumor biology is subject to rapid change, this book will give an overview of the present status of new diagnostic strategies.

We wish to thank all contributors as well as all those who helped us to organize the symposium and to produce this volume.

Uwe Reinhold
Wolfgang Tilgen
Summer 2000 Homburg/Saar, Germany

Contents

I. Biology of Micrometastases and Advances in Methods for Detection

II. Detection of Residual Melanoma Cells in the Peripheral Blood and Bone Marrow

III. Detection of Minimal Residual Disease in Sentinel Nodes

IV. Early Recognition and Monitoring by Serological Markers

V. Clinical Relevance of Micrometastases Detection

VI. Therapeutic Strategies Against Residual Melanoma Cells

List of Contributors*

Aamdal, S.[40]
Abken, H.[249]
Albrecht, J.[204]
Ascierto, P.A.[200]
Assenmacher, M.[51]
Bachter, D.[129]
Balda, B.R.[129]
Barnhill, R.L.[3]
Benez, A.[113]
Bhattacharya, S.[63]
Blaheta, H.-J.[93, 137]
Bock, M.[118]
Bonfrer, J.M.G.[149]
Bosserhoff, A.K.[158]
Botti, G.[200]
Breuninger, H.[137]
Büchels, H.[129]
Buettner, R.[158]
Bystryn, J.-C.[204]
Castello, G.[200]
Christophers, E.[169]
Coit, D.G.[63]
Conrad, A.[204]
Cossu, A.[200]
Curry, B.J.[211]
Deichmann, M.[118]
Dreau, D.[158]
Ellwanger, U.[93]
Faye, R.[40]
Ferrone, S.[231]
Fierlbeck, G.[113]
Fodstad, Ø.[40, 51]
Garbe, C.[93, 137]
Ghossein, R.A.[63]
Gläser, R.[169]
Glass, L.F.[187]
Harris, M.N.[204]
Hauschild, A.[169]
Hein, R.[158]
Herber, M.[51]
Herfarth, C.[181]
Hersey, P.[211]
Heuser, C.[249]
Høifødt, H.K.[40]
Holder, W.D.[158]
Hombach, A.[249]
Hoon, D.S.B.[78]
Hunzelmann, N.[51]
Jäckel, A.[118]
Jung, R.[32]
Keilholz, U.[25]
Knebel Doeberitz, M. von[118]
Koch, M.[181]
Korse, C.M.[149]
Krüger, W.[32]
Lacroix, J.[181]
Landthaler, M.[158]
Li, W.[187]

* The address of the principal author is given on the first page of each contribution.
[1] Page on which contribution begins.

Lin, J.[187]
Lissia, A.[200]
Max, N.[25]
Messina, J.[187]
Michl, C.[129]
Miltenyi, S.[51]
Morton, D.L.[78]
Motti, M.L.[200]
Mozzillo, N.[200]
Myers, K.[211]
Näher, H.[118]
Nakayama, T.[78]
Nestle, F.O.[236]
Neumaier, M.[32]
Nguyen, D.-H.[78]
O'Day, S.J.[78]
Oratz, R.[204]
Otte, M.[14]
Palmieri, G.[105]
Pantel, K.[14]
Pirastu, M.[200]
Rappl, G.[105]
Reinhold, U.[105, 249]
Reintgen, D.S.[187]
Reynolds, S.R.[204]
Rivas, M.C.[204]
Roses, D.F.[204]
Satriano, S.M.R.[200]
Schadendorf, D.[236]
Schiebel, U.[113]
Schittek, B.[93, 137]
Schmitz, J.[51]
Schrödel, A.[181]
Seiter, S.[105]
Shapiro, R.L.[204]
Shivers, S.C.[187]
Siewert, C.[51]
Skovlund, E.[40]
Soondrum, K.[32]
Spike, B.[25]
Stafford, M.[187]
Stall, A.[187]
Strazzullo, M.[200]
Taback, B.[78]
Tanda, F.[200]
Thiel, E.[25]
Tilgen, W.[105]
Ugurel, S.[105]
Vogt, H.[129]
Wacker, J.[118]
Waldmann, V.[118]
Wang, X.[231]
Weitz, J.[181]
Wolf, K.[25]

I. Biology of Micrometastases and Advances in Methods for Detection

The Biology of Melanoma Micrometastases

R. L. Barnhill

Dermatopathology Divisions, Department of Pathology,
Brigham and Women's Hospital, Harvard Medical School, Boston, MA 02115,
USA and the Johns Hopkins Medical Institutions, Baltimore, MD 21239, USA

Abstract

The biology and significance of micrometastases remain poorly understood. Whether such deposits represent hypothetical "dormant" metastases, simply the earliest metastases recognizable, or both has not been resolved. Attempting to answer the latter question among many others, we carried out studies on the rates of proliferation, and microvessel counts in melanoma micrometastases taken from sentinel lymph nodes as compared to conventional melanoma lymph node macrometastases. We found that these micrometastases were not vascularized and had low (and comparable) rates of both proliferation and apoptosis, suggesting a steady or dormant state. On the other hand, the macrometastases were fully vascularized and more proliferative, i.e., they had rates of proliferation that were significantly higher compared to the micrometastases and rate of apoptosis. How micrometastases develop is also poorly understood. Tumor cells are thought to arrive in lymph nodes and other sites through the blood and lymphatic circulation and to extravasate. However, in addition to the latter explanation, another mechanism may be operable which we have proposed as *extravascular migratory metastasis*. In studies of metastatic melanoma we have identified melanoma cells positioned on the surface of endothelial cells both by light and electron microscopy. We have also identified ultrastructurally the presence of an amorphous matrix interposed between the latter two cell types that shows immunostaining for laminin and, recently, the beta-2 chain of laminin. Thus, we currently believe that the latter form of "free" laminin may play a role in this proposed mechanism of metastasis and thus in the formation of micrometastases.

Recent Results in Cancer Research, Vol. 158

Introduction

The biology and significance of micrometastases remain poorly understood. Whether such foci represent hypothetical "dormant" metastases, simply the earliest recognizable metastases, cellular deposits in transit, or all three has not been resolved.

The concept of dormant metastases was hypothesized to explain why solid tumors such as malignant melanoma and breast cancer may develop metastases after disease-free intervals as long as 10–40 years following reaction of the primary tumor and the failure of wide surgical resection margins and elective lymph node dissection to influence prognosis [1–4]. In addition to development of metastases after long periods of time, it has been observed that the subsequent survival of melanoma patients is largely unrelated to disease-free interval; i.e., once melanoma recurs, the subsequent prognosis is fairly predictable, irrespective of the antecedent disease-free interval [1]. The latter observations suggest that microscopic tumor foci may remain quiescent for variable periods of time before some event or events trigger the development of detectable/progressive tumors [1, 2].

Occult or clinically undetectable metastases (micrometastases) have been observed for many years in patients undergoing prophylactic lymph node dissections for various types of solid tumors, including cutaneous melanoma [1, 2]. Recent investigation in animal models has provided evidence that micrometastases do not possess the properties needed for progressive tumor growth; more specifically, these micrometastases are not fully vascularized and are characterized by balanced rates of proliferation and apoptosis suggesting a "dormant" state [5, 6]. The attributes of such micrometastases have never been studied in humans.

Tumor Vascularity, Proliferation, and Apoptosis in Human Melanoma Micrometastases

In recent work, we utilized eight microscopic (clinically undetectable) melanoma metastases obtained from sentinel lymph nodes and 12 macroscopic (clinically palpable) melanoma lymph node metastases to study tumor vascularity, tumor proliferation rate, and rate of apoptosis [7].

Tumor vascularity was quantified using the lectin *Ulex europaeus* agglutinin I to identify microvessels per unit area (7.84×10^{-2} mm^2 at ×400 magnification) with an ocular grid. Melanoma cell proliferation rate was assessed with the MIB-1 antibody (Ki-67) as the number of positive nuclei per total tumor nuclei counted at ×400 magnification.

Apoptosis was quantified using the TdT-mediated dUTP-biotin nick end labeling (TUNEL) method [8]. Positive reactions were detected with a peroxidase-labeled antibody against deoxyuridine triphosphate (dUTP)-digoxigenin.

Table 1. Summary of results

	Mean *n* microvessels	Mean proliferation rate	Mean apoptosis rate
Micrometastases	10.2	2.4%	0.2%
Macrometastases	18.7	18.0	1.6
P	$p=0.0134$	$p=0.0003$	–

Tumor Vascularity

The microvessel counts in the micrometastases ranged from 5 to 22 (mean 10.2) and were not higher compared to the surrounding tissue (Table 1). The macrometastases exhibited significantly higher numbers of tumor microvessels, ranging from nine to 33 (mean 18.7) ($p=0.0134$) compared to micrometastases (Fig. 1 A, B).

Rate of Tumor Cell Proliferation

The proliferation rates for micrometastases ranged from 0.9% to 6.3% (mean 2.4%) and were significantly lower than those for macrometastases (range 5.0% to 35%, mean 18.0%) ($p=0.0003$) (Fig. 1 C, D).

Rate of Apoptosis

The rates of apoptosis were low in both groups of metastases. The micrometastases had apoptotic rates ranging from 0 (for five cases) to 1.0% (mean 0.2%), while the macrometastases had rates ranging from 0.9% to 5.5% (mean 1.6%) (Fig. 1 E, F).

Our findings show that melanoma micrometastases are not vascularized to the degree of clinically detectable macrometastases. In general, the number of tumor microvessels in the micrometastases in general was not increased compared to surrounding tissue, indicating that such metastatic foci have not switched to the angiogenic phenotype and thus are not yet capable of progressive growth. This scenario is directly analogous to that with primary tumors that have not achieved sufficient size and/or shown the transition to the angiogenic phenotype. The capacity of metastases to remain microscopic (and dormant) for long periods of time is hypothetical but supported by clinical observations already mentioned; i. e., the survival of patients after development of metastases is fairly predictable, irrespective of the length of the antecedent disease-free interval.

The micrometastases also exhibited much lower rates of tumor cell proliferation compared to macrometastases. Although the proliferation rate was slightly greater than that of apoptosis, the rates are of comparable magni-

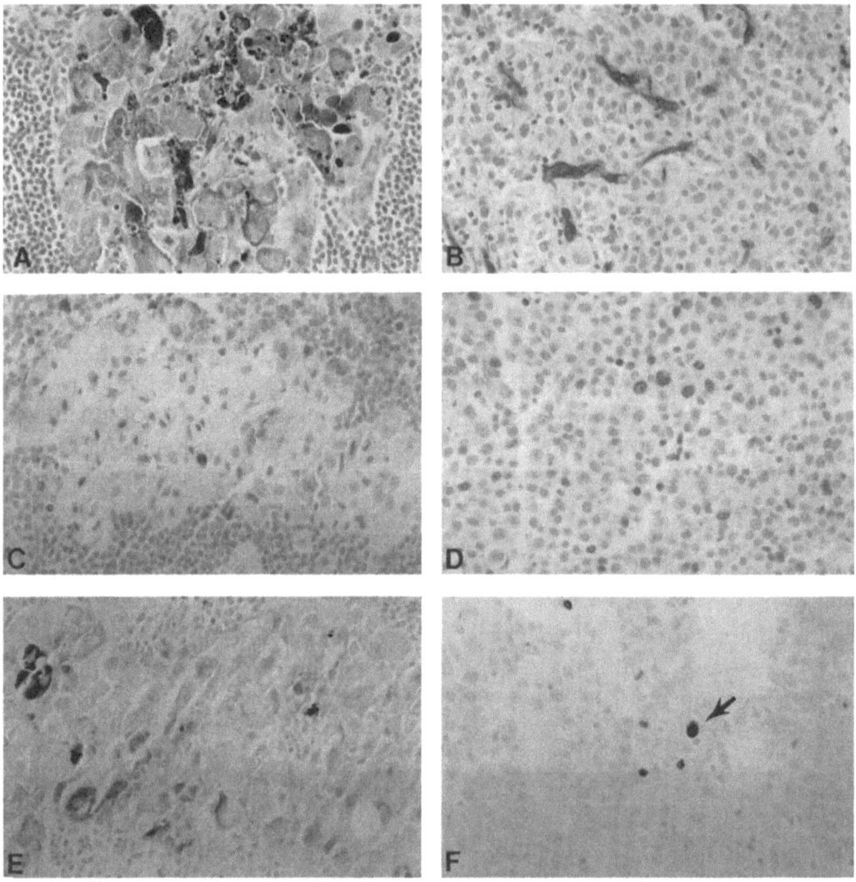

Fig. 1. A Melanoma micrometastasis. Tumor vascularity is not increased compared to background of lymph node. Blood vessels stain red (fast red) with the lectin *Ulex europaeus* agglutinin I. **B** Melanoma macrometastasis. Significantly increased numbers of microvessels as compared to the micrometastasis. **C** Melanoma micrometastasis. Very low rate of cellular proliferation as assessed by the MIB-1 (Ki-67) antibody. Only a few melanoma cells with positive (red) staining. **D** Melanoma macrometastasis. Much higher rate of proliferation as compared to the left. **E** Melanoma micrometastasis. There are no nuclei identified as apoptotic with the TUNEL method (medium brown staining) in this field. The brown pigment is cytoplasmic melanin. **F** Melanoma macrometastasis. Five nuclei are identified as apoptotic (positive brown staining) in this field

tude. Thus, these results seem to indicate that micrometastases exhibit balanced rates of proliferation and apoptosis in a fashion similar to those reported in experimental animal studies [5, 6]. These metastatic foci appear to have achieved a steady state in which tumor size remains small and constant and metabolic demands are not excessive because of relatively low rates of proliferation. Such a state can explain how micrometastases may remain dormant for many years or even indefinitely. On the other hand, the macrometastases showed significantly greater rates of proliferation than apoptosis, consistent with progressive tumor growth and enlargement.

These studies suggest that, as a group, the micrometastases studied herein have not acquired the properties needed for progressive tumor growth, as evidenced by low tumor vascularity and proliferation rates. Our results suggest that these micrometastases may be analogous to dormant metastases described in animal models [5, 6]. However, we realize that some heterogeneity is likely in such a group of microscopic tumor deposits and there is a need to study additional specimens. Nonetheless, this is the first study to analyze the properties of clinically undetectable metastases in humans, and it provides the first data on this unique group of lesions.

Extravascular Migratory Metastasis

How micrometastases develop is also poorly understood. Tumor cells are thought to arrive in lymph nodes and other sites through the blood and lymphatic circulation and to extravasate. However, in addition to the latter explanations, another mechanism may be operable which we have proposed be termed *extravascular migratory metastasis.*

Among the extracellular matrix components, laminin is regarded as playing an essential role in cancer progression [9–13], and tumor cells are capable of secreting laminin. A recent ultrastructural study described a hitherto unrecognized image in human malignant melanoma termed the "angiotumoral complex". In this angio-tumoral complex, tumor cells and endothelium are in contact via an amorphous matrix containing mainly "free" laminin, as opposed to laminin "integrated" into a lamina or basement membrane (Fig. 2) [9]. This distinctive association is absent in melanocytic nevi. This periendothelial laminin may therefore be involved in promoting tumor migration. Because of the small number of cases examined in the latter study and the potential value of such a feature as a marker of invasiveness, we examined 45 additional cases of primary invasive or metastatic melanoma [11]. These tumors were studied by electron microscopy for the presence of this amorphous matrix and by immunohistochemistry to confirm the presence of laminin in this amorphous material.

The 45 cases included consisted of (1) five primary melanomas, (2) two clear cell sarcomas, and (3) 38 melanomas that were recurrent, metastatic, or indeterminate with respect to status, e.g., as to whether they were primary or metastatic. The latter group included 13 tumors from lymph nodes and 25 from various visceral and soft tissue sites.

Among the 45 cases examined by electron microscopy, 28 had paraffin blocks containing sufficient tissue for study by immunohistochemistry.

Electron Microscopy

Among the 45 melanomas examined by electron microscopy, 41 exhibited an amorphous material or matrix between tumor cells and/or in a periendothe-

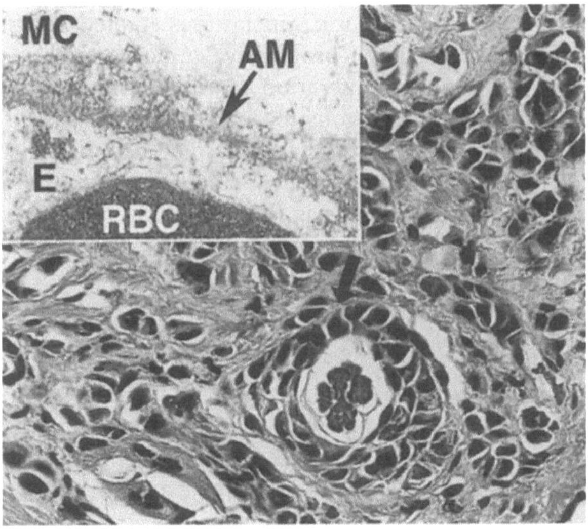

Fig. 2. Primary angiotropic melanoma. Note tumor cells surrounding microvessel in pericytic location. Electron microscopy (*insert*) shows the amorphous matrix (*AM*) between endothelium (*E*) and a melanoma cell (*MC*)

lial location (Fig. 2), depending on the areas examined on the available prints. In the latter case, this matrix was closely opposed to endothelial cells of microvessels, i.e., between endothelial cells and the surrounding cells, whether they were pericytes or tumor cells (Fig. 2). The amorphous material was finely textured and in some cases contained banded collagen fibrils. Except in rare foci, this matrix did not show the architecture of a linear lamina. One case did not exhibit the amorphous matrix and three specimens were equivocal for the latter material.

Immunohistochemistry

Among the 28 cases studied, 24 tumors showed strong immunostaining for laminin localized to the matrix of intratumoral vessels. The latter pattern of laminin immunoreactivity often formed a lattice surrounding the vessels, with radial projections into the adjacent tumor mass (Fig. 3). In some instances, there was also laminin expression by tumor cells. In contrast, the immunostaining for collagen type IV was generally confined to vessels with no expression by tumor cells (Fig. 4). Four melanomas failed to show any immunostaining, due to poor tissue preservation.

In 41 of the 45 cases of malignant melanomas and related tumors, we found an amorphous matrix which, in ultrastructural terms, was not assembled into an organized laminar or basement membrane. In general, immunostaining for laminin showed a distribution similar to that of the amor-

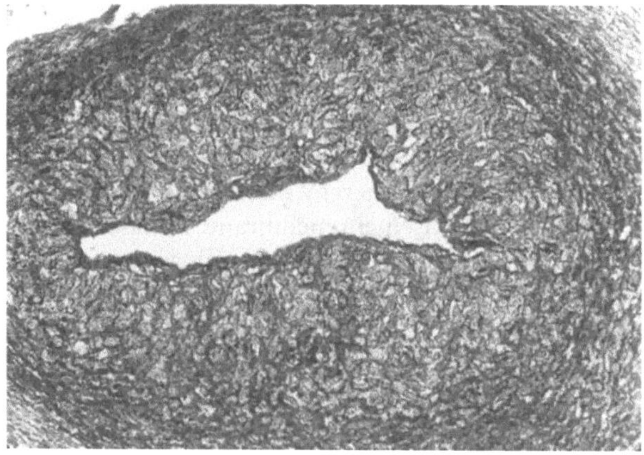

Fig. 3. Melanoma metastatic to a lymph node. The pattern of laminin immunoreactivity forms a lattice surrounding vessels with angiocentric projections into the tumor mass

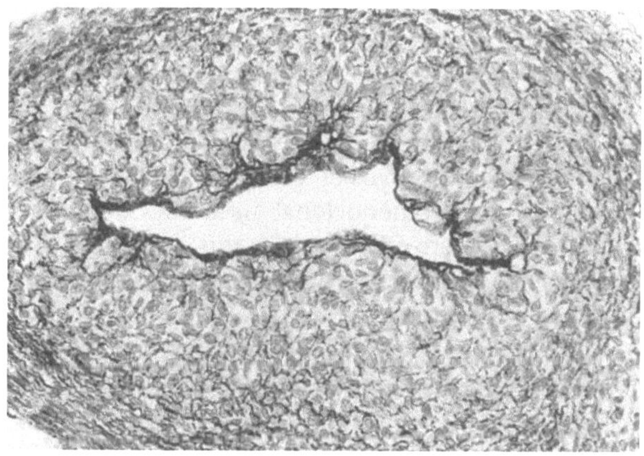

Fig. 4. Melanoma metastatic to a lymph node. Note that collagen type IV immunostaining is more restricted to the main vessel or exhibits a less well developed lattice

phous matrix. The melanoma cells were positive for laminin in some instances but always negative for collagen type IV. The intratumoral vessels were strongly positive for laminin and frequently formed angiocentric projections into the surrounding tumor mass. In contrast, collagen type IV immunostaining was more restricted to the central vessels. Since laminin alone (and most likely free laminin) is secreted by migrating endothelial cells during the early steps of angiogenesis, this angiocentric laminin may correlate to or be associated with angiogenesis at the tumor vascular interface. The interaction between vessels and melanoma cells did not suggest intravasation of tumor cells. These results are in agreement with the description of the angiotumoral complex [9].

The presence of the periendothelial/peritumoral free laminin and its association with the pericytic location of the tumor cells raises the question of its function in metastatic migration. Indeed, given that the activity of pericytes in controlling nontumoral angiogenesis is linked to the constitution of a supramolecular basement membrane, melanoma cells may compete with pericytes for endothelial cell surface, thereby inhibiting locally the reconstitution of the normal supramolecular basement membrane. Because of the function of laminin in migration, the interaction of tumor cells with periendothelial laminin could potentially lead to the exposure and activation of some domains which are masked and inactivated in an organized lamina, as described for a cryptic promigratory site on laminin-5. This activated laminin could promote the migration of melanoma cells over the mesenchymal surface of endothelium and potentially provide another mode of tumor cell spread in addition to the hematogenous mechanism. This intramesenchymal migration may be similar to other recognized forms of migration, such as the migration of neural crest cells in the developing embryo, the neurotropism associated with some melanomas, and the invasion of the brain by glioma cells.

Our current studies are exploring the relative contributions of endothelial cells and tumor cells in the periendothelial secretion of laminin. Furthermore, the expression of particular isoforms of laminin has been correlated to metastatic propensity; thus, in order to identify more precisely the type of LM present in this amorphous periendothelial material, we carried out immunostaining on cryostat sections from 16 human melanoma specimens [12]. Four murine monoclonal antibodies directed against the $\alpha3$, $\beta2$, $\beta3$, and $\gamma2$ LM chains were employed. In this report, we describe our immunohistological results and discuss the potential origin and role of periendothelial LM in tumor migration.

In the melanomas studied, $\alpha3$, $\beta3$, and $\gamma2$ chains showed only minimal focal vascular positivity in 16/16 cases, 12/16 cases, and 14/16 cases, respectively.

In contrast, the $\beta2$ (16/16 cases) LM chain exhibited consistent positivity in an angiocentric pattern around tumor microvessels (Fig. 5). The $\beta2$ LM chain showed angiocentric projections into the surrounding tumor mass, resembling in some cases a lattice between the tumor vessels.

In all melanomas, some tumor cells seemed to spread along the abluminal side of the small vessels, exhibiting a pericytic location. In these cases, tumor cells were seen along the vascular LM staining, particularly along the intratumoral projections formed by the $\beta2$ LM chain.

Recent data have demonstrated the importance of LM in tumor progression but focused principally on the secretion of LM by tumor cells themselves, obviously leading to an increasing diversity of results. The fundamental phenomenon of neoangiogenesis in tumor metastasis could represent a common mechanism leading to active LM secretion when in contact with the surrounding tumor cells. The observation of the $\beta2$ LM chain being localized to microvessels in melanoma could be a first step in identifying common LM chains or isoforms involved in cancer cell migration. This periendothelial

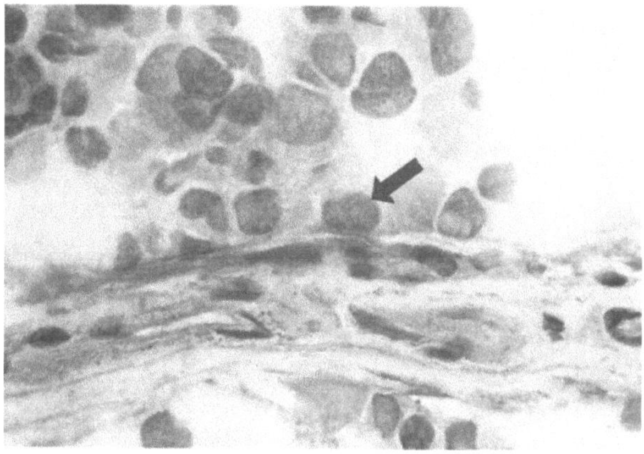

Fig. 5. Immunostaining of metastatic melanoma with an antibody against the beta-2 laminin chain. Note the pericytic location of melanoma cells (*arrow*) along the periendothelial matrix positive for the beta-2 laminin chain

LM chain linked to the pericytic location of the melanoma cells raises the question of their endothelial or tumoral origin. The fact that the chain is expressed in normal vessels from normal skin suggests that it may have an endothelial origin. Furthermore, the $\alpha3$ LM chain, which stained vessels in normal skin, showed very weak staining in the tumor vessels. A recent study using murine tumors derived from two human melanoma cell lines, one secreting and one not secreting LM, showed in both cases the presence of angiotumoral LM, suggesting again an endothelial origin of this LM. However, the intensity of LM staining was much stronger in these angiotumoral areas than around nontumoral vessels. Therefore, we might hypothesize an interaction between tumor cells occupying a pericytic location and activated endothelial cells in stimulating or repressing the expression of particular LM chains, analogous to epithelial-mesenchymal interactions. In addition, pericytes, which stabilize neovessels in nontumoral angiogenesis, can produce collagen IV and LM isoforms. Thus, the pericytic location of tumor cells could interact with the production of some LM chains, possibly preventing pericytes from completing BM formation and stabilizing neovessels.

Studies of Tumor Progression in Murine Brains

In an effort to provide more evidence for the hypothesis of extravascular migratory metastasis, we undertook studies in collaboration with Henry Brem and his colleagues Raymond Haroun and Michael Guarnieri of the Neurosurgery Research Group at Johns Hopkins University. In these preliminary and ongoing studies, approximately 100 tumor cells from each of the B16–F10 melanoma cell lines and a murine glioma cell line were stereotactically inoculated into the brains of 6- to 12-week-old C57/B16 female mice from Har-

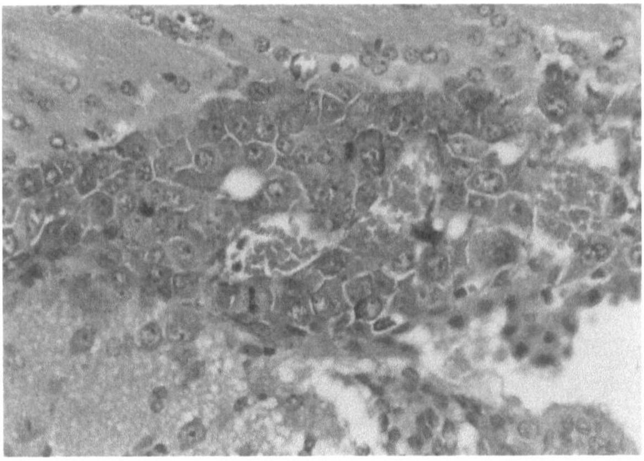

Fig. 6. Section of murine brain at day 10 postinoculation of B16 melanoma cells. There is an aggregate of B16 melanoma cells in an angiotropic pattern

lan Sprague-Dawley (Indianapolis, Ind., USA). The animals were killed on days 10, 15, and 20 following tumor implantation. The murine brains were then harvested and fixed in 10% formalin. Preliminary routine histological examination showed tumor cell aggregates from both cell lines to be localized around microvessels in a periendothelial or angiotropic pattern, suggesting migration of tumor cells along the abluminal surfaces of microvessels (Fig. 6). Preliminary immunostaining revealed greater expression of laminin relative to collagen type IV in periendothelial patterns than in our previous studies. However, much more work must be carried out with this intriguing model and other methods to substantiate this hypothesis.

In summary, we are only beginning to understand the biological properties of micrometastases through some of the studies discussed in this article. Investigation must continue in order to confirm the nature of so-called dormant metastases, if they exist at all, and the mechanisms by which all metastases develop, including circulation through lymphatic and blood vascular channels and/or migration along their and other structures' surfaces.

References

1. Crowley N, Seigler H (1992) Relationship between disease-free interval and survival in patients with recurrent melanoma. Arch Surg 127:1303–1308
2. Meltzer A (1990) Dormancy and breast cancer. J Surg Oncol 43:181–188
3. Piepkorn M, Barnhill RL (1996) A factual, not arbitrary, basis for choice of resection margins in melanoma. Arch Dermatol 132:811–814
4. Piepkorn M, Weinstock MA, Barnhill RL (1997) Theoretical and empirical arguments in relation to elective lymph node dissection for melanoma. Arch Dermatol 133:995–1007
5. Holmgren L, O'Reilly MS, Folkman J (1995) Dormancy of micrometastases: Balanced proliferation and apoptosis in the presence of angiogenesis suppression. Nature Medicine 1:149–153

6. Folkman J (1995) Angiogenesis in cancer, vascular, rheumatoid and other disease. Nature Medicine 1:27–32
7. Barnhill RL, Piepkorn MW, Cochran AJ, Flynn E, Karaoli T, Folkman J (1998) Tumor vascularity, proliferation, and apoptosis in human melanoma micrometastases and macrometastases. Arch Dermatol 134:991–994
8. Gavrieli Y, Sherman Y, Ben-Sasson SA (1992) Identification of programmed cell death in situ via specific labeling of nuclear DNA fragmentation. J Cell Biol 119:493–501
9. Lugassy C, Eyden BP, Christensen L, Escande JP (1997) Angio-tumoral complex in human malignant melanoma characterized by free laminin: ultrastructural and immunohistochemical observations. J Submicrosc Cytol Pathol 29:19–28
10. Lugassy C, Christensen L, LeCharpentier M, Faure E, Escande JP (1998) Ultrastructural and immuno-histochemical observations concerning laminin in B16 melanoma. Is an amorphous form of laminin promoting a non hematogenous migration of tumor cells? J Submicrosc Cytol Pathol 30:137–144
11. Lugassy C, Dickersin GR, Christensen L, Karaoli T, LeCharpentier M, Escande JP, Barnhill (1999) Ultrastructural and immunohistochemical studies of the periendothelial matrix in human melanoma: Evidence for an amorphous matrix containing laminin. J Cutan Pathol 26:78–83
12. Lugassy C, Shahsafaei A, Bonitz P, Busam KJ, Barnhill RL (1999) Tumor microvessels in melanoma express the beta-2 chain of laminin. Implications for melanoma metastasis. J Cutan Pathol 26:222–226
13. Lugassy C, Christensen L, LeCharpentier M, Faure E, Escande JP (1998) Angio-tumoral laminin in murine tumors derived from human melanoma cell lines. Imunohistochemical and ultrastructural observations. J Submicros Cytol Pathol 30:231–237

Disseminated Tumor Cells: Diagnosis, Prognostic Relevance, and Phenotyping

K. Pantel and M. Otte

Molekulare Diagnostik und Therapie, Universitätsfrauenklinik,
UniversitätsKrankenhaus Eppendorf, Martinistrasse 52, 20246 Hamburg, Germany

Abstract

Malignant tumors of epithelial tissue are the most common form of cancer and are responsible for the majority of cancer-related deaths in Western industrialized countries. As a result of progress in surgical treatment of these tumors, lethality is linked increasingly with early metastasis, which is generally occult at the time of primary diagnosis. The decision as to whether systemic adjuvant therapy should be applied for secondary prevention of metastatic relapse following resection of the primary tumor is based solely on the statistical prognosis. For this reason, the direct identification of minimal residual cancer is of particular importance. The studies described below demonstrate the utility of immunocytochemical and molecular analysis in the diagnosis and characterization of minimal residual cancer. These methods give access for the first time to this critical stage of tumor progression and also contribute to the development of new approaches to therapy aimed at preventing manifest metastasis.

Introduction

Research into the molecular basis of tumor metastasis has resulted in the identification of numerous proteins that influence this critical property of tumor cells. The conditions necessary for the growth of epithelial cells that must be present in mesenchymal organs such as bone marrow are extensively unknown. Also unclear are factors determining tumor cell dormancy, i.e., the period between the dissemination of tumor cells and the appearance of clinically manifest metastases, during which time these cells appear to remain latent.

In contrast to solid metastases, isolated micrometastatic tumor cells are appropriate targets for intravenously applied therapeutics because of their accessibility for macromolecules and immunocompetent effector cells. From analyses of single cells, it would appear that most disseminated tumor cells do not proliferate (Pantel et al. 1993). For this reason, forms of treatment

Recent Results in Cancer Research, Vol. 158

aimed at both dormant and proliferating cells are particularly interesting as adjuvant therapy.

Diagnosis and Prognostic Relevance

While even micrometastatic tumor cell aggregates have been identified using conventional histopathological methods (Burkhardt et al. 1980), individual disseminated carcinoma cells in bone marrow have generally resisted clear cytological identification (Schlimok et al. 1987). In the past 15 years, more sensitive immunocytochemical and molecular procedures have been developed that permit the identification of individual disseminated tumor cells in organs remote from the primary tumor on the basis of qualitative features (for review see Pantel et al. 1999). As some epithelial tumors tend to develop skeletal metastases, this relatively easily accessible compartment is particularly amenable to exploration by iliac crest aspiration. In addition, the medullary space is a site of particularly intensive cell exchange between circulating blood and mesenchymal interstitium.

The identification of individual disseminated tumor cells in cytological bone marrow preparations on the basis of cytomorphological criteria is extremely difficult and not very practical because of the lack of sensitivity. Experience to date has shown that cytokeratins (CK), as integral components of the cytoskeleton of epithelial cells, are stably expressed characteristics of tumor cells that can be clearly identified in individual carcinoma cells by means of specific monoclonal antibodies. On the other hand, mucin-like tumor-associated cell membrane proteins are less well suited to analysis due to their expression through hematopoietic cells (Pantel et al. 1994; Braun et al. 1998). Immunohistochemical examinations of bone marrow biopsies have shown that CK-positive tumor cells are mostly situated in interstitial tissue outside the sinusoidal vessels, which indicates that extravasation, one of the last processes in the metastasis cascade, has been successfully completed (Schlimok 1988). Although ectopic or illegitimate mRNA expression of cytokeratins in mesenchymal cells cannot be ruled out (Krismann et al. 1995; Traweek et al. 1993; Zippelius et al. 1997), numerous negative findings in patients with no identifiable malignant processes show that ectopic expression of cytokeratin proteins in bone marrow is very rarely identifiable by immunocytochemistry (Schlimok et al. 1987; Pantel et al. 1994; Pantel et al. 1996). The time-consuming microscopic screening of large amounts of cytological samples could be facilitated in future by automated analysis of stained preparations using an image analysis system (scanner). As an alternative, density gradients and antibody-charged magnetic particles can be used to enrich tumor cells over several logarithmic units (Naume et al. 1997; Martin et al. 1998). However, the reproducibility of these enrichment techniques needs to be confirmed on clinical samples.

Although the prognostic relevance of the immunocytochemical identification procedure has been confirmed in prospective clinical studies by various

Table 1. Immunocytochemical studies of the prognostic relevance of disseminated tumor cells in bone marrow

Type of tumor	Marker, proteins	Detection rate	Prognostic value	Reference
Mammary carcinoma	EMA	89/350 (25%)	DFS, OS	Mansi et al. 1999
	EMA, TAG12, CK	38/100 (38%)	DFS, OS*	Harbeck et al. 1994
	CK	18/49 (37%)	DFS*	Cote et al. 1991
	TAG12	315/727 (43%)	DFS, OS*	Diel et al. 1996
Colorectal carcinoma	CK-18	28/88 (32%)	DFS*	Lindemann et al. 1992
Gastric carcinoma	CK-18	34/97 (35%)	DFS	Schlimok et al. 1991
	CK-18	47/78 (60%)	DFS	Heiss et al. 1995
	CK-18	95/180 (53%)	DFS*	Jauch et al. 1996
Esophagus carcinoma	CK	37/90 (41%)	DFS, OS	Thorban et al. 1996
Bronchial carcinoma (NSCLC)	CK	17/43 (40%)	DFS	Cote et al. 1995
	CK-18	83/139 (60%)	DFS*, OS	Pantel et al. 1996
	CK-18	15/39 (39%)	DFS	Ohgami et al. 1997

EMA, epithelial membrane antigen; CK, cytokeratin; TAG12, tumor-associated glycoprotein 12; DFS, disease-free survival; OS, overall survival; NSCLC, non-small-cell lung cancer.
* Prognostic value as an independent parameter confirmed through multivariate analysis.

working groups (Table 1), doubts have been expressed as to its value (Osborne and Rosen 1994; Funke and Schraut 1998). Closer analysis of these reports shows that the techniques used differ considerably in terms of reproducibility. This might also explain the different detection rates that have been published, ranging for example in mammary carcinoma from 4% to 45% (Osborne, Rosen 1994). It is therefore necessary to define the critical variables in the immunocytochemical method (Pantel et al. 1994) and introduce standardization so as to allow reproducible and more precise determination of residual cancer cell counts (Borgen et al. 1999).

Several studies have confirmed the result of the cytokeratin assay as a prognostic factor unaffected by conventional risk factors (Table 1). The observed correlation to the total relapse rate is of particular interest, as clinically manifest skeletal metastases are very rare in colon carcinoma. It would therefore appear that the presence of epithelial cells in bone marrow is more likely to be an indicator of early systemic tumor cell dissemination, the growth in bone marrow or other organs being determined by the milieu in question. In this context, it is interesting that the repeat identification over a 2-year period of tumor cells in the bone marrow of patients with operable gastric carcinoma had even greater prognostic value than the primary identification of disseminated cells when the primary tumor was resected (Heiss et al. 1995).

Circulating tumor cells can also be identified in peripheral blood. Repeat blood sampling is superior to sequential aspiration of bone marrow as a monitoring procedure. Recent examinations of patients with prostate and colorectal carcinoma and melanomas whose peripheral blood was examined perioperatively by molecular methods (see below) have shown that a temporary intraoperative dissemination of tumor cells in the bed of the vessels can occur (Denis et al. 1996; Eschwège et al. 1995; Hansen et al. 1995; Weitz et al. 1998). Whether these cells reach and survive in secondary organs and form manifest metastases there is as yet unknown.

Early hematogenous tumor cell dissemination is the most common method of metastasis, but a second means, lymphogenous dissemination, is also of great clinical importance for detecting epithelial tumor cells in histopathologically unremarkable lymph nodes of patients with operable non-small-cell lung carcinoma (NSCLC). The antiepithelial antibody BerEp4, which homogeneously stained more than 90% of the primary carcinomas examined, has been used in patients with lung and esophageal cancer (Passlick et al. 1994). More recent experimental studies have shown that BerEp4 recognizes the 17-1 A antigen (Kubuschok et al. 1999). In 15.2% of the carcinoma patients studied, individual tumor cells were identified with the monoclonal antibody BerEp4. Tumor cells were found in lymph nodes, irrespective of established risk factors such as T stage and degree of tumor differentiation. However, a correlation with systemic dissemination in bone marrow could not be established. The autonomy of this lymph node assay as a prognostic aid with respect to total relapse rate and overall survival was confirmed by multivariate analysis ($p = 0.009$) (Kubuschok et al. 1999). The results emphasize the importance of additional verification of lymph node dissemination. The clinical importance of this type of dissemination was recently confirmed in a similar manner for carcinomas of the esophagus (Izbicki et al. 1997) and colon (Lifers et al. 1998).

New Techniques for Detection of Disseminated Tumor Cells

In the past few years, molecular detection procedures have been used increasingly to identify disseminated tumor cells in organs remote from the primary tumor. In principle, cDNA of disseminated tumor cells can be amplified millions of times as a result of the polymerase chain reaction (PCR), so that even the smallest quantities of such tumor cells can be detected (Sidransky et al. 1998; Pantel et al. 1999). For this to happen, however, the tumor cell must show specific changes in its genome or mRNA expression pattern that distinguish it from the surrounding hematopoietic cells. As solid tumors are notable for their extreme genetic heterogeneity, the detection of tumor-specific genomic changes at the single cell level is highly complex. Each individual primary tumor must be genotyped so that the corresponding patient-specific genetic lesion can be identified and the appropriate PCR probes (primers) selected (Hayashi et al. 1995; Tada et al. 1993). This method is currently beyond the means of routine clinical diagnosis.

Table 2. Detection of disseminated tumor cells by molecular methods

Tissue	Tumor organ	mRNA/DNA marker
Bone marrow	Breast tissue	CK-19, CEA
	Colorectum	CEA, CK-19, CK-20
	Stomach	CEA, CK-20
	Pancreas	CEA
	Prostate	PSA, CK-19
	Head and neck	E48
Lymph nodes	Breast tissue	CK-19, MUC1, β-hCG
	Cervix	HPV16, E6/E7
	Colorectum	CEA, CK-19, CK-20, p53 and Ki-ras mutations
	Prostate	PSA, PSM
	Skin (melanoma)	Tyrosinase
	Lung	p53, Ki-ras mutations
	Pancreas	Ki-ras mutations
	Head and neck	p53 mutations
Blood	Breast tissue	CK-19, EGF-R, β-hCG
	Colorectum	Ki-ras mutations, CK-20
	Pancreas	Ras mutations
	Prostate	PSA, PSM
	Skin (melanoma)	Tyrosinase, p97, MUC18, MAGE-3
	Lung	Microsatellite alterations
	Stomach	CK-20
	Liver	α-fetoprotein
	Head and neck	Microsatellite alterations
Liver	Pancreas	Ki-ras mutations
Tumor resection margins	Head and neck	p53 mutations

The detection of tumor-specific expressed mRNA species, on the other hand, appears to present fewer obstacles to more widespread use of the PCR method (Neumaier et al. 1995; Soeth et al. 1997). The cell mRNA is transcribed into cDNA by means of reverse transcriptase (RT), and the cDNA is amplified in the subsequent PCR. Although this method offers great potential for future clinical use, the specificity of tumor cell identification is currently the greatest barrier. Apart from the mRNA of the few tumor cells, the basic material for the PCR also contains the mRNA from the large surplus of hematopoietic cells (in a ratio of 10^6:1), and a false positive result can be obtained even with minimal expression of the corresponding marker mRNA in these hematopoietic cells. Although a series of RT-PCR assays has been developed to detect tumor cells in bone marrow, blood, and lymph nodes (Table 2), a number of reports have questioned the specificity of this method (Krismann et al. 1995; Zippelius et al. 1997; Bostick et al. 1998). Some of the discrepancies could be clarified by methodical comparison in future ring tests for standardization of this extremely interesting detection technique. However, apart from these methodological aspects, the prognostic significance of RT-PCR assays was demonstrated in some studies on smaller

Table 3. Phenotype of cytokeratin-positive cells in bone marrow

Marker	Tumor origin	*N* patients with marker-positive/ CK-negative cells (%)
Growth factor receptors		
erbB2	Breast	48/71 (67.6)
	Colorectum/stomach	14/50 (28.0)
Transferrin receptor	Breast	17/59 (28.8)
	Colorectum	7/41 (41.1)
MHC class I antigens	Breast	9/26 (34.6)
	Colon/stomach	37/65 (56.9)
Adhesion molecules		
EpCAM	Breast	20/31 (64.5)
	Colorectum	4/6
ICAM-1	Lung (NSCLC)	13/31 (41.9)
Placoglobin	Lung (NSCLC)	4/12 (33.3)
	Colorectum	4/13 (30.8)
Proliferation-associated proteins		
Ki-67	Breast	1/12 (8.3)
	Colorectum/stomach	0/21
p120	Breast	1/11 (9.1)
	Colorectum/stomach	9/32 (28.1)

groups of patients with melanomas and various types of carcinomas (Fields et al. 1996; Soeth et al. 1997; Liefers et al. 1998).

Phenotyping

Immunocytochemical double staining methods have been developed for more precise characterization of disseminated tumor cells. In view of the malignant potential of CK-positive cells, a number of tumor-associated characteristics have been identified in this way (Table 3), including expression of Lewis Y blood group precursor antigens, overexpression of the erbB2 oncogene, and deficient expression of MHC class I molecules, which, as restrictive elements, help T lymphocyte-mediated tumor cell recognition (Hämmerling et al. 1989; Wallich et al. 1985). The malignant nature of CK-positive cells in bone marrow has been further confirmed through genomic analysis, which revealed several chromosomal alterations (Klein et al. 1999; Dietmaier et al. 1998) and amplification of the erbB2 gene in these cells (Müller et al. 1996). Extensive cell culture experiments have also shown that cells disseminating into bone marrow have a time-limited proliferative potential at the time of primary tumor diagnosis (Pantel et al. 1995). It may therefore be assumed that, at the primary stage, these cells do not yet proliferate autonomously but are in a latent state known as "dormancy" (Pantel et al. 1993). This observation is consistent with the limited frequency of p53 mutations in CK-positive cells in bone marrow at the time of primary diagnosis (Offner et al. 1999).

The low proliferation rate could explain the relative resistance of micrometastatic tumor cells to chemotherapy (Braun, Kentenich, Janni et al. in press) and would confirm the appropriateness of therapy strategies independent of the proliferation potential, such as antibody therapy (Riethmüller et al. 1998; Braun, Hepp, Kentenich et al. in press).

The low frequency of epithelial tumor cells in bone marrow and their localization in such a well-supplied organ offer ideal conditions for elimination by immunocompetent cells. As the clinical history of epithelial tumor cells shows, however, micrometastatic tumor cells can be ignored for many years by the immune system. In this context, particular attention should be paid to the deficient expression of MHC class I molecules (Table 3). This low regulation could limit the prospects for immunogenetic treatment with tumor cell vaccines (Pardoll 1993). The tumor-killing immunological effect of antibody administration, on the other hand, is independent of MHC antigen expression.

Conclusions and Outlook

Although great progress has been made in oncological surgery in recent decades, minimal residual cancer significantly limits the current prospects for further improvements in lethality rates. Adjuvant therapy should therefore be standard with such residual disease. The statistical risk estimate based on conventional tumor classification gives only a relatively inaccurate assessment of the individual risk to cancer patients. In the past 15 years, immunocytochemical and molecular analysis procedures have therefore been developed to diagnose and characterize minimal residual cancer. Extensive studies are currently in progress to standardize these processes with a view to ensuring reproducibility of the clinically relevant results.

As far as adjuvant therapy is concerned, success or failure can only be assessed after an observation period of several years. It is possible that control examinations of bone marrow and peripheral blood during therapy could provide indications as to the efficacy of the therapeutic approach used. The availability of a surrogate marker for monitoring is of great importance in the development of adjuvant therapy processes. Monitoring procedures of this type would be of considerable value but are not currently available for clinical therapy studies involving solid tumors. Because of their easy accessibility, bone marrow or peripheral blood would be obvious contenders for monitoring controls and would make it possible for the first time for adjuvant therapies to be monitored at the subclinical stage of minimal residual cancer.

Our experience to date indicates that immunocytochemical or molecular monitoring of disseminated cells is possible in principle for individual patients (Pantel et al. 1997; Braun, Hepp, Kentenich et al. in press) although reproducible enrichment of the rare tumor cells would be desirable to reduce the chance factor in such longitudinal studies. In addition, long-term observations are required to establish whether therapy-associated reduction in individual disseminated cells also correlates with improved prognosis. Should tumor cells disseminated in bone marrow or peripheral blood prove suitable as surrogate markers for early assessment of the efficacy of adjuvant therapy, this would have significant influence on future oncological diagnosis and treatment. To achieve this goal, we recently initiated a multicenter randomized trial on patients with nodal positive breast cancer in which bone marrow and peripheral blood are monitored to assess the effect on micrometastatic disease of adjuvant chemotherapy and subsequent therapy with the monoclonal antibody edrecolomab (Panorex) against EpCAM (Table 3).

References

Bostick PJ, Chatterje, S, Chi DD, Huynh KT, Giuliano AE, Cote R, Hoon DS (1998) Limitations of specific reverse-transcriptase polymerase chain reaction markers in the detection of metastases in the lymph nodes and blood of breast cancer patients. J Clin Oncol 16:2632–2640

Braun S, Kentenich ChRM, Janni W, Hepp F, de Waal J, Willegroth F, Sommer HL, Pantel K (2000) Lack of effect of adjuvant chemotherapy on the elimination of single dormant cells in bone marrow of high risk breast cancer patients. J Clin Oncol 18:80–86

Braun S, Hepp F, Kentenich ChRM, Janni W, Pantel K, Riethmüller G, Sommer HL (1999) Monoclonal antibody therapy with Erecolomab in breast cancer patients: Monitoring of elimination of disseminated cytokeratin-positive tumor cells in bone marrow. Clin Cancer Res 5:3999–4004

Braun S, Müller M, Hepp F, Schlimok G, Riethmüller G, Pantel K (1998) Micrometastatic breast cancer cells in bone marrow at primary surgery: prognostic value in comparison with nodal status. J Natl Cancer Inst 90:1099–1100

Borgen E, Naume B, Nesland JM, Kvalheim G, Beiske K, Fodstad Ø, Diel I, Solomayer E-F, Theocharous P, Coombes RC, Smith BM, Wunder E, Marolleau J-P, Garcia J,d Pantel K (1999) Standardization of the immunocytochemical detection of cancer cells in BM and blood: l. etsablishmant of objective criteria for the evaluation of immunostaioned cells. Cytotherapy 1:377–388.

Burkhardt R, Frisch B, Kettner G (1980) The clinical study of micrometastatic cancer by bone biopsy. Bull Cancer 67:291–305

Cote RJ, Rosen PP, Lesser ML, Old MP (1991) Prediction of early relapse in patients with operable breast cancer by detection of occult bone marrow micrometastases. J Clin Oncol 9:1749–1756

Cote RJ, Beattie EJ, Chaiwun B, Shi SR, Harvey J, Chen SC, Sherrod AE, Groshen S, Taylor CR (1995) Detection of occult bone marrow micrometastases in patients with operable lung carcinoma. Ann Surg 222:415–425

Denis MG, Tessier MH, Dréno B, Lustenberger P (1996) Circulating micrometastases following oncological surgery. The Lancet 347:913

Diel IJ, Kaufmann M, Costa SD, Holle R, von Mickwitz G, Solomayer EF, Kaul S, Bastert G (1996) Micrometastatic breast cancer cells in bone marrow at primary surgery: prognostic value in comparison with nodal status. J Natl Cancer Inst 88:1652–1658

Dietmaier W, Hartmann A, Wallinger S, Heinmoller E, Kerner T, Endl E, Jauch K-W, Hofstädter F, Rüschoff J (1999) Multiple mutation analysis in single tumor cells with improved whole genome amplification. Am J Pathol 154:83–95

Eschwège P, Dumas F, Blanchet P, LeMaire V, Benoit G, Jardin A, Lacour B, Loric S (1995) Haematogenous dissemination of prostatic epithelial cells during radical prostatectomy. Lancet 346:1528–1530

Fields KK, Elfenbein GJ, Trudeau WL, Perkins JB, Janssen WE, Moscinski LC (1996) Clinical significance of bone marrow metastases as detected using the polymerase chain reaction in patients with breast cancer undergoing high-dose chemotherapy and autologous bone marrow transplantation. J Clin Oncol 14:1868–1876

Funke I, Schraut W (1998) Meta-analyses of studies on bone marrow micrometastases: an independent prognostic impact remains to be substantiated. J Clin Oncol 16:557–566

Hansen E, Wolff N, Knuechel R, Ruschoff J, Hofstaedter F, Taeger K (1995) Tumor cells in blood shed from the surgical field. Arch Surg 130:387–393

Harbeck N, Untch M, Pache L, Eiermann W (1994) Tumor cell detection in the bone marrow of breast cancer patients at primary therapy: results of a 3-year median follow up. Br J Cancer 69:566–571

Hayashi N, Ito I, Yanagisawa A, Kato Y, Nakamori S, Imaoka S, Watanabe H, Ogawa M, Nakamura K (1995) Genetic diagnosis of lymph-node metastasis in colorectal cancer. The Lancet 345:1257–1259

Hämmerling G, Maschek V, Sturmhöfel K, Momburg F (1989) Regulation and functional role of MHC expression on tumors. In: Melchers F (ed) Prog Immunol, pp 1071–1078. Springer, Berlin

Heiss MM, Allgayer H, Gruetzner KU, Funke I, Babic R, Jauch K-W, Schildberg FW (1995) Individual development and uPA-receptor expression of disseminated tumor cells in bone marrow: A reference to early systemic disease in solid cancer. Nature Medicine, 1:1035–1039

Izbicki JR, Hosch SB, Pichlmeier U, Rehders A, Busch C, Niendorf A, Passlick B, Broelsch CE, Pantel K (1997) Prognostic value of immunohistochemically identifiable tumor cells in lymph nodes of patients with completely resected esophageal cancer. N Engl J Med 337:1188–1194

Jauch KW, Heiss MM, Gruetzner U, Funke I, Pantel K, Babic R, Eissner HJ, Riethmueller G, Schildberg FW (1996) Prognostic significance of bone marrow micrometastases in patients with gastric cancer. J Clin Oncol 14:1810–1817

Klein ChA, Schmidt-Kittler O, Schrad JA, Pantel K, Speicher MR, Riethmüller G (1999) Comparative genomic hybridization, loss of heterozygocity and DNA sequence analysis of single cells. Proc Natl Acad Sci USA, 96:4494–4499

Krismann M, Todt B, Schröder J, Gareis D, Müller K-M, Seeber S, Schütte J (1995) Low specificity of cytokeratin 19 reverse transcriptase-polymerase chain reaction analyses for detection of hematogenous lung cancer dissemination. Journal of Clinical Oncology 13:2769–2775

Kubuschok B, Passlick B, Izbicki J, Thetter O, Pantel K (1999) Disseminated tumor cells in lymph nodes as a determinant for survival in surgically resected non-small cell lung cancer. J Clin Oncol 17:24

Liefers GJ, Cleton JA, d van Hermans VJ, van-Krieken JH, Cornelisse CJ, Tollenaar RA (1998) Micrometastases and survival in stage II colorectal cancer see comments. N Engl J Med 339:223–228

Lindemann F, Schlimok G, Dirschedl P, Witte J, Riethmüller G (1992) Prognostic significance of micrometastic tumor cells in bone marrow of colorectal cancer patients. Lancet 340:685–689

Mansi JL, Gogas H, Bliss JM, Gazet JC, Berger U, Coombes RC (1999) Outcome of primary-breast-cancer patients with micrometastases: a long-term follow-up study. Lancet 354:197–202

Martin VM, Siewert C, Scharl, A, Harms T, Heinze R, Ohl S, Radbruch A, Miltenyi S, Schmitz J (1998) Immunomagnetic enrichment of disseminated epithelial tumor cells from peripheral blood by MACS. Exp Hematol 26:252–264

Müller P, Weckermann D, Riethmüller G, Schlimok G (1996) Detection of genetic alterations in micrometastatic cells in bone marrow of cancer patients by fluorescence in situ hybridization. Cancer Genet Cytogenet 88:8–16

Naume B, Borgen E, Beiske K, Herstad T-K, Ravnas G, Renolen A, Trachsel S, Thrane-Steen K, Funderud S, Kvalheim G (1997) Detection of isolated breast carcinoma cells in peripheral blood or bone marrow by immunomagnetic techniques. J Hematother 6:103–111

Neumaier M, Gerhard M, Wagener C (1995) Diagnosis of micrometastases by the amplification of tissue-specific genes. Gene 159:43–47
Offner S, Schmaus, W, Witter K, Baretton GK, Schlimok G, Passlick B, Riethmüller G, Pantel K (1999) p53 gene mutations are not required for early dissemination of cancer cells. Proc Natl Acad Sci USA 96:6942–6946
Ohgami A, Mitsudomi T, Sugio K, Tsuda T, Oyama T, Nishida K, Osaki T, Yasumoto K (1997) Micrometastatic tumor cells in the bone marrow of patients with non-small cell lung cancer. Ann Thorac Surg 64:363–367
Osborne MP, Rosen PP (1994) Detection and management of bone marrow micrometastases in breast cancer. Oncology 8:25–36
Pantel K, Dickmanns A, Zippelius A, Klein C, Shi J, Hoechtlen-Vollmar W, Schlimok G, Weckermann D, Oberneder R, Fanning E, Riethmüller G (1995) Establishment of micrometastatic carcinoma cell lines: a novel source of tumor cell vaccines. Journal of the National Cancer Institute 87:1162–1168
Pantel K, Izbicki J, Passlick B, Angstwurm M, Häussinger K, Thetter O, Riethmüller G (1996) Prognostic significance of isolated tumor cells in bone marrow of patients with non-small cell carcinomas without overt metastases. Lancet 347:649–653
Pantel K, Enzmann T, Kollermann J, Caprano J, Riethmuller G, Kollermann MW (1997) Immunocytochemical monitoring of micrometastatic disease: reduction of prostate cancer cells in bone marrow by androgen deprivation. Int J Cancer 71:521–525
Pantel K, Schlimok G, Angstwurm M, Weckermann C, Schmaus W, Gath H, Passlick B, Izbicki J, Riethmüller G (1994) Methodological analysis of immunocytochemical screening for disseminated epithelial tumor cells in bone marrow. J Hematother 3:165–173
Pantel K, Schlimok G, Braun S, Kutter D, Schaller G, Funke I, Izbicki J, Riethmüller G (1993) Differential expression of proliferation-associated molecules in individual micrometastatic carcinoma cells. J Natl Cancer Inst 85:1419–1424
Pantel K, Cote RJ, Fodstad Ø (1999) Detection and clinical importance of micrometastatic disease. J Natl Cancer Inst 91:1113–1124
Pardoll DM (1993) Cancer vaccines. Immunol Today 14:310–316
Passlick B, Izbick, JR, Kubuschok B, Nathrath W, Thetter O, Pichelmeier U, Schweiberer L, Riethmüller G, Pantel K (1994) Immunhistochemical assessment of individual tumor cells in lymph nodes of patients with non-small cell lung cancer. J Clin Oncol 12:1827–1832
Riethmüller G, Holz E, Schlimok G, Schmiegel W, Raab R, Hoffken K, Gruber R, Funke I, Pichelmaier H, Hirche H, Buggisch P, Witt J, Pichelmayer R (1998) Monoclonal antibody therapy for resected Dukes' C colorectal cancer: seven-year outcome of a multicenter randomized trial. J Clin Oncol 16:1788–1794
Schlimok G, Funke I, Pantel K, Strobel F, Lindemann F, Witte J, Riethmüller G (1991) Micrometastatic tumour cells in bone marrow of patients with gastric cancer: methodological aspects of detection and prognostic significance. Eur J Cancer 27:1461–1465
Schlimok G (1988) Mikrometastasen epithelialer Tumoren im Knochenmark: Immunzytochemischer Nachweis und in vivo Markierung mit Hilfe monoklonaler Antikörper. Habilitation 1988. Ludwig-Maximilians-Universität München
Schlimok G, Funke I, Holzmann B, Göttlinger HG, Schmidt G, Häuser H, Swierkot S, Warnecke HH, Schneider B, Koprowski H, Riethmüller G (1987) Micrometastatic cancer cells in bone marrow: in vitro detection with anti-cytokeratin and in vivo labeling with anti-17-1A monoclonal antibodies. Proc Natl Acad Sci USA 84:8672–8676
Soeth E, Vogel I, Röder C, Juhl H, Marxsen J, Krüger U, Henne-Bruns D, Kremer B, Kalthoff H (1997) Comparative analysis of bone marrow and venous blood isolates from gastrointestinal cancer patients for the detection of disseminated tumor cells using reverse transcription PCR. Cancer Res 57:3106–3110
Sidransky D (1997) Nucleic acid-based methods for the detection of cancer. Science 278:1054–1059
Tada M, Omata M, Kawai SH, Saisho H, Ohto M, Saiki RK, Sninsky JJ (1993) Detection of ras gene mutations in Pancreatic Juice and Peripheral Blood of patients with pancreatic adenocarcinoma. Cancer Res 53:2472–2474

Traweek ST, Liu J, Battifora H (1993) Keratin gene expression in non-epithelial tissues. Detection with polymerase chain reaction. Am J Pathol 142:1111–1118

Thorban S, Roder JD, Pantel K, Siewert JR (1996) Epithelial tumor cells in bone marrow of patients with pancreatic carcinoma detected by immunocytochemical staining. Eur J Cancer 32 A:363–365

Wallich R, Bulbue N, Hämmerling GJ, Katzav S, Sagl S, Feldman M (1985) Abrogation of metastatic properties of tumor cells by de novo expression of H-2 K antigens following H-2 gene transfection. Nature 315:301–305

Weitz J, Kienle P, Lacroix J, Willeke F, Benner A, Lehnert T, Herfarth C, von-Knebel-Doeberitz (1998) Dissemination of tumor cells in patients undergoing surgery for colorectal cancer. Clin Cancer Res 4:343–348

Zippelius A, Kufer P, Honold G, Riethmüller G (1997) Limitations of reverse-transcriptase polymerase chain reaction analyses for detection of micrometastatic epithelial cancer cells in bone marrow. Journal of Clinical Oncology 15:2701–2708

Nested Quantitative Real Time PCR for Detection of Occult Tumor Cells[1]

N. Max, K. Wolf, B. Spike, E. Thiel, and U. Keilholz

Department of Medicine III, Free University of Berlin, Hindenburgdamm 30, 12200 Berlin, Germany

Abstract

Quantification of tumor mRNA markers expressed by occult circulating tumor cells may be of prognostic value in a variety of neoplasms and disease stages. We therefore developed a novel real time nested polymerase chain reaction (PCR) assay to quantify rare transcripts using the light cycler system. Tyrosinase mRNA expressed by melanocytes and melanoma cells was used as a model. Ten-milliliter samples of ethylenediaminetetra-acetate (EDTA) blood from healthy volunteers were spiked with $10–10^4$ RVH melanoma cells. Following RNA extraction and cDNA synthesis, a nested PCR with specific primers was performed. Resonance energy transfer between fluorescently labeled hybridization probes specific for the amplified portion of the tyrosinase transcript allowed continuous monitoring of the second round of PCR. The number of preamplification cycles in the first round was varied between 20 and 35. Our results show that nested PCR revealed quantitative data, regardless of the number of cycles used in the first round. The range of real time data can span four logs of target mRNA concentrations ($1–10^3$ tumor cells/ml of blood) and the x-intercepts of the log phases were always consistent with the amount of transcripts in the sample. These experiments indicate that nested PCR, which is much more sensitive than single-round PCR, is a useful tool for the quantification of rare transcripts – a result with important implications for the study of minimal residual disease. The assay is currently being adapted for other tumor types including leukemias as well as other solid tumors.

[1] Supported by the Deutsche Krebshilfe, grant no. 70–2459-Ke2, the Sonnenfeldstiftung Berlin, and the EORTC Melanoma Cooperative Group.

Introduction

Reverse-transcriptase polymerase chain reaction (RT-PCR) is a highly sensitive method for detecting rare tumor cell-derived mRNA, allowing the diagnosis of tumor dissemination at early stages. This information may have important prognostic and therapeutic implications, because residual tumor cells that are below the limit of detection using standard diagnostic techniques are nevertheless associated with increased risk for overt clinical relapse [1, 2]. One limitation of RT-PCR assays was the inability to quantitate the transcript amount - an information important for either monitoring tumor progression or assessing the response to therapy in patients who had PCR evidence for circulating tumor cells prior to treatment.

We report the establishment of a system using the light cycler technique to quantitate tyrosinase, a melanocyte-specific gene transcript which is normally not present in blood and therefore a suitable indicator for the presence of circulating melanoma cells [3, 4]. The sensitivity of real time RT-PCR was assessed by blood spiking experiments with a melanoma cell line. The open questions involved whether template amplification by nested RT-PCR is quantitative and within which range quantification is reliable.

Material and Methods

Sample Preparation and RNA Extraction

Ten-milliliter samples of peripheral venous blood collected from healthy volunteers were spiked with cultured melanoma cells (RVH) in dilution series ranging from 10 to 10^4 cells/10 ml blood. Total RNA was isolated by acid guanidinium thiocyanate/phenol chloroform extraction [5] and further purified using the High Pure RNA isolation kit (Roche Diagnostics, Mannheim, Germany). RNA integrity was checked electrophoretically.

Reverse Transcription

Reverse transcription was carried out on 1.5 µg total RNA diluted in a 25 µl mixture containing 0.4 µmol random hexamers, 1 mmol/l dNTP (dATP, dCTP, dTTP, dGTP), 24 U AMV reverse transcriptase, and 40 U Rnasin (Roche Diagnostics). After incubation at 42°C for 1 h, AMV reverse transcriptase was inactivated for 5 min at 95°C and cDNA was stored at -20°C or immediately used for PCR.

Real Time PCR

Two microliters of each cDNA was diluted to a volume of 20 μl of PCR mix (Light Cycler DNA Master hybridization probe kit, Roche Diagnostics) containing a final concentration of 3 mM $MgCl_2$ and 0.5 pmol of primers. For amplification, we used a three-step RT-PCR with 1 s at 95 °C, 12 s at 60 °C, and 7 s at 72 °C for 20, 25, 30, and 35 cycles in the first round and 40 cycles in the second round. For reamplification, 2 μl of the PCR product from the first round of PCR was amplified in a 20 μl reaction volume as detailed above, additionally containing two tyrosinase cDNA-specific oligonucleotide probes (0.2 pmol) with either a donor fluorophore at its 3′ end (Fluorescein) or an acceptor fluorophore (LC Red 605) at the 5′ end. The probe with the acceptor dye was also phosphorylated at the 3′ end to avoid probe extension. Several probe sequences were tested. Primer sequences (Metabion, Munich, Germany) originally described by Smith et al. [6] and the optimal probe sequences (TIB Molbiol, Berlin, Germany) were as follows:
HTYR 1: 5′- TTG GCA GAT TGT CTG TAG CC
HTYR 2: 5′- AGG CAT TGT GCA TGC TGC TT
HTYR 3: 5′- GTC TTT ATG CAA TGG AAC GC
HTYR 4: 5′- GCT ATC CCA GTA AGT GGA CT
Tyr probe 1: 5′- GCG TAA TCC TGG AAA CCA TGA CAA A
Tyr probe 2: 5′- CAC AAC CCC AAG GCT CCC CTC TTC

The outer tyrosinase-specific primers amplify a PCR fragment of 284 bp and the inner primers one of 207 bp. Primers are represented on different exons of the gene, thus prohibiting amplification of tyrosinase genomic DNA. Following target amplification, the specific fluorescent labeled probes annealed to the amplicon in close proximity, enabling fluorescence energy transfer (FRET) between donor and acceptor dye. Acceptor fluorescence emission was measured and continuously monitored during PCR. The fluorescence signals were plotted against crossing points which mark the cycle number when fluorescence becomes significantly different from baseline signal. Specificity of the PCR products was also confirmed electrophoretically.

Precautions

To reduce risk of contamination, thermocycling and post-PCR steps were performed in a different laboratory from that used for RNA extraction, cDNA synthesis, and preparation of the PCR mixture. PCR mixtures were set up in a template tamer (Oncor Appligene). All reagents for RNA synthesis were prepared with diethylpyrocarbonate (DEPC)-treated water. Negative controls were performed for all RT-PCR steps.

Results

Sensitivity

For preclinical sensitivity testing, we performed a tenfold serial dilution experiment with melanoma cells (RVH cell line). The successful establishment of the RT-PCR assay allowed the detection of as few as ten tumor cells in 10 ml of control blood using nested PCR with 35 cycles in the first amplification round. The sensitivity limit of PCRs with 20, 25, or 30 cycles in the first round was 100 tumor cells in 10 ml of blood. With single round PCR, the detection limit was 10000 RVH cells in 10 ml of blood.

Quantification

The amount of PCR product resulting in detectable fluorescence was proportional to the initial number of tumor cells for any given cycle number in the first round of amplification. Theoretically, with 100% efficiency of amplification, in all cycles the crossing point interval between tenfold dilutions should be 3.32 cycles. Under our experimental conditions, the mean crossing point interval between the tenfold dilution steps was 2.9 cycles (Fig. 1), demonstrating high efficiency, reproducibility, and accuracy for this RT-PCR assay. Quantitative nested RT-PCR is linear over the range of 10 to 10000 tumor cells per 10 ml of blood (Fig. 2).

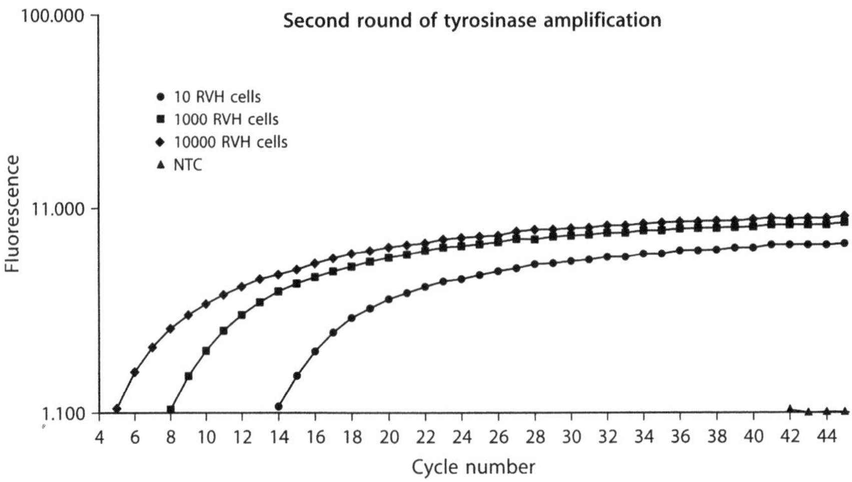

Fig. 1. Sensitivity and quantitation. Fluorescence data of tyrosinase transcripts from serial diluted RVH cells ($10–10^4$) were generated by nested PCR with 35 cycles in the first amplification round. Cycle numbers are plotted versus fluorescence. *Crossing points* mark the beginning of the visibility of the exponential phase

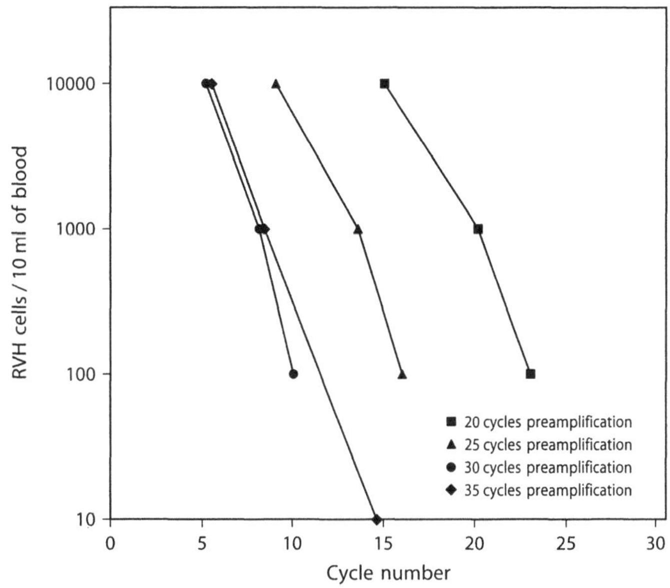

Fig. 2. Reproducibility and accuracy of the tyrosinase RT-PCR. Crossing points of the second round of amplification are plotted versus number of RVH cells. *Curves* represent results after different numbers of preamplification cycles. For any given cycle number in the first amplification round (20, 25, 30, or 35), absolute quantitative data were obtained spanning a linear dynamic range of 3 or 4 orders of magnitude

Specificity

Analyzed electrophoretically, PCR products showed a fragment size of 207 bp, confirming the specificity of the PCR reaction and specific annealing of the hybridization probes (Fig. 3). DNA contaminations can be excluded.

Discussion

Previous investigations attempted to quantify tyrosinase transcripts using either serially diluted and differently sized competitor target molecules [7, 8] or Southern blot analyses standardized to the expression of a housekeeping gene [9]. These methods are laborious as well as time-consuming and provide only semiquantitative data. All these assays reside on close-to-end-point quantitation of transcript amount, which is prone to influencing PCR by rate-limiting reagents and product inhibition. Real time RT-PCR offers for the first time the possibility to quantify melanoma cell-derived tyrosinase transcripts rapidly and accurately using crossing points which mark the early exponential phase. This technique makes quantification much more precise and reproducible, because at the beginning of the exponential phase none of the reagents is rate-limiting and only minimal inhibitory effects occur.

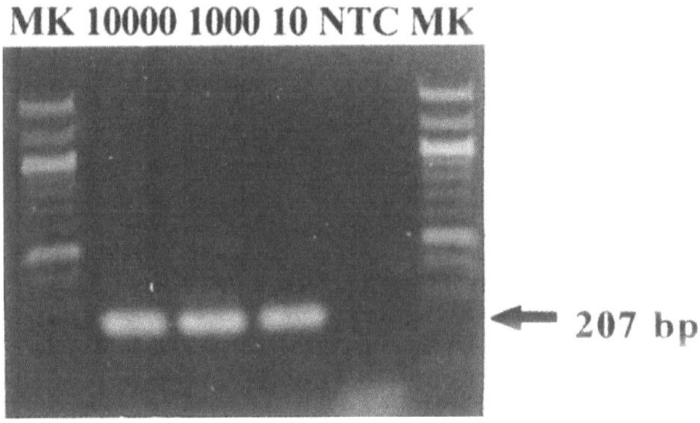

Fig. 3. PCR products after nested PCR with 35 and 45 cycles, size-fractionated (207 bp) in a 1.5% agarose gel containing ethidium bromide. *Top* Number of RVH cells diluted in 10 ml control blood. *NTC* nontemplate control, *MK* 100 bp marker

The dynamic range of quantitation was 4 orders of magnitude with a sensitivity limit of ten melanoma cells (RVH cell line) in 10 ml blood. The sensitivity of this artificial experiment, performed under optimal conditions, must be validated by RT-PCR of blood samples from melanoma patients. As a routine assay, we suggest performing a nested PCR with 35 cycles in the first amplification round to ensure maximal sensitivity.

Furthermore, it is necessary to establish stringent controls to confirm the integrity of RNA and cDNA and to exclude the possibility of false low or negative PCR results due to suboptimal RNA extraction or cDNA synthesis of a given sample. RT-PCR of housekeeping genes such as β2-microglobulin, β-actin, PBGD, or GAPDH is generally used to assess cDNA quality – a procedure which is questionable because housekeeping genes are expressed abundantly and therefore detected even in cDNAs of rather poor quality. With housekeeping gene transcript quantification, it is possible to determine a close range within sufficient cDNA quality can be guaranteed. However, it would be more desirable to work with an internal standard added to the blood sample at low concentration prior to processing, carried throughout the whole process and detected after amplification at a level comparable to that of tyrosinase transcripts [10].

It has to be acknowledged that knowing the amount of tyrosinase transcripts does not allow calculation of the number of circulating tumor cells, since the expression of tyrosinase and other marker genes has been shown to vary interindividually [11, 12] and possibly also in a given patient over time. This is especially important when screening patients undergoing vaccination with melanocyte differentiation proteins. This specific immunologic treatment may lead to a selection of tumor cells with reduced or absent expression of marker genes, as already shown by Scheibenbogen et al. [13] in histologic samples obtained in lesions regressing after nonspecific immunotherapy with interferon (IFN)-α and IL-2.

Quantification of tumor transcripts is a powerful tool for monitoring the course of disease, evaluating the response to chemotherapy in more detail, and identifying patients at high risk of developing hematogenous melanoma metastasis or relapse. If residual tumor cells are detected and the transcript amount of their tumor marker is even quantitated, clinicians could theoretically intervene early with therapy. This would be of potential clinical benefit, because the major problems in clinical management are recurrence and metastasis. Studies on large numbers of patients and with long follow-up periods are needed to evaluate the significance of differences in transcript amount during the course of disease which may predict and correlate with recurrence of disease.

References

1. Battyani Z, Grob J, Xerri L (1995) PCR detection of circulating melanocytes as a prognostic marker in patients with melanoma. Arch Dermatol 131:443–447
2. Mellado B, Colomer D, Castel T (1996) Detection of circulating neoplastic cells by reverse-transcriptase polymerase chain reaction (RT-PCR) correlates with stage and prognosis in malignant melanoma. Proc ASCO, p 433
3. Hoon DSB, Wang Y, Dale PS (1995) Detection of occult melanoma cells in blood with a multiple-marker polymerase chain reaction assay. J Clin Oncol 13:2109–2116
4. Kunter U, Buer J, Probst M (1996) Peripheral blood tyrosinase messenger RNA detection and survival in malignant melanoma. J of Natl Cancer Inst 88:590–594
5. Chomczynski P, Sacchi N (1987) Single step method of RNA isolation by acid guanidinium thiocyanate-phenol-chloroform extraction. Anal Biochem, pp 162, 156
6. Smith B, Selby P, Southgate J (1991) Detection of melanoma cells in peripheral blood by means of reverse transcriptase and polymerase chain reaction. Lancet 338:1227–1229
7. Cross NCP, Feng L, Chase A, Bungey J, Hughes TP, Glodman JM (1993) Competitive polymerase chain reaction to estimate the number of bcr-abl transcripts in chronic myeloid leukemia patients after bone marrow transplantation. Blood, 82:1929–1936
8. Fukuhara T, Hooper WC, Baylin SB, Benson J, Pruckler J, Olson AC, Evatt BL, Vogler WR (1992) Use of the polymerase chain reaction to detect hypermethylation in the calcitonin gene – a new, sensitive approach to monitor tumor cells in acute myelogenous leukemia. Leukemia Res 16:1031–1040
9. Brossert P, Schmier J-W, Krüger S, Willhauck M, Scheibenbogen C, Möhler T, Keilholz U (1995) A polymerase chain reaction-based semiquantitative assessment of malignant melanoma cells in peripheral blood. Cancer Research 55:4056–4068
10. Willhauck M, Vogel S, Keilholz U (1998) Internal control for quality assurance of diagnostic RT-PCR. Biothechniques 25:656–659
11. De Vries T, Fourkour A, Wobbes T, Verkroost G, Ruiter DJ, van Muijen GN (1997) Heterogenous expression of immunotherapy candidate proteins gp100, MART-1, and tyrosinase in human melanoma cell lines and in human melanocytic lesions. Cancer Research 57:3223–3229
12. Chen YT, Stockert E, Tsang S, Coplan KA, Old LJ (1995) Immunophenotyping of melanomas for tyrosinase: implications for vaccine development. Proc Natl Acad Sci USA, 92:8125–8129
13. Scheibenbogen C, Weyers I, Ruiter D, Willhauck M, Bittinger A, Keilholz U (1996) Expression of gp100 in melanoma metastases resected before or after treatment with IFN alpha and IL-2. J. Immunother Emphasis Tumor Immunol 19:375–380

Detection of Micrometastasis Through Tissue-Specific Gene Expression: Its Promise and Problems

R. Jung[1], K. Soondrum[1], W. Krüger[2], and M. Neumaier[1]

[1] Medical Clinic, Department of Clinical Chemistry, University Clinic Hamburg-Eppendorf, 20246 Hamburg, Germany
[2] Medical Clinic, Department of Bone Marrow Transplantation, University Hospital Eppendorf, 20246 Hamburg, Germany

Abstract

The detection of micrometastasis holds great promise for earlier staging of patients with malignant diseases and may ultimately guide therapeutic decisions. So far, reverse-transcriptase polymerase chain reaction (RT-PCR) amplification of genes expressed by the tumor in a tissue-specific manner is the method with the highest diagnostic sensitivity. It is well-established that the identification of single tumor cells is feasible in tissues and bodily fluids in both experimental and clinical samples. However, at present it is difficult to assign clinical significance to results obtained from such tests, primarily because their diagnostic specificity is disputed, both conceptionally and methodologically. For example, amplification of candidate mRNA targets is detectable in non-cancer patients using conditions that generally fail to generate such signals from healthy individuals. We have established that transcription of the tissue-specific genes can be affected by different means. Specifically, some target mRNA species are detectable in peripheral blood nuclear cells as low abundance constitutive-like expression, whereas others are induced through in vitro tissue culturing. In addition, mRNA expression may be distinctly upregulated by different cytokines or growth factors in vivo. Also, background transcription of target mRNAs can occur in different lineages of peripheral blood cells. Finally, expression may be substantially different in tissues such as peripheral blood, bone marrow, or lymph nodes. As a consequence, cancer patients in unrelated clinical situations may present with different levels of background expression, making the diagnostic specificity of test results difficult to assess. To add to this complexity, an increasing body of literature is being generated using various targets for a multitude of malignant diseases. There is a great variety of methods for sampling, specimen processing, nucleic acids recovery, test conditions, and readout formats, making it impossible to compare data. In summary, modalities of quantitative RT-PCR methods and standardization issues should be discussed to address these questions.

Recent Results in Cancer Research, Vol. 158

The Promise in Earlier Diagnosis of Minimal Residual Disease

The prognosis in patients suffering from malignant tumors and metastatically active carcinomas in particular deteriorates rapidly with the spread of the disease. Micrometastatic cells are clinically important (Gusterson 1991). Accordingly, correct staging assessment and early diagnosis of metastatic cells, preferably at the single cell level, could gain importance for rational implementation and/or continuation of anticancer therapy in the future. Correct molecular stratification of patient populations may also provide an incentive for the development of new therapeutic regimens. For example, the German Cancer Aid 17-1A Study Group (Riethmüller et al. 1994) has shown that the administration of monoclonal antibodies specific for tumor-associated antigens may serve as a valid alternative to conventional chemotherapy. Indeed, this group demonstrated that a beneficial effect of their specific immunotherapy was not due to the eradication of pre-existing metastases but rather the prevention of new ones. This suggests that cancer therapies may be effective against micrometastases, making the development of matching laboratory diagnostic procedures to identify these disease states all the more important.

Sensitivity and Specificity of Immunochemical Methods

It has been shown since the early 1980s that detection of single tumor cells in bone marrow by immunocytochemistry is technically feasible (Dearnaley et al. 1983; Dearnaley et al. 1981). Immunocytochemistry has been more broadly applied by using cytokeratins as markers for the presence of epithelial cells and, hence, presumed carcinoma cells in mesenchymal tissues like the bone marrow. Clinical follow-ups generated with this technology (Diel et al. 1992; Lindemann et al. 1992; Pantel et al. 1993) seem to indicate indeed that the presence of cytokeratin-positive cells in the bone marrow is an independent marker for disease-free interval. However, this technology is tedious and difficult to standardize, e.g., with respect to the enrichment of tumor cells from clinical samples, immunochemical staining reactions, and subjective interpretation of positive cells. In particular, the results can hardly be standardized for the high volumes required in routine applications.

Tumor Cell Detection Through Molecular Methods

The goal of molecular biology techniques has been to provide advanced sensitivity and specificity for this field of diagnostics. To this end, three general "classes" of molecular targets exist:

1. Germline mutations in predisposition genes (e.g., familial adenomatous polyposis, hereditary nonpolyposis colonic cancer, or breast cancer) can be assayed for an estimation of individual risk but are not suited for staging purposes.

2. The analysis of tumor-specific gene mutations (e.g., k-ras, adenomatous polyposis coli, or p53) provide grading information with prognostic value (Bergh et al. 1995). However, their complex mutational pattern does not allow for allele-specific amplification, making it difficult to identify mutated alleles in a high background of wild type alleles. However, recent advances show that the detection of these mutations is feasible using capillary electrophoresis (CE). Specifically, it has been demonstrated that, following amplification and heteroduplex formation, the mutated alleles are heteroduplexed, while normal alleles are in homoduplex conformation. After depletion of the homoduplex fraction through CE, the mutated alleles can be analyzed with high sensitivity and specificity. The technology can detect 1/100 000–1/1 000 000 mutated alleles (Coller et al. 1998; Khrapko et al. 1998) and may be sufficient for tumor-specific cell detection in the future.
3. At present, the detection of single tumor cells by amplification of tissue-specific gene expression using the reverse transcriptase polymerase chain reaction (RT-PCR) is the most sensitive technique, using mRNA reverse transcription and amplification of gene expression associated with the tumor cells but not the normal cells in the specimen. Hence, RT-PCR represents the molecular level of tumor markers known in immunochemistry, albeit at higher analytical and diagnostic sensitivity. A multitude of markers and their use in detecting micrometastases have been described in recent years (Battayani et al. 1995; Brossart et al. 1995; Burchill et al. 1994; Cama et al. 1995; Cote et al. 1991; Gomella et al. 1997; Jung et al. 1997; Lehrer et al. 1996; Matsumura et al. 1994; Mattano et al. 1992; Neumaier et al. 1995; Pantel, Riethmüller 1995; Yu et al. 1995; Zippelius et al. 1997). For example, it has been shown that RT-PCR patients with supposedly localized colorectal cancer can be correctly predicted to relapse (Liefers et al. 1998) based on the results of an RT-PCR specific for the carcinoembryonic antigen (CEA) (Gerhard et al. 1994). (See also comment in Lindblom 1998.)

Problems with Molecular Staging by RT-PCR

Recent years have seen an increasing body of literature on the detection of tumor cells using different target mRNAs in tissues and body fluids at sensitivities of 10E-6 or better. However, the clinical significance is still controversial for the following reasons:

1. The assays used are not standardized, leading to results that are difficult to compare. Specifically, positivity rates vary widely, even between patient cohorts of comparable disease status.
2. In the past, assay results have been qualitative or at best semiquantitative, due to the difficulties in quantitative RT-PCR.
3. The diagnostic specificity is controversial for most markers. For example, prostate-specific antigen (PSA)-positive cells have also been demonstrated

Table 1. Preanalytical and analytical factors with critical importance to the validity of RT-PCR results in minimal residual disease detection

Factor		Effects
Preanalytical		
Additives	EDTA, heparin, citrate	Sensitivity
Analyte stability	Native or stabilized material	Sensitivity
Transportation	Shipping time and temperature	Sensitivity
Analytical		
Template recovery	Preparation failure	Sensitivity
Template quality	Degradation of mRNA	Sensitivity
mRNA dependency	Processed pseudogenes	Specificity
Assay robustness	Reagent standardization	Sensitivity
Contamination controls		Specificity
Amplification specificity	Detection of homologous targets	Specificity

in samples from healthy control individuals, patients with nonmalignant diseases, and women with breast cancer (Gomella et al. 1997).

Standardization Issues in RT-PCR

A number of standardization issues appear to be important for enhancing the comparability of results of RT-PCR tests (Table 1). Even taking these into account, two major influential factors are not accounted for and difficult to control: background mRNA expression by normal cells in the specimen and stochastic effects governing the results of single RT-PCR reactions.

Background Transcription of mRNA Targets Used for Cancer Cell Detection

It has been shown that cytokeratin 20 (CK20) mRNA used for detecting gastrointestinal cancer cells can be readily detected in peripheral blood lysates from healthy individuals stabilized with guanidinium isothiocyanate. On the other hand, when these samples had been fractionated into mononuclear cells and polymorphonuclear granulocytes (PMNG), CK20-positive results were obtained in the PMNG fraction but not the mononuclear cell fraction. This demonstrates that CK20 expression does occur in specific nucleated cells in the peripheral blood as a low level background transcript. In contrast, CK18 can be readily detected in mononuclear cells but not the PMNG fraction (unpublished results). In the case of CK20, the background transcription appears to be constitutive. This is not true for other targets. For example, peripheral blood leukocytes cultured in vitro will, after treatment with IFNγ, express CEA mRNA. Other cytokines or growth factors do not induce the CEA message. This is consistent with the fact that CEA positives are found frequently among patients in the acute phase of inflammatory nonmalignant disease (Jung et al. 1998). Apparently, background transcription of mRNA targets can occur constitutively or inducibly.

Stochastic Effects on the Single RT-PCR Test Result

At the sensitivity limit, results obtained from a positive sample will become unpredictable in a single test, depending on whether the method's sensitivity threshold is exceeded. This phenomenon is entirely stochastic and can be assessed using Poisson distribution. In tests for micrometastases, two stochastic processes govern the results of the investigation:

1. If metastatic tumor cells are circulating in the patient, the probability of obtaining a positive sample varies, depending on their density. For example, at a specimen volume of 1 ml, a detection limit of 1 tumor cell/ml, and an intravasal volume of 5,000 ml, the number of circulating cancer cells must well exceed 5,000 at any time to avoid false negative results.
2. When processing positive specimens in the laboratory, a fraction of the mRNA from all the nucleated cells can be assayed at any time for technical reasons. If we accept that the target mRNA is expressed solely in the tumor cell (see above), these molecules are diluted within the mRNA of the normal cells and also fractionated. Depending on assay performance and conditions, the outcome of the single RT-PCR will be uncertain for the same statistical reasons. While we have to accept stochastic influences during sampling, in the analytical phase they may be controlled by increasing the fraction or the sensitivity (Jung et al. 1997).

Promising Solutions

Summing up the main problems of RT-PCR-based detection of minimal residual disease in cancer patients, cutoff values need to be defined for the candidate target mRNAs that take into account the specimen material's reflecting illegitimate transcriptional activity from normal cells. Also, eligibility criteria must be set for patients. Specifically, as observed for some targets, e.g., those induced during acute phase reactions or specific treatments, any background transcription may require postponement of diagnostic RT-PCR tests. To avoid false negative results caused by the stochastics when assaying nonrepresentative specimen fractions, test methods must be devised that allow larger sample fractions and thus the numbers of specific target molecules.

Two recent technical developments allow us to address these major problems:

1. The advent of real time RT-PCR allows researchers readily to develop quantitative PCR amplification tests with a dynamic range of 6–8 orders of magnitude. It can be anticipated that this technology will provide the quantitation necessary to define cutoff values in mRNA copy tests.

2. Enrichment of tumor cells or mRNA target molecules may be obtained using immunobead separation techniques (Eaton et al. 1997; Ghossein et al. 1999; Hardingham et al. 1995) or mRNA adsorption methods to extract the nucleic acids from diluted stabilized specimen materials.

Future Perspectives

So far, RT-PCR methods provide the most sensitive and, from an analytical point of view, most specific way to detect marker molecules expressed by tumor cells. The conflicting reports regarding the positive predictive value of RT-PCR and the clinical importance of detecting single malignant cells perhaps can be partly explained by insufficient standardization among studies. To this end, it will be of utmost importance to develop comprehensive procedures for all assay steps involved. In our experience, most inconsistencies can be avoided by good test design, careful internal quality control of preanalytical interferences, tightly regulated sample preparation and assay procedures, and automated high precision detection formats. It can be foreseen that continued technical improvements will have a major effect on the reliability of RT-PCR assays and the validity of their results. Finally, there is an increasing consensus in the field about the importance of quantitative RT-PCR measurements in light of the growing number of reports on so-called background transcription of candidate molecular markers. According to the literature, it appears that the exquisite sensitivity of tissue-specific gene expression detection has the potential for achieving earlier diagnosis of minimal residual disease. Reassessment of the studies using the new quantitative measurement technologies should help answer the question of the clinical significance of micrometastatic and circulating tumor cells.

References

Battayani Z, Grob JJ, Xerri L, Noe C, Zarour H, Houvaeneghel G, Delpero JR, Birmbaum D, Hassoun J, Bonerandi JJ (1995) Polymerase chain reaction detection of circulating melanocytes as a prognostic marker in patients with melanoma. Arch Dermatol 131:443–447

Bergh J, Norberg T, Sjögren S, Lindgren A, Holmberg L (1995) Complete sequencing of the p53 gene provides prognostic information in breast cancer patients, particularly in relation to adjuvant systemic therapy and radiotherapy. Nature Medicine 1:1029–1034

Brossart P, Schmier JW, Kruger S, Willhauck M, Scheibenbogen C, Mohler T, Keilholz U (1995) A polymerase chain reaction-based semiquantitative assessment of malignant melanoma cells in peripheral blood. Cancer Res 55:4065–4068

Burchill SA, Bradbury FM, Smith B, Lewis IJ, Selby P (1994) Neuroblastoma cell detection by reverse transcriptase-polymerase chain reaction (RT-PCR) for tyrosine hydroxylase mRNA. Int J Cancer 57:671–675

Cama C, Olsson CA, Raffo AJ, Perlman H, Buttyan R, O'Toole K, McMahon D, Benson MC, Katz AE (1995) Molecular staging of prostate cancer. II: A comparison of the application of an enhanced reverse transcriptase polymerase chain reaction assay for the prostate specific antigen versus the prostate specific membrane antigen. J Urol 153:1373–1378

Coller HA, Khrapko K, Torres A, Frampton MW, Utell MJ, Thilly WG (1998) Mutational spectra of a 100-base pair mitochondrial DNA target sequence in bronchial epithelial cells: a comparison of smoking and nonsmoking twins. Cancer Res 58:1268–1277

Cote RJ, Rosen PP, Lesser ML, Old LJ, Osborne MP (1991) Prediction of early relapse in patients with operable breast cancer by detection of occult bone marrow micrometastases. J Clin Oncol 9:1749–1756

Dearnaley DP, Ormerod MG, Sloane JP, Lumley H, Imrie S, Jones M, Coombes RC, Neville AM (1983) Detection of isolated mammary carcinoma cells in marrow of patients with primary breast cancer. J R Soc Med 76:359–364

Dearnaley DP, Sloane JP, Ormerod MG, Steele K, Coombes RC, Clink HM, Powles TJ, Ford HT, Gazet JC, Neville AM (1981) Increased detection of mammary carcinoma cells in marrow smears using antisera to epithelial membrane antigen. Br J Cancer 44:85–90

Diel IJ, Kaufmann M, Görner R, Costa SD, Kaul S, Bastert G (1992) Detection of tumor cells in bone marrow of patients with primary breast cancer: A prognostic factor for distant metastasis. J Clin Oncol 10:1–5

Eaton MC, Hardingham JE, Kotasek D, Dobrovic A (1997) Immunobead RT-PCR: a sensitive method for detection of circulating tumor cells. Biotechniques 22:100–105

Gerhard M, Juhl H, Kalthoff H, Schreiber HW, Wagener C, Neumaier M (1994) Specific detection of carcinoembryonic antigen (CEA)-expressing tumor cells in bone marrow aspirates by PCR. J Clin Oncol 12:725–729

Ghossein RA, Osman I, Bhattacharya S, Ferrara J, Fazzari M, Cordon-Cardo C, Scher HI (1999) Detection of prostatic specific membrane antigen messenger RNA using immunobead reverse transcriptase polymerase chain reaction. Diagn Mol Pathol 8:59–65

Gomella LG, Raj GV, Moreno JG (1997) Reverse transcriptase polymerase chain reaction for prostate specific antigen in the management of prostate cancer [see comments]. J Urol 158:326–337

Gusterson B (1991) Are micrometastases clinically relevant? Br J Hospital Med 47:247–248.

Hardingham JE, Kotasek D, Sage RE, Eaton MC, Pascoe VH, Dobrovic A (1995) Detection of circulating tumor cells in colorectal cancer by immunobead-PCR is a sensitive prognostic marker for relapse of disease. Mol Med 1:789–794

Jung R, Ahmad-Nejad P, Wimmer M, Gerhard M, Wagener C, Neumaier M (1997) Quality management and influential factors for the detection of single metastatic cancer cells by reverse transcriptase polymerase chain reaction. Eur J Clin Chem Clin Biochem 35:3–10

Jung R, Kruger W, Hosch S, Holweg M, Kroger N, Gutensohn K, Wagener C, Neumaier M, Zander AR (1998) Specificity of reverse transcriptase polymerase chain reaction assays designed for the detection of circulating cancer cells is influenced by cytokines in vivo and in vitro. Br J Cancer 78:1194–1198

Khrapko K, Coller HA, Hanekamp JS, Thilly WG (1998) Identification of point mutations in mixtures by capillary electrophoresis hybridization. Nucleic Acids Res 26:5738–5740

Lehrer S, Terk M, Piccoli SP, Song HK, Lavagnini P, Luderer AA (1996) Reverse transcriptase-polymerase chain reaction for prostate-specific antigen may be a prognostic indicator in breast cancer. Br J Cancer 74:871–873

Liefers GJ, Cleton-Jansen AM, van de Velde CJ, Hermans J, van Krieken JH, Cornelisse CJ, Tollenaar RA (1998) Micrometastases and survival in stage II colorectal cancer. N Engl J Med 339:223–228

Lindblom A (1998) Improved tumor staging in colorectal cancer [editorial; comment]. N Engl J Med 339:264–265

Lindemann F, Schlimok G, Dirschedl P, Witte J, Riethmüller G (1992) Prognostic significance of micrometastatic tumour cells in bone marrow of colorectal cancer patients. Lancet 340:685–689

Matsumura M, Niwa Y, Kato N, Komatsu Y, Shiina S, Kawabe T, Kawase T, Toyoshima H, Ihori M, Shiratori Y, et al (1994) Detection of alpha-fetoprotein mRNA, an indicator of hematogenous spreading hepatocellular carcinoma, in the circulation: a possible predictor of metastatic hepatocellular carcinoma. Hepatology 20:1418–1425

Mattano LA, Jr, Moss TJ, Emerson SG (1992) Sensitive detection of rare circulating neuroblastoma cells by the reverse transcriptase-polymerase chain reaction. Cancer Res 52:4701–4705

Neumaier M, Gerhard M, Wagener C (1995) Diagnosis of micrometastases by the amplification of tissue-specific genes. Gene 159:43–47

Pantel K, Izbicki JR, Angstwurm M, Braun S, Passlick B, Karg O, Thetter O, Riethmüller G (1993) Immunocytological detection of bone marrow micrometastasis in operable non-small lung cancer. Cancer Res 53:1027–1031

Pantel K, Riethmüller G (1995) Methods for detection of micrometastatic carcinoma cells in bone marrow, blood and lymph nodes. Onkologie 18:394–401

Riethmüller G, Schneider Gadicke E, Schlimok G, Schmiegel W, Raab R, Hoffken K, Gruber R, Pichlmaier H, Hirche H, Pichlmayr R et al (1994) Randomised trial of monoclonal antibody for adjuvant therapy of resected Dukes' C colorectal carcinoma. German Cancer Aid 17-1A Study Group. Lancet 343:1177–1183

Yu H, Giai M, Diamandis EP, Katsaros D, Sutherland DJ, Levesque MA, Roagna R, Ponzone R, Sismondi P (1995) Prostate-specific antigen is a new favorable prognostic indicator for women with breast cancer. Cancer Res 55:2104–2110

Zippelius A, Kufer P, Honold G, Kollermann MW, Oberneder R, Schlimok G, Riethmüller G, Pantel K (1997) Limitations of reverse-transcriptase polymerase chain reaction analyses for detection of micrometastatic epithelial cancer cells in bone marrow. J Clin Oncol 15:2701–2708

Immunobead-Based Detection and Characterization of Circulating Tumor Cells in Melanoma Patients

Ø. Fodstad[1], R. Faye[1,2], H.K. Høifødt[1], E. Skovlund[2], and S. Aamdal[2]

[1] Department of Tumor Biology, Institute for Cancer Research, The Norwegian Radium Hospital, Oslo, Norway
[2] Department of Oncology, The Norwegian Radium Hospital, Oslo, Norway

Abstract

The presence of circulating tumor cells in bone marrow and peripheral blood of cancer patients may reflect the aggressiveness of the disease. This also applies to cancers that rarely give rise to overt bone marrow metastases. The clinical validity of micrometastasis detection for staging and prognostication depends on the sensitivity and reliability of the detection method. In malignant melanoma, most studies have used reverse transcriptase polymerase chain reaction (RT-PCR) techniques, commonly with tyrosinase mRNA as the target molecule. Unfortunately, highly inconsistent results have been reported, raising doubts about this approach. In a study of 81 melanoma patients with metastatic disease, we used an immunobead rosetting method in which live melanoma cells are selected and identified by binding of paramagnetic beads coated with the 9.2.27 antibody against the high molecular weight melanoma-associated antigen. In bone marrow samples obtained from 60 patients, 14 (23.3%) were positive, compared to only two of 81 in blood. A highly significant correlation ($p = 0.0001$, log rank test) was found between micrometastasis positivity and overall survival from time of removal of the primary tumor. Moreover, in regression analysis it was found that the presence of micrometastatic cells was an independent and the most important indicator of poor prognosis, with a relative risk of 5.38. The immunomagnetic method is simple, rapid, and highly sensitive and will be used in further prospective clinical studies.

Introduction

For a number of different tumor types, relationships have been reported between the presence of micrometastatic cancer cells in bone marrow (BM) and the stage as well as the progression of the disease (review: Pantel et al. 1999). For some tumor types, development of symptom-producing metastases is

Recent Results in Cancer Research, Vol. 158

seen more frequently in bone and BM than at any other site, whereas for other cancers overt metastases in BM are extremely rare (Pittman et al. 1971). In spite of the lack of clinical metastases in the BM of patients with colorectal cancer, for example, micrometastatic tumor cells in BM have been detected at a relatively high frequency (Pantel et al. 1999) and correlations to the malignant behavior of the disease have been observed. Based on the potential of micrometastatis detection to help in disease staging and prognostication, the interest in methods of detection of such cells in the BM and peripheral blood (PB) has grown rapidly during recent years.

In patients with carcinoma, the most common method of identifying circulating cancer cells has been immunocytochemistry, performed on cell smears (Dearnley et al. 1981; Diel et al. 1996) or on cytospin preparations of mononuclear cell (MNC) fractions isolated from BM or blood samples (Pantel et al. 1999). In spite of several advantages, immunocytochemical methods suffer from limitations such as cell loss and the fact that only a limited number of MNCs can be screened, and also that the antibodies and visualization methods used can cause false positive results (Borgen et al. 1998; Fodstad 2000).

In malignant melanoma, most of the published work on micrometastatic detection has concentrated on the use of RT-PCR on blood and BM samples (Hoon et al. 1995; Keilholz 1998; Schitteck et al. 1999; Waldmann et al. 1999). Highly conflicting results have been reported, with positive results ranging from 0% to 100% in patients with disseminated melanoma (Chittek et al. 1999). Related to such discrepancies, the reliability of RT-PCR assays for the detection of circulating tumor cells has been questioned (de Graaf et al. 1997; Keilholz et al. 1998; Bostick et al. 1998; Ruud et al. 1999).

Based on long experience with the use of immunomagnetic beads for purging BM of tumor cells (Kvalheim et al. 1987; Myklebust et al. 1993, 1994), we developed an immunomagnetic method for selection and identification of micrometastatic tumor cells that uses specific binding of immunobeads to target cells, creating "rosettes" for detection (Fodstad et al. 1997; Rye et al. 1998; Fodstad 2000). For melanoma cell detection, superparamagnetic beads were coated with an antibody directed against the 250 K melanoma-associated antigen and tested successfully in model experiments. The advantages of this method are simplicity, the ability to screen up to more than 2×10^7 MNCs, and that the procedure can be completed within 2 h. Here we report data obtained with this method on BM and blood samples from 81 patients with malignant melanoma.

Patients and Methods

Patients

Eighty-one patients previously operated on for primary malignant melanoma were recruited in the period 1994–1998 at admission to our regional cancer hospital for radiotherapy, systemic therapy, or induction of adjuvant treatment.

Twenty-seven female and 54 male patients with a median age of 55.3 years were included. The majority were hospitalized for treatment with chemo- or radiotherapy when the sampling was done. Fifty-nine patients had AJCC melanoma stage IV, 19 had stage III, two had stage II, and one had stage I. The criteria for inclusion were: histologically confirmed primary malignant melanoma and no other known malignancy. Before the sampling, all patients signed written informed consent forms. The study and the patient information form were approved by the regional ethics committee.

The median time from excision of the primary melanoma to enrollment in the study was 2.6 years (range: 0.1–16.0 years). The median observation time after the first sampling was 8.1 months (range: 0–3.4 years).

Sample Collection

Bone marrow samples were drawn from the upper iliac crests by needle aspiration under local anesthesia. A volume of 10–20 ml was drawn into syringes containing 2 ml heparin (1000 IE) per 10 ml of BM. Peripheral blood specimens (40 ml) were collected in heparinized Vacutainer tubes. Samples were brought immediately to the laboratory and kept at 4 °C during transport and laboratory procedures.

Monoclonal Antibodies and Immunobeads

The monoclonal antibody 9.2.27 (Morgan et al. 1981), which recognizes an epitope of the high molecular weight (HMW) melanoma-associated antigen, was kindly provided by Dr. Ralph A. Reisfeld, Scripps Institute, San Diego, Calif., USA. The MOC-31 antiepithelial glycoprotein (EGP2) antibody, obtained from MCA Development, Groningen, The Netherlands, was used as a negative control. The antibodies were directly conjugated to magnetic sheep antimouse IgG M-450 Dynabeads (Dynal, Oslo, Norway) as recommended by the manufacturer. Uncoated SAM M-450 Dynabeads were used as an additional negative control.

Procedure for Detection and Separation of Tumor Cells

The technique for selection and detection of melanoma cells was performed as previously described (Fodstad et al. 1997; Rye et al. 1997). Briefly, the MNC fraction of the patient samples was collected by standard density gradient centrifugation (Lymphoprep, Nycomed, Oslo, Norway), washed in phosphate-buffered saline (PBS), resuspended in PBS with 1% human serum albumin (HSA), and the cells were counted using an electronic particle counter.

Magnetic immunobeads with or without conjugated antibody were added to the MNC fraction in a ratio of one bead to two MNC and incubated with continuous rotation for 30 min at 4 °C. After incubation, cell suspensions were diluted with PBS + 1% HSA and put in a magnet holder for 1–2 min to separate bound, "rosetted," and unbound cells. The cells not bound to immunobeads were decanted off with the tubes still in the magnet holder. Twenty-microliter samples of the positive fraction were pipetted for microscopy and the number of rosetted cells, i.e., those with at least five beads/cell, was counted. A sample was regarded as positive at least two rosettes were found with the 9.2.27 immunobeads and no rosettes with the control beads.

Immunocytochemical staining

In selected cases, part of the MNC fraction prepared from the patient samples was used for preparation of cytospins with 5×10^4 cells per slide and stained with the indirect alkaline phosphatase-anti-alkaline phosphatase (APAAP) method involving HMB45, anti-S-100 or 9.2.27 antibodies or an irrelevant antibody as control. The slides were counterstained with hematoxylin, and the presence of positively stained cells was evaluated by light microscopy.

Statistics

Life-table curves were constructed with the Kaplan-Meier method and distributions were compared by the log rank test. The Cox regression proportional hazards model was applied for multivariate analysis of prognostic factors, calculating relative risk (RR) using SPSS data software, version 6.1.

Results

Bone marrow and peripheral blood specimens were collected from 60 melanoma patients, and PB samples alone were collected in an additional 21 cases. Tumor cells were detected in 14/60 (23.3%) of the BM samples. In blood, only 2 of 81 samples contained tumor cells, one of which was also positive in BM, whereas no BM sample was available in the other.

In one patient, tumor cells were found in the BM aspirate 9 months before distant metastases could be detected by conventional examination with X-ray, CT, or ultrasound examinations.

When survival time from excision of the primary tumor was calculated for patients with (15) and without (66) micrometastatic cells in BM and PB, it was found that the presence of melanoma tumor cells identified with the rosetting method was associated with highly significantly shorter median overall survival (log rank test, $p=0.0001$) (Fig. 1).

Patients with positive immunomagnetic test also showed a clearly shorter median disease-free survival time: 3.8 months compared to 8.5 months in the group with no detectable melanoma cells in BM (not shown). Importantly, multiple regression analysis showed that a positive micrometastasis test was a significant and the most important predictor of overall survival, with a higher calculated relative hazard (RR=5.38) than the depth of growth of the primary tumor, the melanoma morphology, the number of metastatic sites at the time of relapse, and the stage of disease (Table 1).

The depth of invasion at the time of primary excision proved not to be of prognostic significance in the group of patients with metastatic disease detectable by conventional methods (Cox regression, $p=0.81$, RR=1.02). Only two of 17 cases tested so far had melanoma cells detected by immunocytochemistry on cytospins using the 9.2.27, HMB45, and anti-S-100 antibodies.

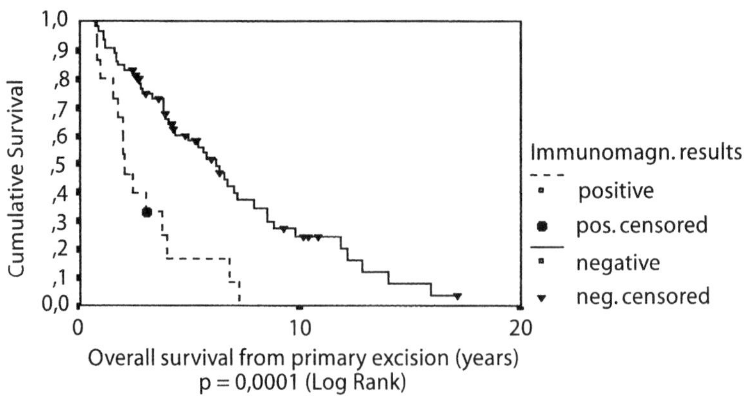

Fig. 1. Kaplan-Meier plot of overall survival of patients with ($n=15$) or without ($n=66$) tumor cells detected in BM or peripheral blood. The difference in survival was highly significant (log rank test, $p=0.0001$)

Table 1. Multiple regression analysis of prognostic parameters. Cox regression analysis was done using "survival from the time of primary excision" as the dependent variable. Twenty-eight cases had missing values and one was censored before the earliest event in a stratum; thus 52 cases were available for analysis

Variables	Relative hazards (exp (B))	95% CI for relative hazards		Significance
		Lower	Upper	
Micrometastasis test	5.38	2.06	14.08	0.0006
Thickness (Breslow)	1.02	0.87	1.20	0.81
Metastatic sites	1.20	0.86	1.67	0.29
Nodular melanoma	0.75	0.31	1.86	0.54
Other melanomas*	2.56	0.73	8.97	0.14

CI, confidence interval.

* Melanoma morphology as a categorical variable was divided into subgroups before analysis. The subgroup "other melanomas" included amelanotic melanomas ($n=1$), lentigo maligna melanomas ($n=1$), acral lentiginous melanomas ($n=1$), and melanomas primarily diagnosed in the lymph nodes ($n=3$) with no known primary cutaneous melanoma. The subgroup "superficial spreading melanomas" was used as the standard for comparison in the morphology category.

Discussion

In the present study of 81 patients with advanced disease, approximately 23% (14/60) of the patients had detectable tumor cells in the BM. The fraction of positive PB samples was strikingly different (2/81). Importantly, survival curves showed a highly significant difference in overall survival from the time of removal of the primary tumor in the groups with and without micrometastatic melanoma cells. Moreover, multiple regression analysis revealed that a positive micrometastasis test was the most important predictor of poor prognosis, independently of the depth of invasion of the primary tumor, the morphology, and the number of metastatic sites at the time of relapse. The data demonstrate that, whereas these other factors give no indication of the future aggressiveness of the disease in advanced cases, the results obtained with the immunomagnetic method do. It was also interesting that, in one case, the findings of micrometastatic disease in BM preceded the detection of relapse with conventional methods by 9 months.

That the detection of tumor cells in the BM was a more important parameter than Breslow tumor depth may seem surprising. However, whereas tumor depth is the most important prognostic indicator at the time of primary excision when the disease is limited to the local or regional stage, its predictive value in advanced disease is fading.

As much as 25 years ago, Einhorn et al. (1974) looked for micrometastatic cells in BM aspirates using conventional cytology. In a large series of stage IV melanoma patients, metastatic disease was found in 9% (24/254) of the cases. In the same study, 96 of the patients were later examined at autopsy, of whom 15 (16%) had BM involvement. With the introduction of immunocytochemical methods, the sensitivity and reliability of detection of melanoma cells in BM and blood increased. Immunocytochemistry is used for micrometastasis detection in most studies on carcinomas (Pantel et al. 1999), although it is known that the method suffers from limitations such as the risk of cell loss and false positive staining (Borgen et al. 1998). Surprisingly few studies applying such techniques on melanoma samples have been published. One explanation may be that available antibodies, such as anti-S-100 and HMB-45, commonly used for immunohistochemical staining of solid melanoma tumors, may not bind to a sufficiently high fraction of circulating melanoma cells. Preliminary data on cytospins prepared from patients in our study showed positive staining in 2 of 17 cases examined so far.

The main advantages of the immunomagnetic method are its high sensitivity, related to the fact that it allows screening of up to 10^8 nucleated cells, its simplicity, and the fact that the results can be produced in 2–3 h. Evidently, this method is also dependent on the use of antibodies with high specificity and that they bind consistently to a very high fraction of target cells. The 9.2.27 anti-HMW melanoma-associated antibody used has been shown to bind to a high proportion of malignant melanoma cell lines and tissues (Morgan et al. 1981; Godal et al. 1992), to have no significant binding to normal BM cells, and can be used for in vivo immunoscintigraphy (Oldham et al. 1984; Hwang et al. 1985). The specificity and efficacy of the rosetting method involving 9.2.27 immunobeads have also been demonstrated in model experiments. Thus, the beads were able to recover a very high percentage of fluorescence-labeled cultivated melanoma cells added to more than 10^7 mononuclear BM or PB cells from healthy volunteers (unpublished results).

The question might still be raised whether some rosetted cells could represent previously unidentified, antigen-expressing normal BM cells or that cutaneous cells could have contaminated the sample. However, several lines of evidence indicate that the rosetted cells are true tumor cells. BM cells from a high number of healthy volunteers and various nonmelanoma patients have consistently been negative with 9.2.27 antibody-coated beads and, in the present study, immunobeads with the anticarcinoma MOC-31 antibody as well as uncoated SAM M450 Dynabeads tested negative in all cases.

In contrast to the RT-PCR results of Waldmann et al. (1999), in our study a low fraction of the patients who tested positive in the BM sample were positive in PB. It is noteworthy that, with our method, the difference between positive samples from BM and blood is much less pronounced for several other tumor types (Fodstad et al. 2000). The low fraction of positive findings in PB of melanoma patients might reflect intermittent shedding of tumor cells and that the BM may act as a reservoir, whereas the blood is a medium for transporting malignant cells from one organ to another. Further studies should include examination of multiple PB samples from the same melanoma patient, especially from those who have tested positive in the BM.

Blood samples from melanoma patients have been intensively studied by a number of research groups during the past 5 years, mainly by means of tyrosinase RT-PCR.

Theoretically, the method should have the potential to detect melanoma cells with high sensitivity. Smith et al. (1991) reported that their assay could detect one single melanoma cell from a cell line in 2 ml of normal blood. Hoon et al. (1995) introduced a multimarker PCR assay and demonstrated that the use of four marker genes was significantly better than using tyrosinase alone. They reported that the risk of relapse within the next 6 months for high risk patients previously treated for node metastases was 3.8 times higher after positive test results than after negative ones. The study by Mellado et al. (1996) was the first tyrosinase RT-PCR study to show a positive test to be an independent prognostic factor ($p=0.002$, multivariate analysis). Brossart et al. (1995) tried to establish a PCR-based semiquantitative assessment of melanoma cells in blood by interpolating the amplified tyrosinase signal strength of patient samples to an equivalent tyrosinase signal of diluted SK-MEL 28 cells. They found that the calculated number of circulating tumor cells correlated with tumor burden.

When evaluating RT-PCR data, it is necessary to remember that this approach also suffers from the risk of false positive and false negative results. False positive RT-PCR results may be due to very low levels of contamination (Lo et al. 1989), real or illegitimate transcription of the target gene in nontarget cells (Chelly et al. 1989), and, in melanoma, to transcription of a pseudotyrosinase gene (Takeda et al. 1991). Glaser et al. (1997) recently performed a comparative analysis of tyrosinase mRNA RT-PCR and found that five studies demonstrated sensitivities in stage III melanoma patients ranging from 13%–50%. Sensitivities of 90% or more in patients in stage III melanoma were reported in three studies. These inconsistent results confirm the need for standardization and quality control of the tyrosinase RT-PCR protocols. The need for such initiatives as well as the technological problems faced with this technique were recently exposed in a study performed by a subgroup of the European Organization for Research and Treatment of Cancer Melanoma Cooperative Group (Keilholz et al. 1998).

Even if the technological difficulties could be mastered, it should be noted that the RT-PCR methods are, with few exceptions, nonquantitative. Importantly, even with semiquantitative methods, the number of mRNA molecules detected does not necessarily reflect the number of live tumor cells. Thus, the mRNA molecule templates for reverse transcription may come from dead or dying cells, and the transcript level may differ between individual cells and tumors.

Both immunological and RT-PCR techniques fail to give information about the metastatic capacity of the melanoma cells. However, our immunomagnetic method isolates intact, live cells, making further characterization of the tumor cells possible. This can be obtained rapidly and directly with a newly developed method in which latex particles containing different fluorochromes are coated with antibodies recognizing various membrane markers and then used to visualize marker expression on individual cells (Fodstad et al. 1998). After immunomagnetic detection, molecular biological methods can also be applied on the cells (Forus et al. 1999), or they can be used for cell cultivation in vitro and in vivo (Rye et al. 1997).

The present work showed that 23% of patients with metastatic malignant melanoma had tumor cells in BM and only 2% in blood. Most previously published studies have used RT-PCR methods and, to our knowledge, only two groups had data previously reported on examination (Ghossein et al. 1998; Waldmann et al. 1999). Recently, Schitteck et al. (1999) reported a relationship between the results obtained with RT-PCR on MelanA mRNA in blood and prognosis. Ghossein et al. (1998) showed the prognostic significance of tyrosinase RT-PCR results. Here we found a highly significant correlation between overall survival and the presence of immunomagnetically detected live melanoma cells in BM. Importantly, the test was an independent and the most important predictor (RR=5.38) of poor prognosis in patients with metastatic disease. The simplicity and sensitivity of the immunomagnetic method, together with the ability to characterize further the selected cells, makes it attractive for further studies on samples from melanoma patients for staging and prognostication, and possibly for monitoring the effect of therapy.

References

1. Borgen E, Beiske K, Trachsl S, Nesland JM, Kvalheim G, Herstad TK, Schlichting E, Qvist H, Naume B (1998) Immunocytochemical detection of isolated epithelial cells in bone marrow: non-specific staining and contribution by plasma cells directly reactive to alkaline phosphatase. J Pathol 185:427–434
2. Bostick PJ et al (1998) Limitations of specific reverse-transcriptase polymerase chain reaction markers in the detection of metastases in the lymph nodes and blood of breast cancer patients. J Clin Oncol 16(8):2632–2640
3. Brossart P, Schmier JW, Kruger S, Willhauck M, Scheibenbogen C, Mohler T et al (1995) A polymerase chain reaction-based semiquantitative assessment of malignant melanoma cells in peripheral blood. Cancer Res 55:4065–4068
4. Chelly J, Concordet JP, Kaplan JC, Kahn A (1989) Illegitimate transcription: transcription of any gene in any cell type. Proc Natl Acad Sci 86:2617–2621
5. de Graaf H, Mælandsmo G, Ruud P, Forus A, Øyjord T, Fodstad Ø, Hovig E (1997) Ecotopic expression of target genes may represent an inherent limitation of RT-PCR assays used for micrometastasis detection – Studies on the epithelial glycoprotein gene EGP-2. Int. J Cancer 72:191–196
6. Dearnaley DP, Sloane JP, Ormerod MG, Steele K, Coombes RC, Clink HM, Powles TJ, Ford HT, Gazet JC, Neville AM (1981) Increased detection of mammary carcinoma cells in marrow smears using antisera to epithelial membrane antigen. Br J Cancer 44:85–90
7. Diel IJ, Kaufmann M, Costa SD, Holle R, von Minckwitz G, Solomayer EF et al (1996) Micrometastatic breast cancer cells in bone marrow at primary surgery: prognostic value in comparison with nodal status. J Natl Cancer Inst 88:1652–1658
8. Einhorn LH, Burgess MA, Vallejos C, Bodey GP Sr, Gutterman J, Mavligit G et al (1974) Prognostic correlations and response to treatment in advanced metastatic malignant melanoma. Cancer Res 34:1995–2004
9. Fodstad Ø, Høifødt HK, Faye R, Marth C, Andresen M, Hovland B, Aamdal S, Bruland Ø (1999) Clinical relevance of immunomagnetically detected micrometastatic cells in bone marrow and peripheral blood. Proc Am Assoc Cancer Res 40:354
10. Fodstad Ø (2000) Immunological methods for detection of minimal residual cancer. Cancer and Metastasis Reviews. In press

11. Fodstad Ø, Trones GE, Forus A, Rye PD, Beiske K, Aamdal S, Høifødt HK (1997) Improved immunomagnetic method for detection and characterization of cancer cells in blood and bone marrow. Proc Am Assoc Cancer Res 38:26
12. Fodstad Ø, Øverli GE, Høifødt HK (1998) New method for phenotypic characterisation of micrometastatic cancer cells. Proc Am Assoc Cancer Res 39:436
13. Forus A, Høifødt HK, Øverli GE, Myklebost O, Fodstad Ø (1999) Sensitive method for FISH characterisation of breast cancer cells in bone marrow aspirates. Molecular Pathol 52:68–74
14. Ghossein RA et al. (1998) Prognostic significance of peripheral blood and bone marrow tyrosinase messenger RNA in malignant melanoma. Clin Cancer Res 4(2):419–428
15. Godal A, Kumle B, Pihl A, Juell S, Fodstad Ø (1992) Immunotoxins directed against the high molecular weight melanoma-associated antigen. Identification of potent antibody-toxin combinations. Int. J Cancer 52:631–635
16. Hoon DS, Wang Y, Dale PS, Conrad AJ, Schmid P, Garrison D et al (1995) Detection of occult melanoma cells in blood with a multiple-marker polymerase chain reaction assay. J Clin Oncol 13:2109–2116
17. Hwang KM, Fodstad Ø, Oldham RK, Morgan AC Jr (1985) Radiolocalization of xenografted human malignant melanoma by a monoclonal antibody (9.2.27) to a melanoma-associated antigen in nude mice. Cancer Res 45:4150–4155
18. Keilholz U et al (1998) Reliability of reverse transcription-polymerase chain reaction (RT-PCR)-based assays for the detection of circulating tumour cells: a quality-assurance initiative of the EORTC Melanoma Cooperative Group. Eur J Cancer 34(5):750–753
19. Kvalheim G, Fodstad Ø, Nustad K, Pharo A, Ugelstad J, Pihl A, Funderud S (1987) Elimination of B-lymphoma cells from human bone marrow: Model experiments using monodisperse magnetic particles coated with primary monoclonal antibodies. Cancer Res 47:846–851
20. Lo YM, Patel P, Wainscoat JS, Sampietro M, Gillmer MD, Fleming KA (1989) Prenatal sex determination by DNA amplification from maternal peripheral blood [see comments]. Lancet 2:1363–1365
21. Mellado B, Colomer D, Castel T, Munoz M, Carballo E, Galan M et al (1996) Detection of circulating neoplastic cells by reverse-transcriptase polymerase chain reaction in malignant melanoma: association with clinical stage and prognosis. J Clin Oncol 14:2091–2097
22. Morgan AC Jr, Galloway DR, Reisfeld RA (1981) Production and characterisation of monoclonal antibody to a melanoma specific glycoprotein. Hybridoma 1:27–36
23. Myklebust AT, Godal A, Pharo A, Juell S, Fodstad Ø (1994) Comparison of two antibody-based methods for elimination of breast cancer cells from human bone marrow. Cancer Res 54:209–214
24. Myklebust AT, Pharo A, Fodstad Ø (1993) Effective removal of SCLC cells from human bone marrow. Use of four monoclonal antibodies and immunomagnetic beads. Br J Cancer 67:1331–1336
25. Oldham RK, Foon KA, Morgan AC, Woodhouse CS, Schroff RW, Abrams PG et al (1984) Monoclonal antibody therapy of malignant melanoma: in vivo localization in cutaneous metastasis after intravenous administration. J Clin Oncol 2:1235–1244
26. Pantel K, Cote RJ, Fodstad Ø (1999) Detection and clinical importance of micrometastatic disease. J Natl Cancer Inst 91(13):1113–1124
27. Pittman G et al. (1971) Metastatic cells in bone marrow; study of 83 cases. Cleve Clin Q 38(2):55–64
28. Rye PD, Høifødt HK, Trones GE, Fodstad Ø (1997) Immunobead-filtration: a novel approach for the isolation and propagation of tumor cells. Am J Pathol 150:99–106
29. Schittek B et al (1999) Amplification of MelanA messenger RNA in addition to tyrosinase increases sensitivity of melanoma cell detection in peripheral blood and is associated with the clinical stage and prognoses of malignant melanoma. Br J Dermatol 141(1):30–36

30. Smith B, Selby P, Southgate J, Pittman K, Bradley C, Blair GE (1991) Detection of melanoma cells in peripheral blood by means of reverse transcriptase and polymerase chain reaction. Lancet 338:1227–1229
31. Takeda A, Matsunaga J, Tomita Y, Tagami H, Shibahara S (1991) Nucleotide sequence of the putative human tyrosinase pseudogene. J Exp Med 163:295–297
32. Waldmann V et al (1999) The detection of tyrosinase-specific mRNA in bone marrow is not more sensitive than in blood for the demonstration of micrometastatic melanoma. Br J Dermatol 140(6):1060–1064

Rapid Enrichment and Detection of Melanoma Cells from Peripheral Blood Mononuclear Cells by a New Assay Combining Immunomagnetic Cell Sorting and Immunocytochemical Staining

C. Siewert[1], M. Herber[1], N. Hunzelmann[2], Ø. Fodstad[3], S. Miltenyi[1], M. Assenmacher[1], and J. Schmitz[1]

[1] Miltenyi Biotec GmbH, Friedrich-Ebert-Str. 68, 51429 Bergisch Gladbach, Germany
[2] Department of Dermatology, University of Cologne, Cologne, Germany
[3] Department of Tumor Biology, The Norwegian Radium Hospital, Oslo, Norway

Abstract

Commonly used methods for detection of melanoma cells in blood, including RT-PCR and immunocytochemistry, display only a limited sensitivity and specificity. Reliable detection of less than one melanoma cell per ml of blood is hardly possible using these methods. To obtain greater sensitivity so that a single melanoma cell in up to 25 ml of blood can be detected (5×10^7 peripheral blood mononuclear cells, or PBMC), we developed a new assay for combined enrichment and immunocytochemical detection of disseminated melanoma cells from PBMC of patients with malignant melanomas. Melanoma cells are directly magnetically labeled using colloidal superparamagnetic microparticles approximately 60 nm in diameter conjugated to the anti-melanoma monoclonal antibody 9.2.27, with no reactivity to normal cells in blood. Magnetically labeled melanoma cells are enriched from PBMC by magnetic cell separation and detected by a new approach for immunocytochemical staining with monoclonal mouse anti-melanoma antibodies (anti-MelanA and HMB-45). The efficiency of this assay was demonstrated in a model system in which 5–500 tumor cells from the melanoma cell line SK-MEL-28 were seeded into PBMC samples from healthy donors containing 5×10^7 leukocytes. Mean recovery of the seeded tumor cells was $47.4 \pm 13.99\%$ ($n = 15$). Applying the assay to 20–50 ml blood samples of patients with stage III–IV malignant melanomas, we were able to detect melanoma cells in two of eight patients (25%).

Introduction

During recent decades, a continually rising incidence of malignant melanoma has been observed. Early metastatic dissemination of the primary tumor is responsible for the poor prognosis and high mortality of this disease. At present, practically no curative therapies exist for late stage metastatic dis-

Recent Results in Cancer Research, Vol. 158

ease. Since it is generally believed that dissemination pathways involve the bloodstream, the detection of single circulating melanoma cells in peripheral blood is considered to be of great prognostic relevance for early micrometastatic disease and may aid in identifying candidate patients for effective adjuvant therapies.

Currently, great effort is being invested in the development of sensitive specific assays for the detection of occult disseminated tumor cells in the peripheral blood of melanoma patients. The main focus is on molecular approaches which are based on the specific amplification of mRNA from melanoma associated markers. Reported sensitivities range from more than one tumor cell per ml of blood to less than one per 10 ml of blood [1–6]. The cause of this variation is largely unclear.

We have developed a cellular assay which combines immunomagnetic enrichment with immunocytochemical detection at a high level of simplicity and rapidity. Combining these two methods, the major limitation of immunocytochemistry, a relatively low sensitivity in the range of one tumor cell per 10^5–10^6 blood cells, is overcome by pre-enriching the melanoma cells from a sample of much larger size. Microscopic analysis of the enriched cell fraction can easily be performed on a single cytocentrifuge slide. Morphological characterization of the target cells can further reduce the frequency of false positive results.

For the enrichment of melanoma cells, PBMC of patients with malignant melanoma are specifically magnetically labeled using colloidal superparamagnetic microparticles approximately 60 nm in diameter (MACS MicroBeads, Miltenyi Biotec GmbH, Bergisch Gladbach, Germany) conjugated to a monoclonal antibody, 9.2.27, with reactivity to a melanoma specific cell surface antigen not found on hematopoietic cells [7–9]. Magnetically labeled cells are enriched in a first round by applying the cells onto a ferromagnetic column (MS^+ column) in the magnetic field of a strong permanent magnet. The enriched cell fraction is eluted and fixed with formaldehyde. The fixed cells are reapplied onto another MS^+ column for further enrichment and for "solid phase" intracellular staining of the magnetically labeled melanoma cells. The latter means that permeabilization and staining steps are performed while the cells are immobilized in the matrix of the column. In this way, washing steps can be performed without centrifugation, which dramatically reduces nonspecific total cell loss. For the detection of disseminated melanoma cells by intracellular staining, we chose monoclonal antibodies that react with MelanA/MART-1 [10] and HMB-45 antigens. Staining of the melanoma cells is done in a doubly indirect way, by incubating the immobilized cells successively with the anti-melanoma antibodies (both IgG-1), FITC-conjugated rat anti-mouse IgG-1, and anti-FITC alkaline phosphatase. After all staining steps, the enriched fraction is eluted and transferred onto slides using a cytocentrifuge. The slides are finally developed by incubation with a substrate for alkaline phosphatase.

The efficiency of the assay was demonstrated in a model system in which defined numbers of a melanoma cell line were deflected into PBMC samples from healthy donors using a flow sorter. After applying the assay, nearly 50% of the seeded cells were recovered on the slides. Applying the assay to blood samples from patients with stage III and IV malignant melanoma, we were able to detect disseminated melanoma cells in two of eight patients.

Materials and Methods

Cells

1. The human melanoma cell line SK-MEL-28 was used for seeding experiments and for positive control samples.
2. PBMC from normal healthy donors were used for seeding experiments and as negative control samples.
3. PBMC from eight patients with stage III–IV malignant melanoma were investigated.

Antibodies

1. Monoclonal mouse anti-human melanoma antibody 9.2.27 conjugated to MicroBeads [7–8].
2. Monoclonal mouse anti-human Melan A antibody (clone: A103, Dako, Glostrup, Denmark).
3. Monoclonal mouse anti-human melanoma antibody HMB-45 (Dako).
4. Monoclonal rat anti-mouse IgG1 antibody conjugated to FITC (clone: X56, Becton Dickinson, San Jose, Calif., USA).
5. Monoclonal mouse anti-FITC antibody conjugated to alkaline phosphatase (Miltenyi Biotec, Bergisch Gladbach, Germany).

Reagents

1. Buffer: phosphate-buffered saline pH 7.2, supplemented with 0.5% bovine serum albumin and 2 mM EDTA. The buffer was degassed by applying vacuum.
2. FcR blocking reagent containing human IgG (Miltenyi Biotec).
3. Inside Fix containing formaldehyde (Inside Stain Kit, Miltenyi Biotec).
4. Inside Perm containing detergent (Inside Stain Kit, Miltenyi Biotec).
5. Phosphate-buffered saline (PBS) pH 7.2.
6. Sigma Fast fast red TR/naphtol AS-MX substrate tablets (Miltenyi Biotec).
7. Meyer's hemalum solution (Merck, Darmstadt, Germany).
8. Kaisers glycerol gelatin (Merck).

Instruments

1. Magnetic cell separator MiniMACS (Miltenyi Biotec).
2. Positive selection columns type MS^+ (Miltenyi Biotec).
3. 30 μm nylon mesh or preseparation filters (Miltenyi Biotec).
4. Cytocentrifuge (Hettich, Tuttlingen, Germany).
5. Slides (Marienfeld, Bad Mergentheim, Germany).
6. Marking pen (Dako).
7. Staining troughs.

Preparation of PBMC

1. Collect 30–40 ml of fresh anticoagulated peripheral human blood.
2. Prepare mononuclear cells by Ficoll Paque density gradient centrifugation.

Seeding of SK-MEL-28 Cells into PBMC Samples

A FACStar cell sorter (Becton Dickinson) was used to deposit single SK-MEL-28 melanoma cells into PBMC samples. We deflected 5, 10, 20, 50, 100, and 500 SK-MEL-28 cells into conical tubes containing 5×10^7 PBMC from healthy donors.

Magnetic Labeling of Melanoma Cells

1. Start with 5×10^7 PBMC resuspended in a total volume of 300 µl of buffer.
2. Add 100 µl of FcR blocking reagent per 5×10^7 total cells and mix well. The final volume is 400 µl per 5×10^7 cells.
3. Add 100 µl of 9.2.27 MicroBeads per 5×10^7 total cells, mix well, and incubate for 30 min at 6–12 °C. The final labeling volume is 500 µl per 5×10^7 cells.
4. Wash cells by adding 10–20 times the labeling volume of buffer, centrifuge at 300 g for 10 min, remove supernatant, and resuspend cell pellet in 500 µl of buffer per 10^8 total cells (for fewer cells, use 500 µl). Proceed to magnetic separation.

Magnetic Separation of Melanoma Cells and "Solid Phase" Intracellular Staining

1. Choose a positive selection column type MS^+ and place the column in the magnetic field of a MiniMACS separator.
2. Prepare column by washing twice with 500 µl of degassed buffer.
3. Pass cells through 30 µm nylon mesh or preseparation filter to remove any clumps. Wet filters with degassed buffer before use.
4. Apply cell suspension onto the column. Let the negative cells pass through. Rinse with 3×500 µl of buffer.
5. Remove column from separator, place column on a suitable collection tube, pipette 500 µl of buffer onto the column, and flush out positive cells using the plunger supplied with the column.
6. Add 500 µl of Inside Fix to the positive fraction and incubate for 20 minutes at room temperature. The final fixation volume is 1 ml.
7. Prepare a new positive selection column type MS^+ by washing twice with 500 µl of degassed buffer.
8. Apply the fixed positive cells onto the new column, let cell suspension completely enter the column matrix, and immediately wash with 2×500 µl of Inside Perm.
9. Apply 100 µl of monoclonal mouse anti-human melanoma antibodies (anti-MelanA and HMB-45 diluted at appropriate titer in Inside Perm) and incubate for 10 min at room temperature.
10. Rinse with 2×500 µl of Inside Perm, apply 100 µl of monoclonal rat anti-mouse IgG1-FITC (diluted at appropriate titer in Inside Perm), and incubate for 10 min at room temperature.
11. Rinse with 2×500 µl of Inside Perm, apply 100 µl of monoclonal mouse anti-FITC alkaline phosphatase (diluted to 1:50 in Inside Perm), and incubate for 10 min at room temperature.

12. Wash column with 500 µl of Inside Perm and 500 µl of PBS.
13. Remove column from separator, place column on a suitable collection tube, pipette 500 µl of PBS onto the column, and flush out positive cells using the plunger supplied with the column.

Immunocytochemical Detection of Melanoma Cells

1. Spin cells from the magnetically enriched fraction onto a slide using a cytocentrifuge. Air-dry slide for 2–18 h at room temperature.
2. Using a marking pen, apply a hydrophobic line around the cell area on slide.
3. Wash slide for 2 min in PBS in a staining trough.
4. Prepare Sigma Fast fast red TR/naphtol AS-MX substrate solution by dissolving the Tris buffer tablet in 1 ml double-distilled water, add substrate tablet, and dissolve by vigorous shaking.
5. Add 50 µl–100 µl of freshly prepared fast red TR/naphtol AS-MX substrate solution to the cell area and incubate for 15 min at room temperature.
6. Wash slide for 2 min in double-distilled water in a staining trough.
7. Optional: counterstain cells for 1 min in filtered Meyer's hemalum solution (diluted to 1:2 in 100 mM Tris-HCl, pH 8.2) in staining trough.
8. Wash slide for 2 min in double-distilled water in a staining trough. Air-dry slide or mount with Kaiser's glycerol gelatin.

Results and Discussion

Enrichment of Melanoma Cells from Mixtures of PBMC and Cells from a Melanoma Cell Line

To evaluate the efficiency of our method for combined magnetic enrichment and immunocytochemical detection of melanoma cells from peripheral blood, the assay was applied to PBMC samples spiked with defined numbers of cells from a melanoma cell line. In two independent experiments using a fluorescence-activated cell sorter, we seeded 5, 10, 20, 50, 100, and 500 tumor cells into samples of PBMC from healthy donors containing 5×10^7 cells. After the enrichment and staining procedures, slides were analyzed in a light microscope and recovery of melanoma cells was determined by counting the number of positively stained cells on the complete cell area. Cells were only judged to be recovered melanoma cells when the positive staining correlated with the morphological characteristics of melanoma cells (size and shape of whole cell and nucleus). Applying the same criteria to negative control samples without melanoma cells, no false positive cells could be detected ($n=18$).

In Fig. 1, the number of seeded melanoma cells is plotted against the number of recovered cells, and Table 1 lists the results for all spiked samples. In experiment 1, the lowest number of melanoma cells seeded into 5×10^7 PBMC was 10. After magnetic enrichment and immunocytochemical staining, 6 cells could be detected in two independent samples. The mean recovery for seven samples with 10, 50, 100, and 500 melanoma cells was

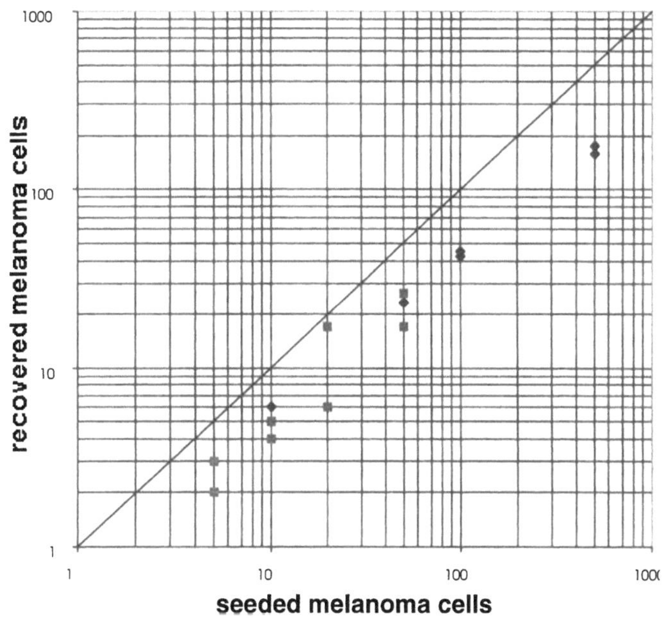

Fig. 1. Recovery of tumor cells enriched from mixtures of PBMC and melanoma cells. Numbers of SK-MEL-28 melanoma cells seeded by FACS into 5×10^7 PBMC from normal healthy donors are plotted against the numbers of SK-MEL-28 cells recovered after twofold enrichment and cytochemical staining (Table 1). The diagonal would correspond to 100% recovery of seeded tumor cells. ◆ Experiment 1, ■ experiment 2

Table 1. Efficiency of immunomagnetic enrichment and immunocytochemical detection of melanoma cells from mixtures of PBMC and SK-MEL-28 cells

Experiment 1	*N* SK-MEL-28 cells seeded[a]	10	10	50	100	100	500	500	
	N SK-MEL-28 cells detected[b]	6	6	23	42	45	175	158	
	Recovery (%)[c]	60	60	46	42	45	32	35	
Experiment 2	*N* SK-MEL-28 cells seeded[a]	5	5	10	10	20	20	50	50
	N SK-MEL-28 cells detected[b]	2	3	4	5	17	6	26	17
	Recovery (%)[c]	40	60	40	50	85	30	52	34

[a] Numbers of SK-MEL-28 cells deflected by flow sorter into healthy donor PBMC samples containing 5×10^7 cells.
[b] Numbers of SK-MEL-28 melanoma cells detected by light microscopy after magnetic enrichment and immunocytochemical staining of samples.
[c] Recoveries calculated on the basis of the numbers of SK-MEL-28 cells added to the PBMC samples and the numbers of SK-MEL-28 cells found in the magnetically enriched fraction.

Table 2. Immunomagnetic enrichment and immunocytochemical detection of melanoma cells in peripheral blood samples from patients with malignant melanoma

Patient ID	Stage	Serum MIA titer[a] (ng/ml)	Blood volume (ml)	*N* of melanoma cells detected[b]
MEL001	IV	n.d.	25	0
MEL002	IV	12.5	25	0
MEL003	IV	160.8	45	55
MEL003	IV	n.d.	25	37
MEL004	III	11.4	50	0
MEL005	IV	7.3	25	0
MEL006	IV	237.5	15	0
MEL007	IV	17.1	20	1
MEL008	IV	4.2	20	0

MIA, melanoma inhibitory activity.
[a] Concentration determined using a MIA ELISA Kit (Roche Diagnostics, Boehringer, Mannheim, Germany).
[b] Number of tumor cells detected by light microscopic analysis of the magnetically enriched and immunocytochemically stained fraction.

45.7%±10.18%. In experiment 2, we seeded between 5 and 50 melanoma cells into 5×10^7 PBMC. From two samples with 5 melanoma cells, we were able to recover 2 and 3 cells, respectively. The mean recovery for eight samples with 5, 10, 20, and 50 melanoma cells was 48.87±16.49%. Considering both experiments, melanoma cells could be reproducibly enriched from PBMC with a recovery of 47.4%±13.99% ($n=15$).

Enrichment and Detection of Melanoma Cells from Peripheral Blood of Patients with Malignant Melanoma

To demonstrate the feasibility of our method for combined immunomagnetic enrichment and immunocytochemical detection on clinical samples, we applied the assay to blood samples from melanoma patients. PBMC were isolated from 20–50 ml of peripheral blood from patients with stages III–IV malignant melanoma. As positive and negative controls, PBMC samples from healthy donors with and without spiked cells from the melanoma cell line SK-MEL-28 were processed in parallel. Table 2 summarizes the results obtained with clinical blood samples ($n=9$). We were able to detect tumor cells in three samples. Two of the positive samples were obtained from the same patient (MEL003) at an interval of 8 days, which demonstrates for clinical samples that the assay is specific and reproducible. Figure 2a shows the light microscopic image of two MelanA positive melanoma cells (red color) which were detected in the magnetically enriched cell fraction from patient MEL003. In the third positive sample (MEL007), we detected one single tumor cell (Fig. 2b) in 2.1×10^7 PBMC, which corresponds to a frequency of 4.76×10^{-8}.

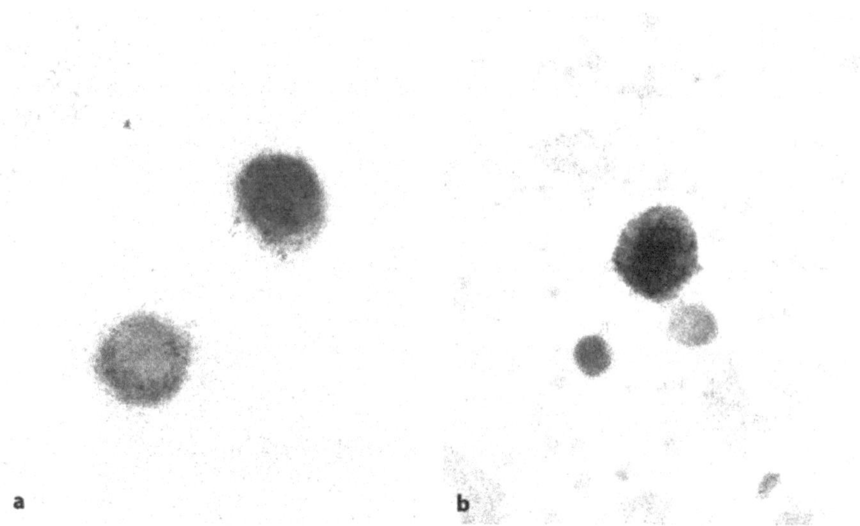

Fig. 2 a, b. Immunocytochemical staining of magnetically enriched melanoma cells from PBMC samples of stage IV malignant melanoma patients. **a** MelanA positive cells (*red*) detected in patient MEL003. **b** MelanA/HMB-45 positive melanoma cell (*red*) detected in patient MEL007 with counterstaining of nuclei using hemalum solution (*blue*)

In summary, the described assay for enrichment and detection of melanoma cells from PBMC has proven to be a powerful tool for highly sensitive detection of extremely rare occult melanoma cells in hematopoietic tissue. Using a model system in which PBMC were spiked with defined numbers of cells from a melanoma cell line, tumor cells could be detected with recoveries of about 50%. Samples with as few as 5 melanoma cells in 5×10^7 PBMC could reliably be shown to be tumor cell-positive. For clinical blood samples from melanoma patients, the feasibility of the assay was demonstrated by detecting melanoma cells in two of eight patients, one patient being analyzed twice with similar results at an interval of 8 days. The assay is also applicable to mononuclear cells from bone marrow and lymphoid tissue.

References

1. Mellado B, Colomer D, Castel T, Munoz M, Carballo E, Galan M, Mascaro JM, Vives Corrons JL, Grau JJ, Estape J (1996) Detection of circulating neoplastic cells by reverse-transcriptase polymerase chain reaction in malignant melanoma: association with clinical stage and prognosis. J Clin Oncol 14:2091–2097
2. Gläser R, Rass K, Seiter S, Hauschild A, Christophers E, Tilgen W (1997) Detection of circulating melanoma cells by specific amplification of tyrosinase complementary DNA is not a reliable tumor marker in melanoma patiens: a clinical two-center study. J Clin Oncol 15:2818–2825

3. Reinhold U, Lüdtke-Handjery HC, Schnautz S, Kreysel HW, Abken H (1997) The analysis of tyrosinase-specific mRNA in blood samples of melanoma patients by RT-PCR is not a useful test for metastatic tumor progression. J Invest Dermatol 108:166–169
4. Keilholz U, Willhauck M, Rimoldi D, Brasseur F, Dummer W, Rass K, de Vries T, Blaheta J, Voit C, Lethe B, Burchill S (1998) Reliability of reverse transcription-polymerase chain reaction (RT-PCR)-based assays for the detection of circulating tumour cells: a quality-assurance initiative of the EORTC melanoma cooperative group. Eur J Cancer 34:750–753
5. Curry BJ, Myers K, Hersey P (1998) Polymerase chain reaction detection of melanoma cells in the circulation: relation to clinical stage, surgical treatment, and recurrence from melanoma. J Clin Oncology 16:1760–1769
6. Farthmann B, Eberle J, Krasagakis K, Gstöttner M, Wang N, Bisson S, Orfanos CE (1998) RT-PCR for tyrosinase-mRNA-positive cells in peripheral blood: evaluation strategy and correlation with known prognostic markers in 123 melanoma patients. J Invest Dermatol 110:263–267
7. Morgan AC, Galloway DR, Reisfeld RA (1981) Production and characterization of monoclonal antibody to a melanoma specific glycoprotein. Hybridoma 1:27–35
8. Bumor TF, Reisfeld RA (1982) Unique glycoprotein-proteoglycan complex defined by monclonal antibody on human melanoma cells. Proc Natl Acad Sci USA 79:1245–1249
9. Pluschke G, Vanek M, Evans A, Dittmar T, Schmid P, Itin P, Filardo EJ, Reisfeld RA (1996) Molecular cloning of a human melanoma-associated chondroitin sulfate proteoglycan. Proc Natl Acad Sci USA 93:9710–9715
10. Chen YT, Stockert E, Jungbluth A, Tsang S, Coplan KA, Sanlan MJ, Old LJ (1996) Serological analysis of Melan-A (MART-1), a melanocyte-specific protein homogeneously expressed in human melanomas. Proc Natl Acad Sci USA 93:5915–5919

II. Detection of Residual Melanoma Cells in the Peripheral Blood and Bone Marrow

Reverse Transcriptase Polymerase Chain Reaction (RT-PCR) Detection of Melanoma-Related Transcripts in the Peripheral Blood and Bone Marrow of Patients with Malignant Melanoma. What Have We Learned?

R.A. Ghossein[1], S. Bhattacharya[1], and D.G. Coit[2]

[1] Department of Pathology, Memorial Sloan-Kettering Cancer Center, New York, NY 10021, USA
[2] Department of Surgery, Memorial Sloan-Kettering Cancer Center, New York, NY 10021, USA

Abstract

The detection of circulating tumor cells (CTC) and bone marrow micrometastases (BMM) by reverse transcriptase polymerase chain reaction (RT-PCR) may help predict recurrence and survival in malignant melanoma (MM). Since the appearance of the original article by Smith et al. in 1991 (Lancet 338:1227), several groups have attempted the detection of CTC and BMM in MM using RT-PCR for melanocytic specific markers, mainly tyrosinase mRNA. Most studies show that tyrosinase is not present in the PB and BM of control individuals without MM. The PCR positivity rates in MM are extremely variable, ranging from 0% to 100%. There was a correlation between RT-PCR and stage in some but not all of the studies. These disparate findings could in part be explained by differences in RNA extraction and blood separation techniques, to unrecognized contamination leading to false positive results, or differences in patient selection. Despite these discrepancies, we and others have shown that RT-PCR for tyrosinase mRNA in PB is able to predict overall survival (OS) and disease-free survival (DFS) in a statistically significant manner. In AJCC stage II–IV patients rendered surgically free of disease, we found that blood tyrosinase positivity was an independent predictor of OS and DFS. We also found that BM tyrosinase positivity is an independent predictor of DFS in the same group of patients. RT-PCR may help identify subgroups of patients at high risk for early relapse for more aggressive adjuvant therapy. Large prospective studies and interlaboratory quality assurance initiatives are necessary to confirm the accuracy and prognostic value of these RT-PCR assays.

Recent Results in Cancer Research, Vol. 158

Introduction

The detection of circulating tumor cells (CTC) and bone marrow micrometastases (BMM) may help predict recurrence and survival in malignant melanoma. The detection of CTC and micrometastases has been attempted in this century using cytological examination and immunocytochemical analysis [1–4]. Both techniques have significant limitations. Morphologic examination of blood specimens for CTC was attempted in the late 1950s and early 1960s on thousands of cancer patients. The technique was, however, soon shown to have a very low sensitivity rate (in the order of 1%) [1]. Immunocytochemical assays were shown to identify BM disease with much greater sensitivity than conventional techniques [3–4]. Indeed, these immunocytological tests were able to detect a single tumor cell seeded among 10 000–100 000 mononuclear cells. Despite evidence of the prognostic value of this determination in some studies [4–7], the detection of micrometastases by immunocytochemistry was not routinely used in cancer staging protocols [8]. This was due to a combination of factors such as the absence of clinical significance in some studies [9–12], loss of antigen expression in poorly differentiated tumors, and reports of antigen false positivity [13, 14]. In the meantime, there was hope for development of an even better method for the detection of occult tumor cells using DNA and RNA analysis. This hope was realized with the advent in the late 1980s of the highly sensitive polymerase chain reaction (PCR) technique, which has greatly facilitated the detection of CTC and micrometastases. Since 1987, a variety of PCR-based techniques have been devised for the identification of occult tumor cells in leukemias, lymphomas, melanomas, neuroblastomas, and various types of carcinomas [15–20]. This article focuses on the use of RT-PCR for the detection of CTC and BMM in malignant melanoma. We start with a general description of PCR and its power and limitations in the detection of CTC and BMM and then concentrate on the results obtained in melanoma patients.

The PCR Technique

Polymerase chain reaction is an in vitro method that enzymatically amplifies specific DNA sequences using oligonucleotide primers (short DNA sequences) that flank and therefore define the region of interest in the target DNA [21]. The procedure consists of a repetitive series of cycles, each of which consists of template denaturation, primer annealing, and extension of the annealed primers by a thermostable DNA polymerase to create the exponential accumulation of a specific DNA fragment whose ends are determined by the 5′ ends of the primers [21]. After 20 cycles, the amplification is about 10^6- to 10^8-fold [21]. PCR amplification can be accomplished using RNA as the starting material. This procedure, known as reverse transcriptase PCR (RT-PCR) is similar to DNA PCR, with the modification that PCR amplification is preceded by reverse transcription of RNA into cDNA. Figure 1 shows

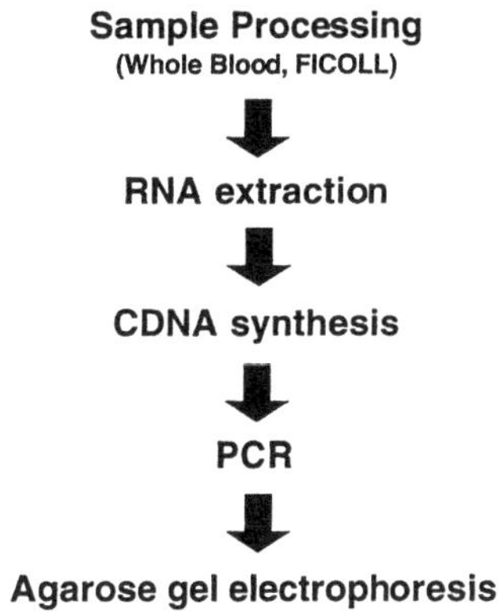

Fig. 1. Different steps involved in the RT procedure for detecting circulating tumor cells and micrometastases. RNA is extracted from whole blood or from density gradient separated white cells. This is followed by cDNA synthesis, PCR amplification, and agarose gel detection of the RT-PCR product

the different steps involved in the RT-PCR detection of melanoma-related markers in blood.

One major strategy for the detection of occult tumor cells is the PCR amplification of tumor-specific abnormalities present in the DNA or mRNA of these cells. This approach was mostly used for the detection of minimal residual disease (MRD) in hematological malignancies. It was first applied to the detection of the t(14;18) translocation associated with follicular lymphomas [19]. The primers used hybridize to the region flanking the translocation and will therefore only amplify the DNA when the translocation is present. If the translocation is not present, the primers anneal to different chromosomes and PCR is impossible.

The other PCR strategy for the detection of occult tumor cells involves amplification of tissue-specific mRNA by RT-PCR. This has been mainly used for the detection of CTC and micrometastases in solid tumors. This approach is based on the fact that malignant cells often continue to express markers that are characteristic of their tissue of origin. Tyrosinase mRNA, for example, has become a useful marker for the detection of CTC in melanoma. In principle, PCR amplification of tissue-specific mRNA offers several advantages over the protein-based assay. Firstly, RNA is very unstable in the extracellular environment; therefore its detection should indicate the presence of tumor cells in the examined tissue. Secondly, although monoclonal antibody assays are becoming increasingly sensitive, they are not expected to approach the single-molecule detection capability of PCR tests. Thirdly, tissue-specific mRNA can indicate the presence of tumor cells despite a negative protein-based assay. For example, prostatic specific antigen (PSA) transcripts have been detected in poorly differentiated prostatic carcinoma cells that do not express the PSA protein [22]. From a technical standpoint, RT-PCR detection of any tissue-specific marker requires knowledge of its gene sequence and specifically of intron-exon junctions, which facilitates the selection of oligonucleotide primers for RT-PCR. Using primer sets spanning introns allows discrimination between RT-PCR products from mRNA targets

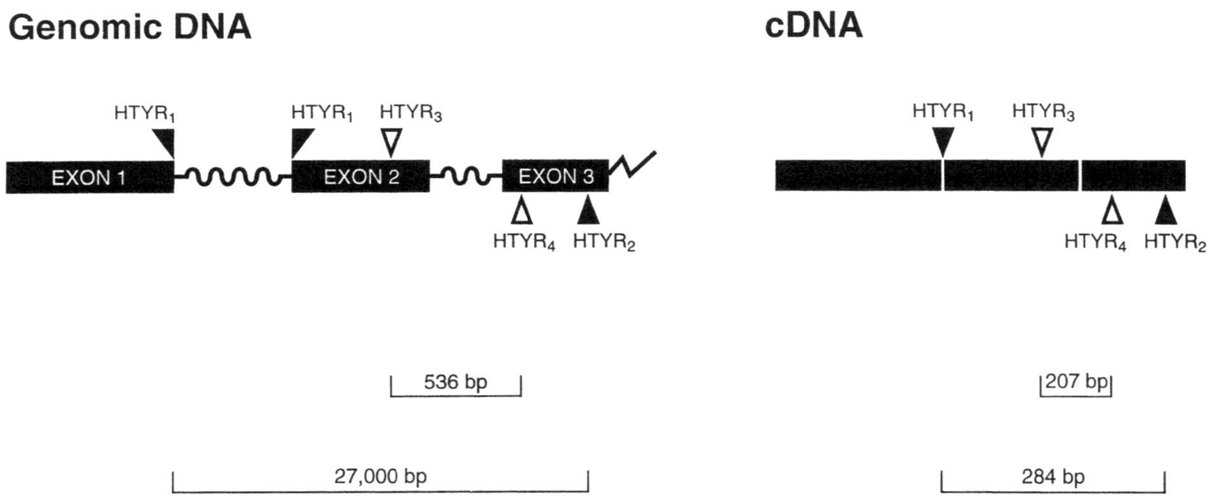

Fig. 2. Tyrosinase primers and PCR products: the outer primers (HTYR1, HTYR2) and the nested primers (HTYR3, HTYR4) span long intronic sequences. Therefore, genomic DNA either could not be amplified or would generate a PCR product of much greater length (*left*) than those derived from cDNA (*right*). The outer primers generate a 284-bp RT-PCR product, and the nested primers generate a 207 bp diagnostic RT-PCR product (*right*). (Adapted with permission from: Smith et al. (1991). Detection of melanoma cells in peripheral blood by means of reverse transcriptase and polymerase chain reaction. Lancet 338:1227–1229)

and PCR products resulting from DNA amplification (Fig. 2). This prevents the occurrence of false positives generated from a small amount of genomic DNA present in the sample.

Limitations of PCR Technology

False Positive PCR Results

The power of PCR resides in the extreme sensitivity of the technique. Current publications report the detection of one tumor cell diluted with 1 million to 10 million normal cells [18, 23]. It is this extreme sensitivity that confers an inherent tendency to produce false positive results if sufficient precautions are not taken to prevent contamination of samples. Meticulous laboratory techniques have been developed to prevent this contamination [21]. The most important rule is to keep the pre- and post-PCR reactions separate [21]. Indeed, the product output of PCR confers high contamination potential, since a single aerosol particle of a solution of PCR products may transfer 100 to 1000 million copies of amplified DNA [21]. In addition, every PCR reaction should include a negative PCR control (containing all the reagents except the template) to monitor for contamination of the reagents by amplifiable nucleic acids. False positives could be due to the general process of illegitimate transcription (i.e., transcription of any gene in any cell type). Although the number of these transcripts in inappropriate cells is very low (estimated at one mRNA molecule per 100 to 1000 cells) [24], it can result in false positives because of the high sensitivity of RT-PCR. For example, a neuronal specific marker, neuroendocrine protein gene product (PGP 9.5) was shown to be present in scant amounts in normal bone marrow cells [25]. However, even in the presence of such a phenomenon, it is sometimes possible to design specific RT-PCR assays by optimizing the PCR thermocycling conditions, as has been shown for tyrosinase mRNA [26]. Pseudogenes can also give rise to false positive results. Since they lack an intronic sequence, RT-PCR amplification of pseudogenes will lead to PCR products indistinguishable from those generated from the mRNA. Because most markers of CTC and micrometastases in solid tumors are tissue-specific (i.e., expressed in tumor and their normal tissue of origin), the mechanical introduction of normal or benign cells in the circulation after invasive procedures may lead to false positive PCR results. For example, many studies showed that a significant number of patients hemoconverted from RT-PCR negative to RT-PCR positive after radical prostatectomy [27]. However, the percentage of RT-PCR negative patients hemoconverting after less invasive procedures (e.g., transrectal ultrasound, prostatic core biopsy) was much lower. These false positive PCR results can be averted by timing the RT-PCR tests several weeks after any invasive procedure. Venipuncture by itself could in theory cause false positive results by RT-PCR. However, we encountered no false positives while PCR-testing peripheral blood (PB) and BM for melanocytic tissue specific markers in a control population which included dark-skinned individuals [28]. If false positives occur because of venipuncture, this can be avoided by discarding the first few milliliters of PB that are collected, which may harbor rare epidermal or melanocytic cells.

False Negative PCR Results

Inhibitors present in some tissues and fluids can diminish PCR sensitivity and lead to false negative results. Therefore, careful controls are necessary to ensure there is amplifiable RNA or DNA in the sample. This is accomplished by demonstrating amplification of a constitutively present transcript such as beta-actin or beta-globin. Unfortunately, some of these housekeeping genes are so widely expressed that they can be detected even in samples containing poor quality RNA not suited for sensitive detection of transcripts from rare CTC several orders of magnitude lower. The reader should be aware that the in vitro sensitivity reported in all articles on CTC and micrometastases (often expressed in number of cell line-derived tumor cells detected per million of white cells) does not necessarily reflect the in vivo sensitivity of PCR. The latter is most probably lower than the in vitro sensitivity because of inhibitors of the PCR reaction present in tissues and body fluids and because the tumor cell lines chosen for the in vitro sensitivity experiments strongly express the marker of interest. In contrast, the tumor cells in tissues and body fluids do not necessarily express the marker of interest. Technical errors (e.g., omission of one of the reagents) could lead to false negatives. This can be solved by the inclusion of a positive control of low to moderate intensity in every PCR reaction. False negative results could also be due to a sampling problem, since only a few milliliters of peripheral blood are analyzed at a certain time, or to intermittent shedding of tumor cells in the circulation. These problems could be overcome by sequential sampling, defined as the analysis of multiple blood samples at different timepoints. False negative results could also be caused by downregulation of the target gene by therapy (e.g., hormonal treatment) or the presence of poorly differentiated subclones that do not express the tissue-specific marker being tested. For example, PSA mRNA expression was shown to be decreased by antiandrogen therapy [29] and in poorly differentiated prostatic carcinoma [22]. The use of multiple marker assays will help diminish this type of false negatives.

Quantitative PCR

It is possible to quantify the amount of target nucleic acids present in a given sample using RT-PCR. This can be done by the addition of differently sized competitor target molecules [30–32] or the use of serial dilutions [33]. These techniques are, however, quite cumbersome. An automated real time quantitative RT-PCR assay is now available and user-friendly [34]. These quantitative PCR methods are unfortunately not able to estimate the number of tumor cells present in a sample, since the transcription rate (i.e., the amount of target mRNA) varies between individual tumor cells [35]. This fact significantly limits the value of quantitative PCR in detecting occult tumor cells.

Quality Control and Other Technical Considerations

There is an urgent need for quality assurance in any PCR-related procedure, especially in melanoma, where discrepant results were reported between various laboratories. An interesting collaborative quality control study was conducted by the European Organization for Research and Treatment of Cancer (EORTC) Melanoma Cooperative Group [36]. In this study, nine laboratories performed tyrosinase RT-PCR assays on a series of blind samples containing various amounts of melanoma cells. These laboratories had approximately 50% of false negative results occurring at the level of 10 cells in 10 ml of blood. This is definitely less sensitive than most articles, which claimed a sensitivity of one melanoma cell in 1–10 ml of blood. Consistent results were obtained between all laboratories when cDNA samples were amplified, while variable results occurred when whole blood or mononuclear cells were used as starting material [36]. This demonstrates that sample preparation, RNA extraction, and cDNA synthesis rather than PCR protocols may account for the heterogeneous results. Indeed, different sample preparation procedures (i.e., cell separation techniques) can lead to different sensitivities. For example, RNA extraction from whole blood may decrease the quality and purity of isolated RNA but minimize tumor cell loss, which is a concern for density gradient separation techniques like the Ficoll method. Lack of RNA amplification was also reported in this study, as well as false positives. In order to circumvent all these problems, a series of controls were recommended for diagnostic RT-PCR [36] (Table 1).

Detection of CTC and BMM in Melanoma Patients

Currently, the main criteria for assessing prognosis in malignant melanoma are the histopathological features of the primary tumor and the clinical presentation. However, these factors are of limited value, especially in the advanced stages of the disease [37]. There is therefore a need for a better prognostic marker in such patients. The molecular detection of CTC and BM micrometastases has the potential of predicting outcome in patients with malignant melanoma. Smith et al. were the first to propose that melanoma cells could be detected in the PB using RT-PCR for tyrosinase mRNA [26]. Tyrosinase is a key enzyme in melanin biosynthesis that catalyzes the conversion of tyrosine to dopa and of dopa to dopaquinone. This test is presumed to detect circulating melanoma cells, since tyrosinase is one of the most specific markers of melanocytic differentiation [38] and melanocytes are not known to circulate. Furthermore, most studies show that tyrosinase mRNA is not present in the PB of healthy individuals [28, 37, 39–41] (Table 2). Since the

Table 1. Suggested controls for melanoma RT-PCR. RNA quantification is used to control for variability in RNA extraction from sample to sample. Minus RT (i.e., PCR without addition of RT) is used to control for pseudogene amplification. Housekeeping genes widely expressed in all cells, like beta-actin, are used to control for amplifiable RNA. Negative control PCR includes all the reagents except the template in order to check for reagent contamination

Control procedure	Item controlled for
RNA quantification (spectrophotometry, agarose gel)	Variability in RNA extraction
Without RT	Pseudogenes
Housekeeping gene	Amplifiable RNA
Duplicate analysis of target markers	Reproducibility of RT-PCR
Healthy donor	Marker specificity
Negative control PCR	Contamination of reagents
Positive control	Efficiency of RT-PCR

RT, reverse transcriptase; PCR, polymerase chain reaction.

Table 2. RT-PCR positivity rates for melanoma related markers in blood and BM of control subjects without melanoma. Controls without melanoma included healthy subjects and individuals with malignancies other than melanoma. All false positives listed occurred in healthy subjects including individuals with surgically removed benign nevi

Author	Marker	Sample type	Positive/total
Brossart et al. [41]	Tyrosinase	Blood	0/56
Glaser et al. [47]	Tyrosinase	Blood	0/35
Battayani et al. [37]	Tyrosinase	Blood	0/14
Kunter et al. [40]	Tyrosinase	Blood	0/9
Ghossein et al. [28]	Tyrosinase	Blood	0/12
	Tyrosinase	BM	0/13
Hoon et al. [39]	Tyrosinase	Blood	0/39
	P97	Blood	0/39
	MAGE-3	Blood	0/39
	Muc-18	Blood	2/39 (5%)
Curry et al. [45]	Tyrosinase	Blood	0/50
	MART-1	Blood	0/50
	P97	Blood	FP
	Muc-18	Blood	FP
	gp100	Blood	FP
Schitteck B et al. [49]	Tyrosinase	Blood	0/40
	MART-1	Blood	0/40
	gp100	Blood	FP
	Muc-18	Blood	FP
Muhlbauer et al. [52]	MIA	Blood	2/44 (5%)
Kuo et al. [55]	Beta 1–4GalNac-T	Blood	0/37
Cheung et al. [54]	GAGE	BM	0/31
	GAGE	Blood	1/17 (6%)

RT-PCR, reverse transcriptase polymerase chain reaction; BM, bone marrow; FP, false positives (exact number of cases unknown).

original study by Smith et al., several groups have attempted the detection of CTC in malignant melanoma using mainly tyrosinase mRNA [28, 37, 39–47]. As shown in Table 3, the PCR positivity rates are extremely variable, ranging from 0% to 100%. These discrepant results could in part be explained by differences in sample processing, RNA extraction, and transcription (see quality control section). These disparate findings could also be due to unrecognized contamination leading to false positive results [38]. Indeed, Foss et al. acknowledged the presence of significant technical problems due to carryover contamination that took 1 year to overcome [42]. These large variations in tyrosinase positivity rates have lead researchers to question the reproducibility of these assays.

In order to analyze reproducibility, de Vries et al. tested 109 samples from 68 melanoma patients for CTC using RT-PCR for tyrosinase and MART 1 [48], a melanocytic tissue-specific marker that was detected by RT-PCR in the PB of melanoma patients [45, 49]. In de Vries' article, each blood specimen was assayed 4 times for each marker in order to study RT-PCR reproducibility [48]. A minority of patients were positive in all determinations for tyrosinase or MART 1. Variable results (1–3 times positive) were therefore found in the majority of positive cases. By using real time quantitative RT-PCR for tyrosinase and MART-1, a low amount of melanoma tumor cell equivalents was found in the blood of melanoma patients with variable results and a higher number of equivalents in the group with a consistently positive result [48]. The authors also found that mRNA quality is similar among all positive cases. They concluded therefore that low reproducibility of a repeated assay for the detection of melanoma cells is caused by a low number of melanoma-related transcripts in the sample and not differences in mRNA quality [48].

There was a correlation between RT-PCR detection of melanoma transcripts and clinical stage in some but not all of the studies (Table 3). Despite these discrepancies, we and others have shown that RT-PCR for tyrosinase mRNA in PB is able to predict overall survival and disease-free survival in a statistically significant manner [28, 37, 40, 44–45] (Table 4). We were also able specifically to detect tyrosinase transcripts in the BM of patients with American Joint Committee on Cancer (AJCC) stage II–IV melanoma (stage II, primary tumor >1.5 mm in thickness with no metastases; stage III, regional lymph node metastases; stage IV, distant metastases) [28]. In patients with thick and advanced melanoma who were surgically rendered free of disease (AJCC stage II–IV), we found that BM positivity for tyrosinase mRNA is an independent predictor of poorer disease-free survival [50]. In this same patient population (median follow up of 18.3 months), blood RT-PCR positivity for tyrosinase was shown to be an independent predictor of poorer overall and disease-free survival [50]. In an effort to improve the clinical value of RT-PCR for tyrosinase mRNA, Brossart et al. developed a semiquantitative RT-PCR assay [51]. According to these authors, the amount of tyrosinase transcripts increases with tumor burden in patients with metastatic disease and decreases in patients responding to immunotherapy. These observations may have important clinical implications. RT-PCR may help define subsets of patients with poor prognosis for whom toxic

Table 3. Detection of CTC in the peripheral blood of patients with cutaneous malignant melanoma using RT-PCR. Number of RT-PCR positive patients/total number of patients tested (%) according to AJCC stage

Author	I–II	III	IV
Brossart et al. [41]	1/10 (10%)	6/17 (35%)	29/29 (100%)
Hoon et al. [39][a]	13/17 (76%)	31/36 (86%)	63/66 (95%)
Battayani et al. [37]	2/10 (20%)	22/51 (43%)	16/32 (50%)
Foss et al. [42]	–	–	0/6 (0%)
Pittman et al. [43]	–	–	3/24 (12.5%)
Kunter et al. [40]	0/16 (0%)	0/16 (0%)	9/34 (26%)
Mellado et al. [44]	8/44 (18%)	2/13 (15%)	–
Curry et al. [45][b]	48/160 (30%)	60/116 (52%)	–
Farthman et al. [46]	6/46 (13%)	7/41 (17%)	16/36 (44%)
Schitteck B et al. [49][b]	28/119 (24%)	14/48 (29%)	30/58 (52%)
Cheung et al. [54]	5/17 (29%)	4/54 (7%)	4/27 (15%)

CTC, circulating tumor cells; RT-PCR, reverse transcriptase polymerase chain reaction; Pos, positive; AJCC, American Joint Committee on Cancer; AJCC stage I, primary tumor < 1.5 mm in thickness with no metastases; AJCC stage II, primary tumor > 1.5 mm in thickness with no metastases; AJCC stage III, lymph node metastases; AJCC stage IV, distant metastases.

[a] In this study, the peripheral blood was analyzed for 4 markers (tyrosinase, p97, Muc-18, MAGE-3).

[b] In both reports, the samples were tested for tyrosinase and MART-1.

In all three articles [39, 45, 49], RT-PCR positivity was defined as positivity for any of the markers. In Cheung's article [54], GAGE was used as melanoma marker. In all the other studies listed, tyrosinase alone was used as a marker for melanoma cells.

forms of adjuvant therapies are justified. This test may help improve the stratification of patients for clinical trials into more homogeneous groups. This assay could also be used to measure treatment response in patients on current or novel therapeutic regimens like vaccine therapy.

Recently, a new marker termed “melanoma inhibitory activity” (MIA) was used for RT-PCR detection of circulating melanoma cells [52]. MIA is a malignant melanoma-derived growth regulatory protein highly expressed in melanomas but found at extremely low levels in keratinocytes, fibroblasts, melanocytes, and lymphocytes when a standard single-round RT-PCR is used [52]. Muhlbauer et al. found an increase in RT-PCR positivity with tumor burden in patients with metastatic disease and a decrease after adjuvant therapy [52]. Our group recently tested another marker termed GAGE for the detection of CTC and micrometastases in melanoma. GAGE belongs to a family of genes that encodes distinct tumor associated antigens present on melanoma cells and recognized by autologous cytolytic T lymphocytes [53]. These tumor-associated antigens are expressed in human tumors of diverse histological types but are silent in normal adult tissue except the testis and placenta [54]. In this study, 133 patients with melanoma (21 AJCC clinical stage II, 74 AJCC clinical stage III, and 38 AJCC clinical stage IV) had a single marrow and/or blood sample drawn immediately before surgery. There was a statistically significant correlation between GAGE positivity in BM and/or blood and overall survival among all patients and within the stage III

Table 4. Molecular prognosis in melanoma using RT-PCR. The relative risk was not available in all references. However, in each study, RT-PCR positivity correlated with poorer survival time. Only those studies using Kaplan-Meier survival analysis are included in this table. In Curry's article [45], the samples were tested for tyrosinase and MART-1. RT-PCR positivity was defined as positivity for any of the markers. In Cheung's article [54], RT-PCR positivity in blood and/or BM was considered as indicative of the presence of occult tumor cells. In Coit's study [50], the patients were followed after being rendered surgically free of disease

Author	AJCC Stage	Marker	Sample	Endpoint	*P* value
Mellado et al. [44]	I–III	Tyrosinase	Blood	DFS	0.003
	I–III	Tyrosinase	Blood	OS	0.001
Kunter et al. [40]	IV	Tyrosinase	Blood	OS	<0.0006
Ghossein et al. [28]	II	Tyrosinase	Blood	OS	0.01
	II	Tyrosinase	BM	OS	0.06
	III	Tyrosinase	Blood	OS	0.02
Curry et al. [45]	I–III	Tyrosinase/ Mart 1	Blood	DFS	0.0022
Coit et al. [50]	II–IV	Tyrosinase	Blood	OS	0.01
	II–IV	Tyrosinase	Blood	DFS	0.0001
	II–IV	Tyrosinase	BM	DFS	0.02
Cheung et al. [54]	II–IV	GAGE	Blood/BM	OS	0.01
	III	GAGE	Blood/BM	OS	0.01

RT-PCR, reverse transcriptase polymerase chain reaction; AJCC stage I, primary tumor <1.5 mm in thickness with no metastases; AJCC stage II, primary tumor >1.5 mm in thickness with no metastases; AJCC stage III, regional lymph node metastases; AJCC stage IV, distant metastases; OS, overall survival; DFS, disease free survival; BM, bone marrow.

category. In multivariate analysis, RT-PCR for GAGE in blood was an independent prognostic variable for survival [54].

Other markers were used (Table 5) for RT PCR detection of melanoma cells [39, 55], such as gp100 (a melanocytic tissue-specific marker whose antibody, HMB45, is widely used in diagnostic surgical pathology), p97, MUC 18, and MAGE 3. The latter three molecules are tumor-associated antigens. Like GAGE, MAGE has been found in melanomas but not in normal tissues, except the adult testes. Transcripts from gp100, p97, MUC 18, and MAGE 3 were detected in the blood of normal subjects using RT-PCR, despite the use of a range of PCR conditions and several different primer sets [45] (Table 2). Beta 1–4-N-acetylgalactosaminyltransferase (beta 1–4GalNac-T), an enzyme involved in ganglioside synthesis, has been used for the detection of circulating melanoma cells [55]. According to Kuo et al., this transcript is specific for melanoma cell detection in the PB and more frequently found in advanced tumors [55].

Because of the limitations of PCR (e.g., contamination of samples and the inability to quantify tumor cells or perform functional assays), it is now clear that other techniques should be used as an adjunct for the detection of occult tumor cells. In the past year and a half, we and others have used immunomagnetic separation technology to improve the detection of CTC [56–58]. In this technique, the specimen is incubated with magnetic beads coated

Table 5. Molecular markers used for RT-PCR detection of CTC and BMM in melanoma patients

Marker	Marker type
Tyrosinase	Tissue-specific
MART-1	Tissue-specific
MIA	Tumor-associated
GAGE	Tumor-associated
Muc-18	Tumor-associated
MAGE-3	Tumor-associated
gp 100	Tissue-specific
Beta 1–4 galNac-T	Tumor-associated

RT-PCR, reverse transcriptase polymerase chain reaction; CTC, circulating tumor cells; BMM, bone marrow micrometastases; MIA, melanoma inhibitory activity; beta 1–4 GalNac-T, beta 1-4-N-acetylgalactosaminyltransferase.

with antibodies directed against antigens present on the surface of specific tumor cell types (e.g., Ber-EP4 antibody directed against epithelial cells). The tumor-rich magnetic fraction can be used for downstream RT-PCR, flow cytometry, or immunocytochemical analysis. The sample used for RT-PCR will therefore be considerably enriched in tumor cells with a minimal background of non-neoplastic cells. Tumor cell enrichment using magnetic beads will render RT-PCR much more sensitive and specific. Multicolor flow cytometry and immunocytochemical analysis of the sample will allow quantification of the tumor cells [57], their functional analysis, and their assessment for various markers of disease progression. The molecular characterization of CTC and micrometastases will help monitor the effect of targeted therapy. This therapeutic approach is aimed at specific molecular targets overexpressed in tumor cells like the monoclonal antibody against HER-2, commercially known as Herceptin. The clinical value of occult tumor cell detection in melanoma will be greatly enhanced by the combined use of RT-PCR, flow cytometry, and immunocytochemistry.

In view of the correlation between RT-PCR positivity for tyrosinase and outcome, RT-PCR assays for the detection of CTC and micrometastases in melanoma seem very promising. However, to define clearly the clinical usefulness of RT-PCR for occult melanoma cells, large prospective studies and methodological issues must be addressed using interlaboratory studies [59].

References

1. Christopherson W (1965) Cancer cells in the peripheral blood: A second look Acta Cytol 9:169–174
2. Moss TJ, Sanders DG (1990) Detection of neuroblastoma cells in blood. J Clin Oncol 8:736–740
3. Redding, WH, Coombes RC, Monaghan P, Clink HM, Imrie SF, Dearnaley DP, Ormerad MG, Sloane JP, Gazet JC, Powles TJ, Munro Neville A (1983) Detection of micrometastases in patients with primary breast cancer. Lancet 2:1271–1273

4. Stahel RA, Mabry M, Skarkin AT, Speak J, Bernal SD (1985) Detection of bone marrow metastasis in small-cell lung cancer by monoclonal antibody. J Clin Oncol 3:455–456
5. Diel IJ, Kaufman M, Goerner R, Costa SD, Kaul S, Bastert G (1992) Detection of tumor cells in bone marrow of patients with primary breast cancer: a prognostic factor for distant metastasis. J Clin Oncol 10:1534–1539
6. Pantel K, Izbicki J, Passlick B, Angstwurm M, Haussinger K, Thetter O, Riethmüller G (1996) Frequency and prognostic significance of isolated tumor cells in bone marrow of patients with non-small cell lung cancer without overt metastases. Lancet 347:649–653
7. Lindemann F, Schlimock G, Dirschedl P, Witte J, Riethmüller G (1992) Prognostic significance of micrometastatic tumor cells in bone marrow of colorectal patients. Lancet 340:685–689
8. Pelkey TJ, Frierson HF, Bruns DE (1996) Molecular and immunological detection of circulating tumor cells and micrometastases from solid tumors. Clin Chem 42:1369–1381
9. Kirk SJ, Cooper GG, Hoper M, Watt PC, Roy AD, Odling-Smee W (1990) The prognostic significance of marrow micrometastases in women with early breast cancer. Eur J Surg Oncol 16:481–485
10. Salvadori B, Squicciarni P, Rovini D, Orefice S, Andreola S, Rilke F, Barletta L, Menard S, Colnaghi MI (1990) Use of monoclonal antibody Mbr1 to detect micrometastases in bone marrow specimens of breast cancer patients. Eur J Cancer 26:865–867
11. Singletary SE, Larry L, Tucker SL, Spitzer G (1991) Detection of micrometastatic tumor cells in bone marrow of breast carcinoma patients. J Surg Oncol 47:32–36
12. Courtemanche DJ, Worth AJ, Coupland RW, MacFarlane JK (1991) Detection of micrometastases from primary breast cancer. Can J Surg 34:15–19
13. Miettinen M (1991) Keratin subsets in spindle cell sarcomas. Keratins are widespread but synovial sarcoma contains a distinctive keratin polypeptide pattern and desmoplakins. Am J Pathol 138:505–513
14. Thomas P, Battifora H (1987) Keratins versus epithelial membrane antigen in tumor diagnosis-an immunohistochemical comparison of five monoclonal antibodies. Hum Pathol 18:728–734
15. Campana D, Pui CH (1995) Detection of minimal residual disease in acute leukemias: Methodological advances and clinical significance. Blood 85:1416–1434
16. Cave H, Guidal P, Rohrlich P, Delfau MH, Broyart A, Lescoeur B, Rahimy C, Fenneteau O, Monplaisir N, d'Auriol L, Elion J, Vilmer E, Grandchamp B (1994) Prospective monitoring and quantitation of residual blasts in childhood acute leukemias by polymerase chain reaction of delta and gamma T-cell receptor genes. Blood 83:1892–1902
17. Miyajama Y, Kato K, Numata S, Kudo K, Horibe K (1995) Detection of neuroblastoma cells in bone marrow and peripheral blood at diagnosis by the reverse transcriptase-polymerase chain reaction for tyrosine hydroxylase mRNA. Cancer 75:2757–2761
18. Gerhard M, Juhl H, Kalthoff H, Schreiber HW, Wagener C, Neumaier M (1994) Specific detection of carcinoembryonic antigen-expressing tumor cells in bone marrow aspirates by polymerase chain reaction. J Clin Oncol 12:725–729
19. Lee MS, Chang KS, Cabanillas F, Freireich EJ, Trujillo JM, Stass SA (1987) Detection of minimal residual cells carrying the t(14;18) by DNA sequence amplification. Science 237:175–178
20. Komeda T, Fukuda Y, Sando T, Kita R, Furukawa M, Nishida N, Amenomori M, Nakao K (1995) Sensitive detection of circulating hepatocellular carcinoma cells in peripheral venous blood. Cancer 75:2214–2219
21. Eeles RA, Janssen JGW (ed) (1993) Polymerase chain reaction. The technique and its applications. RG Landes Cie, Austin TX
22. Qiu SD, Young CY, Bilhartz DL, Prescott JL, Farrow GM, He WW, Tindall DJ (1990) In situ hybridization of prostatic-specific antigen mRNA in human prostate. J Urol 144:1550–1556
23. Ghossein RA, Scher HI, Gerald WL, Kelly WK, Curley T, Amsterdam A, Zhang ZF, Rosai J (1995) Detection of circulating tumor cells in patients with localized and metastatic prostatic carcinoma prostatic carcinoma: Clinical implications. J Clin Oncol 13:1195–1200

24. Kaplan JC, Kahn A, Chelly J (1992) Illegitimate transcription: Its use in the study of inherited disease. Hum Mutat 1:357–360
25. Mattano LA, Moss TJ, Emerson SG (1992) Sensitive detection of rare circulating neuroblastoma cells by the reverse transcriptase-polymerase chain reaction. Cancer Res 52:4701–4705
26. Smith B, Selby P, Southgate J, Pittman K, Bradley C, Blair GE (1991) Detection of melanoma cells in peripheral blood by means of reverse transcriptase and polymerase chain reaction. Lancet 338:1227–1229
27. Olsson CA, de Vries GM, Buttyan R, Katz AE (1997) Reverse transcriptase-polymerase chain reaction for prostate cancer. Urol Clin Noth Am 24:367–378
28. Ghossein RA, Coit D, Brennan M, Zhang ZF, Wang Y, Bhattacharya S, Houghton A, Rosai J (1998) Prognostic significance of peripheral blood and bone marrow tyrosinase mRNA in malignant melanoma. Clin Cancer Res 4:419–428
29. Young CYF, Montgomery BT, Andrews PE, Qui SD, Bilhartz DL, Tindall DJ (1991) Hormonal regulation of prostate-specific antigen messenger RNA in human prostatic adenocarcinoma cell line LNCaP. Cancer Res 51:3748–3752
30. Fukuhara T, Hooper WC, Baylin SB, Benson J, Pruckler J, Olson AC, Evatt BLL, Vogler WR (1992) Use of the polymerase chain reaction to detect hypermethylation in the calcitonin gene-a new, sensitive approach to monitor tumor cells in acute myelogenous leukemia. Leukemia Res 16:1031–1040
31. Cross NC, Feng L, Chase A, Bungey J, Hughes TP, Goldman JM (1993) Competitive polymerase chain reaction to estimate the number of bcr-abl transcripts in chronic myeloid leukemia patients after bone marrow transplantation. Blood 82:1929–1936
32. Meijerink JP, Smetsers TF, Raemaekers JM, Bogman MJ, De Witte T, Mensink EJ (1993) Quantitation of follicular non-Hodgkin's lymphoma cells carrying t(14;18) by competitive polymerase chain reaction. Br J Haematol 84:250–256
33. Brisco MJ, Condon J, Hughes E, Neoh SH, Sykes PJ, Seshadri R, Toogood I, Waters K, Tauro G, Ekert H, Morley AA (1994) Outcome prediction in childhood acute lymphoblastic leukemia by molecular quantification of residual disease at the end of induction. Lancet 343:196–200
34. Heid CA, Stevens J, Livak KJ, Mickey Williams P (1996) Real time quantitative PCR. Genome Res 6:986–994
35. Johnson PWM, Burchill SA, Selby PJ (1995) The molecular detection of circulating tumor cells. Br J Cancer 72:268–276
36. Keilholz U, Willhauck M, Rimoldi D, Brasseur F, Dummer W, Rass K, de Vries T, Blaheta J, Voit C, Lethe B, Burchill S (1998) Reliability of reverse transcription polymerase chain reaction (RT-PCR) based assays for the detection of circulating tumor cells: a quality assurance initiative of the EORTC melanoma cooperative group. Eur J Cancer 34:750–753
37. Battayani Z, Grob JJ, Xerri L, Noe C, Zarour H, Houvaeneghel G, Delpero JR, Birmbaum D, Hassoun J, Bonerandi JJ (1995) Polymerase chain reaction detection of circulating melanocytes as a prognostic marker in patients with melanoma. Arch Dermatol 131:443–447
38. Buzaid AC, Balch CM (1996) Polymerase chain reaction for detection of melanoma in peripheral blood: Too early to assess clinical value. J Natl Cancer Inst 88:569–570
39. Hoon DSB, Wang Y, Dale PS, Conrad AJ, Schmid P, Garrison D, Kuo C, Foshag LJ, Nizze AJ, Morton DL (1995) Detection of occult melanoma cells in blood with a multiple-marker polymerase chain reaction assay. J Clin Oncol 13:2109–2116
40. Kunter U, Buer J, Probst M, Duensing S, Dallmann I, Grosse J, Kirchner H, Schluepen EM, Volkenandt M, Ganser A, Atzpodien J (1996) Peripheral blood tyrosinase messenger RNA detection and survival in malignant melanoma. J Natl Cancer Inst, 88:590–594
41. Brossart P, Keiholz U, Willhauck M, Scheibenbogen C, Mohler T, Hunstein W (1993) Hematogenous spread of malignant melanoma cells in different stages of disease. J Invest Dermatol 101:887–889
42. Foss AJ, Guille MJ, Occleston NL, Hykin PG, Hungerford JL, Lightman S (1995) The detection of melanoma cells in peripheral blood by reverse transcriptase polymerase chain reaction. Br J Cancer 72:155–159

43. Pittman K, Burchill S, Smith B, Southgate J, Joffe J, Gore M, Selby P (1996) Reverse transcriptase-polymerase chain reaction for expression of tyrosinase to identify malignant melanoma cells in peripheral blood. Ann Oncol 7:297–301
44. Mellado B, Guttierrez L, Castel T, Colomer D, Fontanillas M, Castro J, Estape J (1999) Prognostic significance of the detection of circulating malignant cells by reverse transcriptase-polymerase chain reaction in long-term clinically disease-free melanoma patients. Clin Cancer Res 5:1843–1848
45. Curry BJ, Myers K, Hersey P (1998) Polymerase chain reaction detection of melanoma cells in the circulation: Relation to clinical stage, surgical treatment, and recurrence from melanoma. J Clin Oncol 16:1760–1769
46. Farthman B, Eberle J, Krasagakis K, Gstottner M, Wang N, Bisson S, Orfanos CE (1998) RT-PCR for tyrosinase mRNA positive cells in peripheral blood: Evaluation strategy and correlation with known prognostic markers in 123 melanoma patients. J Invest Dermatol 110:263–267
47. Glaser R, Rass K, Seiter S, Hauschild A, Christophers E, Tilgen W (1997) Detection of circulating melanoma cells by specific amplification of tyrosinase complementary DNA is not a reliable tumor marker in melanoma patients: A clinical two-center study. J Clin Oncol 15:1218–2825
48. de Vries TJ, Fourkour A, Punt CJ, van de Locht LT, van den Bosch S, de Rooij MJ, Mensink EJ, Ruiter DJ, van Muijen GN (1999) Reproducibility of detection of tyrosinase and MART-1 transcripts in the peripheral blood of melanoma patients: a quality control study using a real-time quantitative RT-PCR. Br J Cancer 80:883–891
49. Schitteck B, Bodingbauer Y, Ellwanger U, Blaheta HJ, Garbe C (1999) Amplification of Melan A messenger RNA in addition to tyrosinase increases sensitivity of melanoma cell detection in peripheral blood and is associated with the clinical stage and prognosis of malignant melanoma. Br J Dermatol 141:30–36
50. Coit D, Ghossein RA, Vlamis V, Satagopan J, Livingston P, Rosai J, Houghton A. Prognostic significance of detection of tyrosinase mRNA in the peripheral blood and/or bone marrow of melanoma patients rendered surgically free of disease. Presented at the 1998 annual meeting of the American Society of Clinical Oncology, Los Angeles CA [Abstract #1981]
51. Brossart P, Schmier JW, Kruger S, Willhauck M, Scheibenbogen C, Mohler T, Keilholz U (1995) A polymerase chain reaction based semi-quantitative assessment of malignant melanoma cells in peripheral blood. Cancer Res 55:4065–4068
52. Muhlbauer M, Langenbach N, Stolz W, Hein R, Landthaler M, Buettner R, Bosserhoff AK (1999) Detection of melanoma cells in the blood of melanoma patients by melanoma-inhibitory activity (MIA) reverse transcription PCR. Clin Cancer Res 5:1099–1105
53. Van den Eynde B, Peeters O, De Backer O, Gaugler B, Lucas S, Boon T (1995) A new family of genes coding for an antigen recognized by autologous cytolytic T lymphocytes on a human melanoma J Exp Med 182:689–698
54. Cheung I, Cheung NKV, Ghossein RA, Satagopan JM, Bhattacharya S, Coit DG (1999) Association between molecular detection of *GAGE* and survival in patients with malignant melanoma: A retrospective cohort study. Clin Cancer Res 5:2042–2047
55. Kuo CT, Bostick PJ, Irie RF, Morton DL, Conrad AJ, Hoon DSB (1998) Assessement of messenger RNA of beta1-4-N-Acetylgalactosaminyltransferase as a molecular marker for metastatic melanoma. Clin Cancer Res 4:411–418
56. Martin VM, Siewert C, Scharl A, Harms T, Heinze R, Ohl S, Radbruch A, Miltenyi S, Schmitz J (1998) Immunomagnetic enrichment of disseminated epithelial tumor cells from peripheral blood by MACS. Exp Hematol 26:252–264
57. Racila E, Euhus D, Weiss AJ, Rao C, McConnell J, Terstappen LW, Uhr JW (1998) Detection and characterization of carcinoma cells in blood. Proc Natl Acad Sci USA 95:4589–4594
58. Ghossein RA, Osman I, Bhattacharya S, Ferrara J, Fazzari M, Cordon-Cardo C, Scher HI (1999) Detection of prostatic specific membrane antigen mRNA using immunobead reverse transcriptase polymerase chain reaction. Diagn Mol Pathol 8:59–65
59. Keilholz U (1998) New prognostic factors in melanoma: mRNA tumor markers. Eur J Cancer 34:(Suppl3) S37–41

The Clinical Utility of Multimarker RT-PCR in the Detection of Occult Metastasis in Patients with Melanoma*

B. Taback, D.L. Morton, S.J. O'Day, D.-H. Nguyen, T. Nakayama, and D.S.B. Hoon

Department of Molecular Oncology, John Wayne Cancer Institute, 2200 Santa Monica Blvd., Santa Monica, CA 90404, USA

Abstract

Cutaneous melanoma is characterized by a high propensity for metastasis. Currently, surgical intervention remains the mainstay of therapy. This approach has proven most beneficial when the diagnosis is of early stage primary lesions. Likewise, patients undergoing resection for a solitary site of metastasis have shown a survival advantage. Identification of metastatic disease depends predominantly on radiographic techniques requiring the presence of significant tumor burdens for successful imaging. However, at that time, the role of surgery and/or biochemotherapy may be of limited value. Techniques to identify minimal disease states may permit more accurate assessment of prognosis. The detection of occult tumor cells by RT-PCR in the blood, lymph nodes, and bone marrow of melanoma patients provides one such approach to monitor tumor progression. Single-marker RT-PCR has been used as one such approach but is noted to have limitations in sensitivity and specificity based on the heterogeneity of tumor marker expression among tumors as well as within an individual tumor lesion or among multiple lesions in individual patients. We employed a multimarker reverse transcriptase polymerase chain reaction assay that demonstrates improved sensitivity over a single-marker approach. Currently, the consequences of detecting systemic subclinical metastasis remain unknown pending longer-term follow-up. The detection of occult melanoma cells using molecular techniques in conjunction with known clinicopathologic prognostic factors may provide a novel and efficient approach in monitoring tumor progression and further identify high-risk patients diagnosed early in the disease course.

* The work reported here was supported in part by NIH PO1 grants CA 12582 and CA 1038, Roy E. Coats Research Foundation, Los Angeles, CA, USA

Recent Results in Cancer Research, Vol. 158

Introduction

Metastatic melanoma presents a formidable diagnostic challenge to the clinician. Despite a full complement of diagnostic modalities including standard radiography, computed tomography, and magnetic resonance imaging, the ability to diagnose metastatic melanoma at a stage where therapeutic intervention may still have some success is limited. The addition of positron emission tomography (PET) has improved the detection of early metastasis. A recent study revealed that 23 of 87 (26%) patients without clinical evidence of metastatic disease had abnormal PET scans, and 18 of them (72%) subsequently developed overt clinical metastasis within 6 months [1]. Historical data suggest that, from the time when clinical evidence of disseminated disease becomes apparent, less than 2% of patients will survive beyond 2 years. Currently, only two pathological parameters, Breslow thickness and the presence of regional lymph node metastasis correlate with staging and thus impact prognosis and survival [2]. The identification of markers expressed early in the disease course, which promises significant prognostic value for clinical outcome, would provide the clinician with an invaluable tool. Most tumors disseminate through a hematogenous route. Thus, sampling the blood for a particular tumor marker provides a logistically accessible site to monitor the status of a malignancy. In addition, since blood is in constant contact with the tumor, it provides an ideal source for monitoring changes that occur during disease progression as well as the tumor's response to therapy.

Malignant melanoma is distinguished by its high propensity for metastasis characterized by an unpredictable pattern of end organ involvement. Molecular methods that identify subclinical metastasis, not amenable to detection by conventional radiographic modalities, provide an attractive approach in complementing current staging procedures. Furthermore, they offer the theoretical advantage of permitting earlier therapeutic interventions with the potential of improving patient survival.

Protein/Carbohydrate Tumor Markers

Early studies in the elucidation of micrometastatic disease attempted to detect circulating tumor cells in the bloodstream using standard cytologic techniques. However, the level of cancer cells in the peripheral blood is usually low (less than 1 in 10^6 cells) in patients with limited metastatic disease [3]. Identifying metastasis using a microscope and staining procedures is time-consuming and operator-dependent, and the associated morphological distortions limit efficiency, sensitivity, and accuracy [4].

Since tumor metastasis is the primary cause of death in cancer patients, investigators have focused their efforts on identifying tumor-associated markers elaborated from a malignancy which, when monitored, would provide valuable diagnostic and prognostic information. One approach involves quantifying proteins associated with a cellular phenotype that characterizes metastasis. These may include proteins or enzymes expressed by tumor cells which affect angiogenesis (inhibitors and stimulators), local invasion (attachment molecules, proteolytic enzymes), and/or cell cycle regulation [5].

Melanoma cells are derived from neuroectodermal primordial cells. Initial pathologic studies have attempted to capitalize on this association as an aid to the histologic diagnosis of melanoma, particularly in variants that are amelanotic [6]. Subsequently, investigators attempted to employ these distinct features (enzymes and their substrate products) as specific tumor markers for metastatic melanoma [7, 8]. Unfortunately, in vivo these enzymes, proteins, and substrate products were found to be more difficult to identify than anticipated, limiting their sensitivity [9]. Furthermore, protein/enzyme levels are noted to fluctuate significantly in response to inflammatory, infectious, and other unrelated nonspecific disease states, thereby limiting their specificity and reliability. One of the first reports investigated neuron-specific enolase (NSE), an enzyme specific for melanocytes and other cells of the amine precursor uptake and decarboxylase family. Initial studies found that less than 50% of patients with advanced disease (stage III and IV) expressed this marker, and serum levels were noted to vary widely within this group [10, 11].

In an attempt to differentiate tumor cells from normal cells, researchers have found a higher concentration of sialic acid-containing lipids, namely gangliosides, on cancer cells as compared to their normal counterparts. Some have suggested that shedding of these glycolipids in the serum of cancer patients may be valuable as a tumor marker for monitoring disease [12]. Unfortunately, this marker may be elevated in a wide variety of acute inflammatory states, thus contributing to its low specificity and reduced diagnostic accuracy in patients with melanoma [13, 14].

More recently, investigators have attempted to correlate S100 levels with the staging of melanoma [15–17]. S100 is a low molecular weight (21 Kda) calcium-binding protein composed of two subunits (α and β) which can form three isomers, $\alpha\alpha$, $\beta\beta$, and $\alpha\beta$. In 1980, Gaynor isolated S100 protein from melanoma cells in culture and postulated its potential value as a tumor marker [18, 19]. Thereafter, S100B has been identified in Langerhans' cells as well as melanocytes and currently is a major immunodiagnostic marker for melanoma cells in pathology [20, 21]. Initial protein assay studies in patients with malignant melanoma were hampered by their low sensitivity [22]. The advent of radioimmunoassays has improved the sensitivity and permits widespread clinical testing in patients with melanoma. However, there remains considerable discrepancy in the literature, which prevents a universal endorsement of common reference standards for clinical application. Numerous studies evaluating the utility of various protein markers as an aid in the detection of occult metastasis have failed to show consistent results in large series of patients with melanoma at any stage of disease [23, 24]. Factors pertaining to the exclusivity of tumor cell expression and antibody specificity remain as major variables for the reliable detection of occult metastasis using protein assays [25].

The mRNA Tumor Markers

Numerous protein/carbohydrate markers have been pursued in melanoma patients to provide similar clinical utility as carcinoembryonic antigens and prostate-specific antigens in colon and prostate carcinomas, respectively. Since various protein assays for melanoma have been criticized for their low specificity, these markers have not gained widespread acceptance as an adjunct in the detection of occult circulating cancer cells. In addition, their sensitivity during the early stages of disease, i.e., those associated with low tumor burdens, have been inconsistent [16, 26]. Polymerase chain reaction (PCR) technology has been suggested to enhance the sensitivity of tests employed in the detection of the rare tumor cells circulating in the bloodstream. Amplification of genetic sequences uniquely associated with a distinct tumor type would significantly improve the specificity and sensitivity of prospective markers, particularly at low tumor volumes, where detecting occult metastasis would have a more profound impact on treatment options and thus potentially alter the disease course. One advantage of reverse transcriptase polymerase chain reaction (RT-PCR) is its potentially higher specificity and sensitivity, compared to protein assays.

Initially, Smith et al. demonstrated in 1991 the ability to identify tyrosinase mRNA in a sample of blood obtained from several patients with metastatic melanomas [27]. Tyrosinase is one of several major enzymes involved in melanin biosynthesis. Refinements of the PCR technique by various investigators have confirmed the specificity of the marker using normal donors as well as those with other tumors. Currently, tyrosinase is the most commonly employed mRNA marker assayed in melanoma.

In the early 1990s, researchers began to investigate the clinical utility of RT-PCR in the detection of tumor-associated molecular markers in cancer patients at various stages of disease (Table 1) [28–33]. Despite these initially encouraging results, a majority of the more recent literature demonstrates a disparity between PCR positivity and clinical staging [34–36]. In patients with stage IV disease, where tumor volume and circulating malignant cells are expected to be the greatest, positive PCR results have ranged from 0–100% [28, 30]. Glaser and others have further questioned the credibility of tyrosinase mRNA as a marker of disease progression when they demonstrated variably low rates of expression, albeit with less disparity, in the early stages of melanoma [34]. In patients with advanced disease, Reinhold demonstrated that sample positivity varied from day to day as well as within the same day [35]. This confirms speculation that metastatic cells may be transiently shed into the systemic circulation, and therefore random samples may be not truly representative of patients' clinical status. Many studies have implicated an assortment of factors contributing to low positive PCR results, including methods of RNA extraction and purification, cycling and PCR setup, quality control standards, endpoint analysis of PCR product, and data interpretation. Other differences among the various studies may reflect biases depending on the time point at which blood was sampled, i.e., early or late

Table 1. Tyrosinase mRNA expression in published series

Author	Total patients	Stage	Positive patients/ total patients (%)
Smith (1991)	7	III	1/2 (50)
		IV	3/5 (60)
Brossart (1993)	56	I, II	1/10 (10)
		III	6/17 (35)
		IV	29/29 (100)
Battayani (1995)	93	I, II	2/10 (20)
		III	8/18 (44)
		IV	16/32 (50)
Foss (1995)	6	IV	0/6 (0)
Kunter (1996)	64	I, II	0/16 (0)
		III, IV	9/48 (19)
Pittman (1996)	24	IV	3/24 (13)
Mellado (1996)	91	I	4/17 (23)
		II	10/22 (45)
		III	7/17 (40)
		IV	32/35 (94)
Glaser (1997)	102	I, II	1/43 (2.3)
		III	0/15 (0)
		IV	12/44 (27.3)
Ghossein (1997)	73	II	2/16 (12.5)
		III	6/40 (15)
		IV	1/17 (6)
Jung (1997)	50	IV[a]	13/50 (26)
		IV[b]	5/50 (10)
Reinhold (1997)	65	I, II	0/31 (0)
		III	1/21 (5)
		IV	5/13 (39)
Curry (1998)	276	I	5/31 (15)
		II	43/129 (34)
		III	60/116 (60)
Farthmann (1998)	123	I, II	6/16 (13)
		III	7/41 (17)
		IV	16/36 (44)
Kuo (1998)	89	I, II	6/18 (33)
		III	21/35 (60)
		IV	19/36 (53)
Mellado (1999)	57	I	2/11 (18)
		II	6/33 (19)
		III	2/13 (15)

[a] Density gradient; [b] whole blood.

within the same stage of disease, preoperative, or postoperative, and fluctuations in the time frame during which blood is obtained within the same day. Curry showed that the timing of surgery may influence PCR results by demonstrating 15 of 23 (65%) patients with positive results preoperatively converted to a negative status postoperatively [37]. More importantly, 62% converted to negative for unknown reasons 3 to 6 months after surgery. Additional studies consisting of longer follow-up with clearly defined endpoints (time to disease recurrence, time to death) are required to determine which patients are truly positive. Studies using serial sampling will further identify those time points which most closely correlate with recurrence and the significance of conversion to the patient's outcome. Investigators have tried to use single-marker RT-PCR testing as a highly predictive indicator of disease progression. However, the literature is filled with results demonstrating conflicting reproducibility. Fundamentally, some of the major problems of the assay system pertain to the lack of standard operating procedures for analysis. If an assay is to be correlated with clinical parameters, it must be rigorously performed under a standard procedure and data must be verified using objective criteria. Metastasis is a complex and dynamic event, and single-marker RT-PCR may not satisfy the diverse requirements of this system.

Mellado showed that PCR positivity correlated with stage of disease and that PCR-positive patients had a higher rate of relapse than PCR-negative patients in the same stage [33]. Inexplicably, these findings only applied to patients in stages II and IV. However, in an additional study these same authors found no correlation between PCR and stage, demonstrating the variability of results even within the same laboratory [36]. Nevertheless, consistent to both studies was that PCR-positive patients experienced recurrences more frequently and positive PCR results were significantly associated with lower 2-year disease-free and overall survival rates. A similar correlation was found by Battayani, who showed that stage III and stage IV patients who converted to a positive PCR status were at significantly increased risk of disease progression within the ensuing 6 months [29]. Once again, PCR sensitivity ranged more broadly in the advanced stage (IV), compared to other stages. This may be attributed to the sites (organs) of metastasis and the overall tumor volume, which is not distinguished at this stage [29, 31, 34]. In other words, not all stage IV patients may behave in the same way and PCR status may identify those subsets.

More recently, melanoma inhibiting activity (MIA), characterized as a small soluble protein with yet unknown function isolated from in vitro melanoma cell lines, has been shown to correlate with disease progression [38]. When quantitative RT-PCR studies were performed in patients with melanoma, there was 13% expression of this marker in stage I and 23% expression in stage II patients versus 100% expression in both stage III and stage IV patients. These authors found MIA levels of expression to have a higher sensitivity than S100 and intracellular adhesion molecules (ICAM), a protein product associated with a metastatic phenotype. In serial assessments of 350 patients with stage I and II melanomas, 32 developed a positive MIA result and 16 of those proceeded to develop clinical evidence of metastatic disease. However, a longer follow-up period to determine the outcome of the other 50% of patients who are MIA-positive yet clinically free of recurrence at the termination of this study is necessary to determine the true power of MIA as a prognostic marker. In contrast, a study evaluating mRNA MIA from blood samples of 154 patients with various stages of melanoma showed no difference in expression between stages I/II and III/IV – 26.8% versus 28.4%, respectively [39]. This study concluded that amplification of MIA mRNA had little value as a marker for clinical staging or the detection of metastatic disease.

It is generally accepted that RT-PCR, through the amplification of a tumor-specific mRNA sequence, allows for increased sensitivity in the detection of occult malignant cells from a particular sampling site. However, the lack of consistency in its reliability as reported throughout the literature is the single greatest obstacle in the widespread acceptance of RT-PCR as a surrogate marker for clinical staging or as a prognosticator of impending disease progression. Numerous factors may contribute to these reported inconsistencies. They may include procedural variations which involve differences in sample procurement and RNA extraction methods, variations in thermocycling techniques, and meticulous attention to preventing cross contamination. Additional factors which must be considered are inherent to the biology of cancer and involve the intermittent shedding of tumor cells into the bloodstream, identification of clones which do not produce the marker being assessed, mRNA stability, and dilutional effects of additional cellular mRNA transcripts concomitantly extracted.

Multimarker RT-PCR

Blood

Originally, we developed a multimarker RT-PCR assay using four melanoma-associated antigens to improve sensitivity in the detection of occult melanoma tumor cells. Initially, these included tyrosinase, P97, Mage-3, and MUC-18 [40]. Further refinement identified five antigens: tyrosinase, tyrosinase-related proteins 1 (TRP-1) and 2 (TRP-2), Pmel 17/gp 100, and MART-1/MelanA. A few of these markers are involved in the melanin biosynthesis pathway, but all were found to be expressed in 100% of cultured melanoma cell lines and are immunogenic in humans [41].

These antigens are highly specific for detecting occult disease, as their expression has not been found in normal tissues except for those of neuroectodermal origin [42, 43]. We found that 74% of tumors biopsied, 43% of regional lymph nodes with foci of metastasis, and 47% of patient blood samples expressed all five markers (Table 2). In 86% of the specimens assayed, at least one marker was expressed. The specificity of the markers for detecting melanoma was confirmed by their absence of expression in normal tissue and/or blood samples.

Table 2. Expression of mRNA markers in various tissues in patients with melanoma

Number of mRNA markers expressed[a]	Tumor $n=23$	Regional lymph nodes $n=28$	Blood $n=35$
5	17 (74%)	12 (43%)	15 (43%)
4	2 (9%)	9 (32%)	7 (20%)
3	1 (4%)	2 (7%)	7 (20%)
2	2 (9%)	3 (4%)	2 (6%)
1	1 (4%)	1 (4%)	4 (11%)
0	0 (0%)	1 (4%)	0 (0%)

[a] The mRNA markers tyrosinase, TRP-1, TRP-2, Pmel 17/gp100, and MART-1/Melan A were assessed using RT-PCR and Southern blot in tumor tissues, histologically positive lymph nodes, and blood specimens from AJCC stage I–IV melanoma patients.

Table 3. Level of mRNA marker expression in tumor tissues, histologically positive lymph nodes, and blood specimens from AJCC stage I–IV melanoma patients using RT-PCR and Southern blot analysis

mRNA marker	Expression		
	Tumor $n=23$	Lymph node $n=28$	Blood $n=35$
Tyrosinase	23 (100%)	26 (93%)	30 (86%)
TRP-1	18 (78%)	18 (64%)	20 (57%)
TRP-2	19 (83%)	20 (71%)	26 (74%)
Pmel 17/gp100	21 (91%)	22 (79%)	30 (86%)
MART-1/MelanA	20 (87%)	24 (86%)	29 (83%)

Tyrosinase was the most commonly expressed marker in tumor tissue (100%), regional lymph nodes (93%), and blood samples (86%) (Table 3). We postulate that the lack of expression of a single marker from all samples may be attributed to a variety of factors, including a low level of mRNA expression, dilution of a marker among normal cellular RNA, and/or that a marker may not reflect all metastatic phenotypes. Furthermore, a marker may not be expressed until late in the course of disease progression, which would limit its prognostic utility. One potential advantage of multimarker RT-PCR is that it allows one to monitor the transcribed result of specific genetic events that occur during the evolution of a malignancy [44]. For instance, a variety of different markers may be expressed at various time points throughout the sequence of disease progression, invasion, and metastasis. Expression of unique markers may characterize critical events or time points in cancer progression (i. e., loss of cell cycle control, unrestrained proliferation, metastatic potential, etc.) where detection may be more indicative of specific clinical correlations. Furthermore, multimarker RT-PCR may provide the clinician with an expanded armamentarium to allow specific feedback and periodic assessments of the efficacy of various chemotherapeutic, immunologic, or genetic therapies which may impact the tumor through different pathways.

Lymph Nodes

More recently, we employed multimarker RT-PCR in the detection of occult metastasis in the regional lymph nodes (sentinel nodes) of patients with early stage melanoma. Regional lymph node involvement often occurs prior to disseminated disease and is a reliable predictor of patient prognosis. The ability to detect metastasis at an early stage has significant clinical implications and may aid in the decision on further therapy. The addition of adjuvant therapy early in the disease course, when the tumor burden is low but the risk of metastasis is increased, has important value. Identification of lymph node micrometastasis in this setting may enhance the efficiency of adjuvant therapeutic interventions.

Single-marker RT-PCR has been utilized in the identification of occult metastasis in lymph nodes not otherwise detected using conventional hematoxylin and eosin (H&E) or immunohistochemical (IHC) techniques [45]. We have shown the procedure of sentinel lymphadenectomy (SLND) to predict accurately the pathologic status of lymph nodes draining a primary tumor site. In our experience, when the sentinel lymph node is negative by standard staining techniques (H&E and IHC), regional lymph nodes will be involved with tumor in less than 1% of cases [46]. This is particularly advantageous in patients with early stage disease, where significant prognostic information can be obtained based solely on the status of the sentinel node, as opposed to performing a full nodal dissection, which subjects patients to increased morbidity. Methods that yield the greatest information from modest amounts of sample provide a less invasive alternative with lower complications and have a higher benefit: risk ratio for the patient. With these goals in mind, we applied multimarker RT-PCR to sentinel lymph nodes in high-risk patients with early stage melanoma [47]. We were able to upstage 20 of 55 patients (36%) with histopathologically negative sentinel nodes by demonstrating the expression of two or more mRNA markers. Furthermore, patients with negative sentinel nodes by IHC yet positive by multimarker RT-PCR were at a significant risk of disease recurrence ($p=0.02$), compared to patients whose sentinel lymph nodes expressed one or no markers. Lymph nodes are difficult to assess by RT-PCR, particularly for a single marker, because of the greater probability of contaminating cell types being present. In our study, single markers such as tyrosinase were not as efficient as multimarker combinations. These results clearly demonstrate the greater accuracy of molecular techniques in detecting occult metastasis and their potential application for clinical correlation.

The combination of RT-PCR and SLND may improve detection of subclinical metastasis and further identify those patients at high risk for recurrence (local or distant). One approach to identifying patients at high risk for recurrent disease is the use of RT-PCR to detect residual tumor cells in the surgical wound following resection. We recently employed RT-PCR to wound drainage fluid (seroma) obtained from axillary, inguinal, or neck lymph node dissections in 23 patients with AJCC stage III and IV melanomas. Forty-eight hours following surgery, tyrosinase mRNA and TRP-1 mRNA were noted in 61% and 52% of seroma samples, respectively, and the combination of markers improved detection to 70%. This represents an additional source for assessing local residual disease which may play a role in identifying patients at risk for local failure.

Bone Marrow

Likewise, investigators have attempted to identify occult malignant cells in the bone marrow of patients without clinical evidence of such metastasis as a way of predicting future patient outcome [48, 49]. Investigators have postulated that identifying these patients early in their disease course would enable therapeutic intervention at a time when the disease burden is low and therefore have greater impact on the disease course.

Ghossein showed a higher expression of tyrosinase mRNA expression in the bone marrow of patients with various stages of melanoma as compared to blood samples, 16.5% versus 12%, respectively [50]. Ironically, despite its lower overall expression rate as compared to bone marrow, the positive expression of tyrosinase in the blood correlated more closely with overall survival but not clinical stage of disease. Clinically significant melanoma metastasis to bone is not a frequent event and may contribute to these discrepancies. This point raises an interesting dilemma: what does a positive PCR result from a metastatic site represent – a true metastasis, a significant metastasis, or a false positive result? This study further demonstrates the divergence among individual studies. Furthermore, levels of mRNA expression may vary within the same patient with respect to the site biopsied – the concordance rate for blood and bone marrow was 19%. Multimarker RT-PCR may permit the identification of various clones from distinct metastatic sites that represent a range of potential for lethality. This approach provides a mechanism to address genetic instability and heterogeneity of the tumor occurring during disease progression.

We performed additional studies to determine the validity of multimarker RT-PCR in detecting subclinical skeletal metastasis in patients with isolated AJCC stage IV melanomas with no evidence of disseminated disease as noted by conventional radiographic methods. We found the frequency of mRNA marker expression from the bone marrow of ribs incidentally resected in 26 patients who underwent surgical procedures for a single isolated thoracic or abdominal visceral metastasis as follows: tyrosinase 58%, TRP-1 27%, Pmel 17 54%, and MUC-18 38% (Table 4). Seventeen of 26 (65%) bone marrow samples expressed two or more mRNA markers (Table 5). In patients with matched blood and bone marrow samples, the correlation of marker expression was: tyrosinase 29%, TRP-1 19%, Pmel 17/gp100 38%, and MUC-18 10% (Table 6).

In 66% of the bone marrow samples, there was expression of at least one marker indicating the presence of residual disease not detected with cur-

Table 4. Comparison of mRNA marker expression in bone marrow (obtained from a surgically resected segment of rib), tumor tissues, and blood specimens from AJCC stage IV melanoma patients with a single visceral metastasis using RT-PCR and Southern blot analysis, tumors, and blood samples of melanoma patients

Specimen source	Expression			
	Tyrosinase	TRP-1	Pmel 17/gp100	MUC-18
Bone marrow $n=26$	15/26 (58%)	7/26 (27%)	14/26 (54%)	10/26 (38%)
Tumor $n=17$	14/17 (82%)	10/17 (59%)	14/17 (82%)	12/17 (70%)
Blood $n=21$	9/21 (43%)	5/21 (24%)	14/21 (67%)	7/21 (33%)

Table 5. Number of melanoma mRNA markers expressed in bone marrow (BM) obtained from a surgically resected segment of rib and from AJCC stage IV melanoma patients with a single visceral metastasis, using RT-PCR and Southern blot analysis for the following mRNA markers: tyrosinase, TRP-1, Pmel 17/gp100, and MUC-18

Number of melanoma mRNA markers expressed	Number of BM specimens expressing mRNA/ total BM specimens
4	4/26 (15%)
3	3/26 (11%)
2	10/26 (39%)
1	1/26 (4%)
0	8/26 (31%)

Table 6. Melanoma mRNA marker expression in bone marrow (obtained from a surgically resected segment of rib) and blood samples from AJCC stage IV melanoma patients ($n=21$) with a single visceral metastasis, using RT-PCR and Southern blot analysis

Sample source	mRNA marker expression			
	Tyrosinase	TRP-1	Pmel 17/gp100	MUC-18
Bone marrow	13 (62%)	6 (29%)	12 (57%)	6 (29%)
Blood	10 (48%)	6 (29%)	14 (67%)	7 (33%)
Bone marrow and blood	6 (29%)	4 (19%)	8 (38%)	2 (10%)

rently available clinical modalities. The implications of these findings are potentially significant. These findings are in contrast to a previous study which showed much lower rates of PCR positivity in bone marrow (10%) and blood samples (6%) of patients with AJCC stage IV melanoma. Furthermore, the correlation between bone marrow and blood was 11% for the single-marker tyrosinase as compared with our findings of 29%. Although 15 of 28 (58%) of our bone marrow samples expressed tyrosinase mRNA, the addition of supplemental markers to our assay further increased the sensitivity to 69%. This is the first report demonstrating the molecular detection of melanoma micrometastasis at a skeletal site other than those associated with the traditional approach of iliac aspiration for bone marrow analysis. Moreover, we have shown that bone marrow expression exceeds that of the blood. The bloodstream is a harsh environment for tumor cell survival and these studies provide molecular results that support Paget's original theory that certain local environmental factors promote the establishment of metastasis [51]. Additionally, variations in tumor marker expression may be a result of local factors which promote proliferation of a certain tumor clone or select for the expression of a distinct array of mRNA transcripts. Therefore, efforts must focus not only on the absolute presence or absence of micrometastasis as seen by the expression of mRNA in the blood but also on the significance of those sites which may harbor metastatic foci. For instance, what do bone marrow melanoma metastases detected solely by PCR represent: true micrometastasis, cells in transit, or incidental melanoma cells? Do certain metastases have different prognostic importance? Investigations in the understanding of local environmental factors that promote metastasis versus those which suppress it may provide insight into the behavior of micrometastasis and potential future therapies. Finally, because not all tumors are similar, complementary markers may have more prognostic value than single marker assays.

We have shown a higher rate of marker expression in melanoma cells in culture as compared to tissue samples obtained in vivo, which may correspond to an expression bias promoted by growth factors unique to an in vitro milieu. The expression of a particular mRNA marker may represent a clonal selection and/or epigenetic influences of the organ environmental conditions as well as host selective pressures (i.e., immune response). Factors exclusive to cell culturing conditions may not accurately reflect the heterogeneity of cells and their respective markers which compose a tumor mass in the host environment. In either event, these results suggest that current approaches using single marker RT-PCR to detect occult malignant cells in an effort to enhance clinical staging may be limited and that the addition of multimarker RT-PCR may improve the sensitivity of this methodology. Finally, serial sampling may further improve the accuracy of mRNA markers in the detection of micrometastasis in an in vivo environment, where dynamic interactions between tumor cells and their surroundings are not static but continuously occurring. These relationships may significantly influence and alter the cellular expression of a variety of mRNA transcripts throughout the evolution of a malignant process. If mRNA markers are to be utilized in the diagnosis of disease, detection of progression, and response to various therapeutic interventions, these concepts should be considered in future investigations. Caution is advised when interpreting the detection of tumor cells using RT-PCR techniques and in the clinical application of these methods. The establishment of metastasis is not an efficient process of tumor cells in the blood. As previously described, there are many factors that can abort the metastatic process at any stage. The detection of tumor cells in the blood by RT-PCR should be used as a tool in combination with other known clinicopathologic factors to predict disease progression. Recently we have demonstrated that the presence of multimarkers in the blood of disease-free patients can be used as an independent prognostic factor for disease recurrence. Future applications of this assay may be utilized to diagnose disease as well. However, one should not criticize the efficiency of the test itself unless operating procedures strictly adhere to standard protocols. The development and validation of clinical detection assays require significant efforts, which is well-documented for current cancer diagnostic testing in use today.

References

1. Hsueh EC, Gupta RK, Glass EC et al (1998) Positron emission tomography plus serum TA90 immune complex assay for detection of occult metastatic melanoma. J AM Coll Surg 187:191–197
2. Eton O, Legha SS, Moon TE et al (1998) Prognostic factors for survival of patients treated systemically for disseminated melanoma. J Clin Oncol 16:1103–1111
3. Liotta L, Stetler-Stevenson G (1991) Tumor invasion and metastasis: an imbalance of positive and negative regulation. Cancer Res 51:5054–5059
4. Goldblatt SA, Nadel FM (1965) Cancer cells in the circulating blood: a critical review II. Acta Cytol 9:6–20
5. Woodhouse EC, Chuaqui RF, Liotta LA (1997) General mechanisms of metastasis. Cancer (Supp) 80:1529–1537
6. Dhillon AP, Rode J, Leathem A (1982) Neurone specific enolase: an aid to the diagnosis of melanoma and neuroblastoma. Histopathology 6:81–92
7. Horikoshi T, Ito S, Wakamatsu K et al (1994) Evaluation of melanin-related metabolites as markers of melanoma progression. Cancer 73:629–636
8. Letellier S, Garnier JP, Spy J et al (1997) Determination of the L-DOPA/L-tyrosine ratio in human plasma by high-performance liquid chromatography. Usefulness as a marker in metastatic melanoma. J Chrom B Biomed Sci Appl 696:9–17
9. Hasegawa M, Takata M, Hatta N et al (1997) Simultaneous measurement of serum 5-S-cysteinyldopa, circulating intercellular adhesion molecule-1 and soluble interleukin-2 receptor levels in Japanese patients with malignant melanoma. Melanoma Res 7:243–251
10. Wibe E, Paus E, Aamdal S (1990) Neuron specific enolase (NSE) in serum of patients with malignant melanoma. Cancer Lett 52:29–31
11. Buzaid AC, Sandler AB, Hayden CL et al (1994) Neuron-specific enolase as a tumor marker in metastatic melanoma. Am J Clin Oncol 17:430–431
12. Hoon DSB, Irie RF, Cochran AJ (1988) Gangliosides from human melanoma immunomodulate response of T cells to interleukin-2. Cellular Immun 111:410–419
13. Schutter EM, Visser JJ, van Kamp GJ et al (1992) The utility of lipid-associated sialic acid (LASA or LSA) as a serum marker for malignancy. A review of the literature. Tumour Biol 13:121–132
14. Miliotes G, Lyman GH, Cruse CW et al (1996) Evaluation of new putative tumor markers for melanoma. Ann Surg Oncol 3:558–563
15. Guo HB, Stoffel-Wagner B, Bierwirth T et al (1995) Clinical sinificance of serum S100 in metastatic malignant melanoma. Eur J Cancer 31 A:1898–1902
16. Schultz ES, Diepgen TL, Driesch P (1997) Clinical and prognostic relevance of serum S100B protein in malignant melanoma. Br J Derm 138:426–430
17. Hauschild A, Engel G, Brenner W et al (1999) S100B protein detection in serum is a significant prognostic factor in metastatic melanoma. Oncology 56:338–344
18. Gaynor R, Irie R, Morton D et al (1980) S100 protein is present in cultured human malignant melanomas. Nature 286:400–401

19. Gaynor R, Herschman HR, Irie R et al (1981) S100 protein: a marker for human malignant melanomas? Lancet 1:869–871
20. Cochran AJ, Lu HF, Li PX et al (1993) S100 protein remains a practical marker for melanocytic and other tumors. Melanoma Res 3:325–330
21. Nakajima T, Watanabe S, Sato Y et al (1982) Immunohistochemical demonstration of S100 protein in malignant melanoma and pigmented nevus, and its diagnostic application. Cancer 50:912–918
22. Fagnart OC, Sindic CJ, Laterre C (1988) Particle counting immunoassay of S100 protein in serum. Possible relevance in tumors and ischemic disorders of the central nervous system. Clin Chem 34:1387–1391
23. Seregni E, Massaron S, Martinetti A et al (1998) S100 protein serum levels in cutaneous malignant melanoma. Oncol Rep 5:601–604
24. Buer J, Probst M, Franzke A et al (1997) Elevated serum levels of S100 and survival in metastatic malignant melanoma. Br J Cancer 75:1373–1376
25. Braun S, Muller M, Hepp F et al (1998) Re: Micrometastatic breast cancer cells in bone marrow at primary surgery: Prognostic value in comparison with nodal status (correspondence). J Natl Cancer Inst 90:1099–1100
26. Bonfrer JMG, Korse CM, Nieweg OE et al (1998) The luminescence immuoassay S-100: A sensitive test to measure circulating S-100B: its prognostic value in malignant melanoma. Br J Cancer 77:2210–2214
27. Smith B, Selby P, Southgate J et al (1991) Detection of malanoma cells in peripheral blood by means of reverse transcriptase and polymerase chain reaction. The Lancet 338:1227–1229
28. Brossart P, Keilholz U, Willhauck M et al (1993) Hematogenous spread of malignant melanoma cells in different stages of disease. J Invest Derm 101:887–889
29. Battayani Z, Grob JJ, Zerri L et al (1995) Polymerase chain reaction detection of circulating melanocytes as a prognostic marker in patients with melanoma. Arch Derm 131:443–447
30. Foss AJE, Guille MJ, Occleston NL et al (1995) The detection of melanoma cells in perpheral blood by reverse transcription-polymerase chain reaction. Br J Cancer 72:155–159
31. Kunter U, Buer J, Probst M et al (1996) Peripheral blood tyrosinase messenger RNA detection and survival in malignant melanoma. J Natl Cancer Inst 88:590–594
32. Pittman K, Burchill S, Smith B, et al (1996) Reverse transcriptase polymerase chain reaction for expression of tyrosinase to identify malignant melanoma cells in peripheral blood. Ann Oncol 7:297–301
33. Mellado B, Colomer D, Castel T et al (1996) Detection of circulating neoplastic cells by reverse-transcriptase polymerase chain reaction in malignant melanoma: Association with clinical stage and prognosis. J Clin Oncol 14:2091–2097
34. Glaser R, Rass K, Seiter S et al (1997) Detection of circulating melanoma cells by specific amplification of tyrosinase complementary DNA is not a reliable tumor marker in melanoma patients: A clinical two-center study. J Clin Oncol 15:2818–2825
35. Reinhold U, Ludtke-Handjery H-C, Schnautz S et al (1997) The analysis of tyrosinase-specific mRNA in blood samples of melanoma patients by reverse transcriptase polymerase chain reaction is not a useful test for metastatic tumor progression. J Invest Derm 108:166–169
36. Mellado B, Gutierrez L, Castel T et al (1999) Prognostic significance of the detection of circulating malignant cells by reverse transcriptase polymerase chain reaction in long-term clinically disease-free melanoma patients. Clin Cancer Res 5:1843–1848
37. Curry BJ, Myers K, Hersey P (1998) Polymerase chain reaction detection of melanoma cells in the circulation: Relation to clinical stage, surgical treatment, and recurrence from melanoma. J Clin Oncol 16:1760–1769
38. Bosserhoff A-K, Kaufmann M, Kaluza B et al (1997) Melanoma-inhibiting activity, a novel serum marker for progression of malignant melanoma. Cancer Res 57:3149–3153

39. Muhlbauer M, Langenbach N, Stolz W et al (1999) Detection of melanoma cells in the blood of melanoma patients by melanoma-inhibitory activity (MIA) reverse transscription-polymerase chain reaction. Clin Cancer Res 5:1099–1105
40. Hoon DSB, Wang Y, Dale PS et al (1995) Detection of occult melanoma cells in blood with a multiple-marker polymerase chain reaction assay. J Clin Oncol 13:2109–2116
41. Sarantou T, Chi DD, Garrison DA et al (1997) Melanoma-associated antigens as messenger RNA detection markers for melanoma. Cancer Res 57:1371–1376
42. Hoon DSB, Garrison D, Chi DDJ et al (1996) Molecular detection of tumor-associated antigens shared by human melanomas and gliomas. FASEB J 10:1414
43. Chi DDJ, Merchant RE, Rand R et al (1997) Molecular detection of tumorassociated antigens shared by human cuntaneous melanomas and gliomas. Am J Path 150:2143–2152
44. Kuo CT, Bostick PJ, Irie RF et al (1998) Assessment of messenger RNA of β1->4-*N*-acetylgalactosaminyltransferase as a molecular marker for metastatic melanoma. Clin Cancer Res 4:411–418
45. Shivers SC, Wang X, Li W et al (1998) Molecular staging of malignant melanoma: Correlation with clinical outcome. JAMA 280:1410–1415
46. Morton DL, Wen DR, Wong JH et al (1992) Technical details of intraoperative lymphatic mapping for early stage melanoma. Arch Surg 127:392–399
47. Bostick PJ, Morton DL, Turner RR et al (in press) Prognostic significance of occult metastasis detected by sentinel lymphadenectomy and RT-PCR in clinical stage I melanoma patients. J Clin Oncol
48. Zippelius P, Kufer P, Honold G et al (1997) Limitations of reverse-transcriptase polymerase chain reaction analysis for detection of micrometastasic epithelial cancer cells in bone marrow. J Clin Oncol 15:2701–2708
49. Putz E, Witter K, Offner S et al (1999) Phenotypic characteristics of cell lines derived from disseminated cancer cells in bone marrow of patients with solid epithelial tumors: Establishment of working models for human micrometastasis. Cancer Res 59:241–248
50. Ghossein R, Coit D, Brennan M et al (1998) Prognostic significance of peripheral blood and bone marrow tyrosinase messenger RNA in malignant melanoma. Clin Cancer Res 4:419–428
51. Zetter BR (1990) The cellular basis of site-specific tumor metastasis. N Engl J Med 322:605–612
52. Hoon DSB, Bostick P, Kuo C et al (2000) Molecular markers in blood as surrogate prognostic indicators of melanoma recurrence. Cancer Res 60:2253–2257

Polymerase Chain Reaction in the Detection of Circulating Tumour Cells in Peripheral Blood of Melanoma Patients

B. Schittek, H.-J. Blaheta, U. Ellwanger, and C. Garbe

Section of Dermatologic Oncology, Department of Dermatology,
Eberhard Karls University, Liebermeisterstraße 25, 72076 Tübingen, Germany

Abstract

Conflicting results were obtained by various research groups using the tyrosinase reverse transcription polymerase chain reaction (RT-PCR) for detecting melanoma cells circulating in peripheral blood. Whereas 100% positivity was initially reported for stage IV patients, more recent investigations reported positive detection rates between 30% and 50% in patients with disseminated melanoma. While the high detection rate initially reported in metastatic melanoma may be explained by contamination problems, methodological differences in different steps of the technical procedure of RT-PCR may account for the differences reported in more recent examinations. Major differences may result from the kind of blood preparation, the RNA isolation method, the kind of RT enzyme used, and the gene targeted by PCR primers. In our experience, blood purification by a Ficoll gradient increased melanoma cell detection rates compared to RNA extraction from total blood or after erythrocyte lysis. Amplification of MelanA in addition to tyrosinase resulted in a 30% enhanced sensitivity of melanoma cell detection compared to amplification to tyrosinase alone, whereas gp100/pMel17 and MUC18 gene products were already detected in blood from nonmelanoma patients. These findings are in agreement with those of other groups. Currently, an increase in the sensitivity for detection of circulating tumour cells to more than 50% of patients with disseminated melanoma seems to be unlikely. It is interesting that between 15% and 30% positive results and sometimes more have already been obtained from patients with primary melanoma. So far, there is no data for judging the prognostic significance of the detection of circulating tumour cells in patients without clinically recognisable metastases. Our limited experience shows that staging examinations in these patients reveal no proof of macrometastasis. Therefore, it is presently unclear whether these positive findings are associated with long-term prognosis or if they merely reflect false positive findings in this highly sensitive RT-PCR technique.

Recent Results in Cancer Research, Vol. 158

Introduction

The application of reverse transcription polymerase chain reaction (RT-PCR) for the detection of micrometastatic cells in peripheral blood or bone marrow of tumour patients has been used as a highly sensitive test for the amplification of tumour-specific genes in patients with neuroblastoma (Naito et al. 1991; Mattano, Jr. et al. 1992), breast cancer (Datta et al. 1994), prostate cancer (Moreno et al. 1992; Seiden et al. 1994), hepatocarcinoma (Matsumura et al. 1995; Hillaire et al. 1994), gastrointestinal tumour (Gerhard et al. 1994), and malignant melanoma (Buzaid, Balch 1996). Using this method, a sensitivity of one tumour cell in 10^6 to 10^7 blood cells was achieved in blood spiking experiments in several tumour systems (Ghossein, Rosai 1996). Using RT-PCR, the detection of metastasising cells in peripheral blood of tumour patients may facilitate the identification of patients at increased risk of recurrence.

For the detection of tumour cells in peripheral blood of melanoma patients, a number of groups have used the RT-PCR for tyrosinase, a key enzyme of melanin biosynthesis. The tyrosinase gene is actively expressed only in melanocytes and melanoma cells (Kwon et al. 1987) and, since melanocytes cannot be detected in the systemic circulation, the detection of tyrosinase mRNA indicates the presence of melanoma cells. However, the results of different research groups using RT-PCR for tyrosinase varied considerably, most likely due to different sample processing and RT-PCR protocols used (Battayani et al. 1995; Brossart et al. 1994, 1993, 1995; Curry et al. 1996; Foss et al. 1995; Hoon et al. 1995; Mellado et al. 1996; Smith et al. 1991; Kunter et al. 1997; Glaser et al. 1997; Jung et al. 1997; Reinhold et al. 1997; Farthmann et al. 1998; Curry et al. 1998; Muhlbauer et al. 1999; Pittman et al. 1996; de Vries et al. 1999; Mellado et al. 1999; Palmieri et al. 1999; Waldmann et al. 1999; Schittek et al. 1999a; Alao et al. 1999; Berking, Schlupen 1999). Therefore, a main goal is to provide a standardised RT-PCR protocol and increase the sensitivity of the assay without producing false positive results. In this report we summarise the results of the different research groups using RT-PCR from peripheral blood and discuss factors which influence the sensitivity of the assay.

Influence of the RT-PCR Protocol on the Sensitivity of Melanoma Cell Detection

For the detection of a limited number of circulating tumour cells in the blood of melanoma patients, a highly sensitive standardised and reproducible method is required. Most research groups using RT-PCR for the detection of melanoma cells in peripheral blood used different experimental conditions for blood purification, RNA extraction, or PCR analysis (Table 1). This might account for most of the heterogeneity in the results of these research groups.

Table 1. The different protocols used for tyrosinase RT-PCR

Reference	Blood amount	Blood preparation	RNA amount	cDNA primer	PCR amount	PCR cycles
Smith et al. 1991	2–10 ml EDTA	Total	?	Tyr	1/2	2′30
Brossart et al. 1993, 1994, 1995	10 ml heparin	Total	1 μg	Hexamer	1/10	2′30
Foss et al. 1995	2–3 ml EDTA	Total	6–12 μg	10-mer	1/3	1) 35; 2) 25
Battayani et al. 1995	15–25 ml	Ficoll	2 μg	Oligo-dT	1/80	2′30
Hoon et al. 1995	15 ml EDTA	Ficoll	3 μg	Oligo-dT	All	2′40
Mellado et al. 1996	15–20 ml EDTA	Ficoll	1 μg	Tyr	1/2	2′30
Kunter et al. 1996	? ml heparin	Total	?	Tyr	1/2	2′30
Reinhold et al. 1997	10 ml heparin	Ficoll	All	Oligo-dT	1/2	2′35
Gläser et al. 1997	9 ml EDTA	Lysis	1–5 μg	Oligo-dT	1/25–1.25 μg	1) 20; 2) 35
Jung et al. 1997	20 ml EDTA	Ficoll and total	1 μg	Hexamer	1/4	1) 35; 2) 30
Farthmann et al. 1998	10 ml EDTA	Lysis	1 μg	Hexamer	1/4	1) 35; 2) 29
Curry et al. 1998	10 ml heparin	Total	2–8 μg	Oligo-dT	1/6	2′40
Ghossein et al. 1998	10–15 ml EDTA	Ficoll	800 ng	Tyrosinase	All	1) 33; 2) 30
De Vries et al. 1999	5 ml citrate	Vacutainer (BD)	2 μg	Hexamer	1/4	1) 60; 2) 30
Palmieri et al. 1999	5 ml EDTA	Ficoll	1 μg	Hexamer	1/2	2′30
Waldmann et al. 1999	10 ml heparin	Ficoll	1 μg	Hexamer	1/12	2′30
Schittek et al. 1999	10 ml EDTA	Ficoll	3 μg	Hexamer	1/10	2′35
Berking et al. 1999	10 ml heparin or 3 ml EDTA	Total	2.5 μg	Hexamer	1/10	1) 30; 2) 40
Alao et al. 1999	10 ml heparin	Histopaque	10–40 μg	Hexamer	1/8	2′30

EDTA, ethylenediaminetetraacetate.

We analysed the influence of different parameters of sample processing on the sensitivity of the tyrosinase RT-PCR using peripheral blood spiked with defined numbers of SKMEL28 melanoma cells. Purification of the mononuclear cell fraction with a Ficoll gradient with a density of 1.077 g/ml prior to RNA isolation resulted in the highest sensitivity. Increasing the density of the gradient to 1.090 g/ml or extracting the RNA from whole blood or from erythrocyte-lysed blood resulted in loss of most of the melanoma cells (Schittek et al. 1999b). These data are in agreement with a study by Jung et al. (1997) which showed that processing blood with a density gradient method before RNA isolation results in higher sensitivity than by extracting RNA from whole-blood cells (Jung et al. 1997). Whereas Gläser et al. (1997) observed no differences in detection levels of tyrosinase RT-PCR of blood samples prepared by either erythrocyte lysis or Ficoll gradient separation, the sensitivity of whole blood preparation was also lower compared to the other methods (Glaser et al. 1997).

Not only the method of blood preparation but also the RNA isolation method and the kind of RT enzyme used had a significant effect on the sensitivity and reproducibility of tyrosinase detection, whereas variations in the PCR conditions had only a minor influence (Schittek et al. 1999b). Nevertheless, we found that in 20% of the samples with 20 SKMEL28 cells and 40% of the blood samples with 2 SKMEL28 cells, tyrosinase transcripts were still not detected. This might be due to several factors which influence the detection of melanoma cell transcripts: (a) not all melanoma cells can be recovered from the gradient, (b) the SKMEL28 cells express different levels of tyrosinase, (c) RNA is lost during the preparation, and (d) the RT reaction is not efficient enough to detect all transcripts. The efficiency of the RT-reaction may be indeed the rate-limiting step - depending on the enzyme used for reverse transcription, only high abundant messages (GAPDH) or transcripts from only a few cells in the sample (tyrosinase) can be detected (Schittek et al. 1999b).

Markers for Melanoma Cell Detection in Peripheral Blood

The use of multiple markers might improve the sensitivity of the RT-PCR (Hoon et al. 1995; Palmieri et al. 1999). Genes like MelanA/MART-1, gp100/pMEL17, TRP-1, and TRP-2 were found to be expressed specifically in cells of melanocytic origin, and the tumour progression markers MUC18 and MAGE-3 were shown to be expressed by melanoma cells (Coulie et al. 1994; Gaugler et al. 1994; Jimbow et al. 1994a; Jimbow et al. 1994b; Kawakami et al. 1994; Luca et al. 1993; Shih et al. 1994; Van den Eynde et al. 1995).

In our study, amplification of MelanA in addition to tyrosinase enhanced sensitivity of melanoma cell detection, whereas gp100/pMel17 and MUC18 gene products were already detected in blood from nonmelanoma patients (Schittek et al. 1999b). MAGE-3 was not analysed, since approximately 30% of melanomas do not express this gene; it seems to be expressed only in low amounts in the tumour cells and the level of detection is likely to be very low (Hoon et al. 1995).

MelanA/MART-1 is specifically expressed in melanocytes, melanoma cells, melanoma tumours, and in the retina (Chen et al. 1996; Coulie et al. 1994; Kawakami et al. 1994; Kawakami et al. 1997). The majority of melanoma tumours and cell lines analysed express this gene. In other tumours or tissues, MelanA/MART-1 expression was not detected (Coulie et al. 1994; Kawakami et al. 1994; Kawakami et al. 1997). Amplification of MelanA in addition to tyrosinase for the detection of melanoma cells in peripheral blood has also recently been used in three other studies and was shown to increase sensitivity (Curry et al. 1998; Palmieri et al. 1999; de Vries et al. 1999).

GP100/pMEL17 and MUC18 transcripts are already detectable in blood samples from most healthy individuals (Schittek et al. 1999b). GP100 and pMEL17 are encoded by a single gene and generated by alternative splicing (Adema et al. 1994). This gene encodes a melanosomal matrix protein involved in melanogenesis and expressed preferentially in pigment cells (Kwon et al. 1987; Adema et al. 1994). However, recent evidence suggests that posttranscriptional mechanisms regulate the restricted protein expression in melanocytic cells, since the mRNA for this gene is found in many different cell types analysed (Brouwenstijn et al. 1997). Therefore, RT-PCR for gp100 is nonspecific and unsuitable for detecting melanoma cells in peripheral blood.

The MUC18 protein, a member of the immunoglobulin superfamily and related to several adhesion molecules, shows an expression pattern in human malignant melanoma which is closely associated with tumour progression and the onset of metastasis (Luca et al. 1993). The MUC18 protein is present not only on melanoma cells but also on the endothelia of blood vessels penetrating primary and metastatic melanomas and on activated T cells (Sers et al. 1994; Pickl et al. 1997). Therefore, it is not surprising that in most peripheral blood samples from healthy donors we detect mRNA for MUC18, demonstrating that RT-PCR for MUC18 is also nonspecific and unsuitable for the detection of melanoma micrometastasis. A high number of false positives in the RT-PCR for MUC18 was also reported recently (Palmieri et al. 1999). However, Hoon et al. (1995) found MUC18 transcripts in only two out of 39 analysed blood samples from healthy individuals.

The p97 gene encodes a glycoprotein that is a tumour-associated antigen on melanoma referred to as melanotransferrin. Palmieri et al. (1999) showed that a multimarker RT-PCR assay including MelanA and p97 improves the sensitivity of detection of metastatic melanoma cells (Palmieri et al. 1999). In two studies, p97 was not detected by RT-PCR in the blood of healthy controls (Hoon et al. 1995; Palmieri et al. 1999). However, Curry et al. (1998) did detect mRNA for p97 in peripheral blood of healthy control subjects (Curry et al. 1998). Therefore, it is unclear whether p97, in addition to tyrosinase and MelanA, is a suitable candidate for a multimarker RT-PCR.

Factors That May Influence the Sensitivity of Melanoma Cell Detection in Peripheral Blood

Why do the results of the different research groups performing RT-PCR for tyrosinase differ so much? We analysed 340 peripheral blood samples from 225 patients in different clinical stages for the presence of tyrosinase and MelanA/MART1 mRNA (Table 2) and found that the following parameters influence detection levels of melanoma cell transcripts: the numbers of specific genes amplified, blood samples analysed, and PCR analyses performed:

A. Since tumour cells tend to lose parts of their chromosomes, it may be that the gene of interest, e.g., tyrosinase, is not expressed by the tumour cells and cannot be amplified. Therefore, the use of multiple markers might improve the sensitivity of the RT-PCR (Hoon et al. 1995; Curry et al. 1998; Palmieri et al. 1999). We were able to demonstrate that the additional analysis of MelanA increased the sensitivity of melanoma cell detection in the circulation by 30% (Table 2) (Schittek et al. 1999a).

B. Melanoma cells are not continuously present in the circulation and presumably are shed intermittently from tumours (Reinhold et al. 1997).

Table 2. RT-PCR results and stage of disease

	Total number	Stage I	Stage II	Stage III	Stage IV
Blood samples	340	78	48	80	134
Patients	225	74	45	48	58
Tyrosinase+patients	50	13	8	8	21
MelanA+patients	38	5	6	7	20
Tyrosinase or MelanA+patients (evaluation of first blood sample per patient)	59 (26%)	12 (16%)	14 (30%)	10 (22%)	23 (40%)
Tyrosinase or MelanA+patients (evaluation of all blood samples per patient)	72 (32%)	14 (19%)	14 (31%)	14 (29%)	30 (52%)

Therefore, the chance of detecting tumour cells in the sample depend on the blood volume and the number of samples analysed per patient. In the majority of RT-PCR-positive patients in stages III and IV, we found that the first blood sample was already positive for tyrosinase and MelanA transcripts. However, the additional analysis of a second or more blood samples increases the chance of detecting melanoma cells in peripheral blood. Recently it was shown that the analysis of a second blood sample per patient increases detection rates of tyrosinase mRNA by 25% (Farthmann et al. 1998).

C. In some cases, only a few tyrosinase or MelanA transcripts might be present in the samples, which implies that the chance of detection should increase when more PCR analyses are performed per sample and primer pair. We showed that in 30–40% of our positive samples, tyrosinase or MelanA was detected only in the second or third PCR performed. Only a few patients are reproducibly positive in the RT-PCR for tyrosinase and MelanA (27 of 72 patients, or 38%) (Schittek et al. 1999a). Similar findings were also shown by Farthmann et al. (1998). Furthermore, de Vries et al. (1999) demonstrated a low reproducibility of tyrosinase and MelanA RT-PCR and concluded in repeated assays for the detection of circulating melanoma cells that it is not caused by differences in mRNA quality between the samples but by low numbers of amplifiable target mRNA molecules (de Vries et al. 1999).

Despite these major factors influencing sensitivity, RNA degradation may be responsible for negative findings in an unknown percentage of examinations, since RNA is very unstable in the extracellular environment and a rapid processing of samples is necessary. In addition, the type of blood sample preparation (i.e., gradient separation or erythrocyte lysis) has an influence on the quality of the RNA and recovery of the tumour cells (Schittek et al. 1999b).

Furthermore, excessive sensitivity or an amplification of genes nonspecific for the tumour cells often leads to an overestimation of the number of patients with circulating tumour cells. This has been described for the carcinoembryonic antigen (CEA) gene in colorectal cancer patients (Zippelius et al. 1997). We showed that two other genes expressed by melanoma cells and already used in melanoma cell diagnostics - gp100 and MUC18 - are not specific for this cell type. Especially for gp100, it was recently shown that small amounts of transcripts can be detected by RT-PCR in cell types other than melanoma cells, whereas the expression of the protein is restricted to melanoma cells (Brouwenstijn et al. 1997). Furthermore, the extreme sensitivity confers an inherent tendency to produce false positive results if sufficient precautions are not taken to prevent contamination of samples. This could also result in the percentage of RT-PCR-positive patients being exaggerated, since it is the most likely reason for the 100% detection level in the studies by Brossart et al. (1993, 1995).

Clinical Impact of the RT-PCR in Peripheral Blood

Most research groups performing RT-PCR for tyrosinase found either no or very low numbers of patients in early stages of the disease with a positive RT-PCR result and only between 21% and 38% of tyrosinase- or tyrosinase/MelanA-positive patients in patients with disseminated metastases (Table 3) (Glaser et al. 1997; Buzaid, Balch 1996; Reinhold et al. 1997). The authors concluded that the RT-PCR may be unsuited to detecting micrometastatic cells in peripheral blood due to its low sensitivity. On the other hand, four groups have already described the prognostic significance of the RT-PCR in melanoma patients. In a study by Kunter et al. (1996), only 28% of melanoma patients in stage IV were positive for tyrosinase; however, those patients had more rapid tumour progressions and poorer clinical outcomes compared to tyrosinase-negative patients (Kunter et al. 1997).

Ghossein et al. (1998) showed by multivariate analyses that the blood RT-PCR for tyrosinase mRNA is an independent predictor of survival in stage II–III (Ghossein et al. 1998). In a study by Mellado et al. (1996), tyrosinase expression was an independent prognostic factor for recurrence and could be detected in 23% of stage I, 45% of stage II, 40% of stage III, and 94% of stage IV patients (Mellado et al. 1996). These detection rates are similar to ours for stages I, II, and III (Table 2) but are higher than ours for stage IV patients, with 52% tyrosinase- or MelanA-positive patients. Interestingly, a decrease in the percentage of tyrosinase-positive stage III patients was observed, similar to our study. In a recent report, this group assessed the prognostic significance of the detection of circulating melanoma cells by tyrosinase RT-PCR in long-term clinically disease-free melanoma patients. They could show that the presence of late circulating melanoma cells in this group of patients was significantly associated with a subsequent high risk of relapse and death (Mellado et al. 1999). In a study by Battayani et al. (1995), tyrosinase detection in peripheral blood was also a marker of rapid disease progression: 50% of patients with visceral metastases were tyrosinase-positive and had more rapid disease progression (Battayani et al. 1995). In stage I pa-

Table 3. Studies using tyrosinase RT-PCR for the detection of tumour cells in peripheral blood of patients with cutaneous melanoma

Reference	Markers	RT-PCR-positive patients (AJCC stage)			
		Stage I	Stage II	Stage III	Stage IV
Smith et al. 1991	Tyrosinase	–	–	–	4/7 (57%)
Brossart et al. 1993	Tyrosinase	0/4	1/6 (17%)	6/17 (35%)	29/29 (100%)
Brossart et al. 1994	Tyrosinase	–	–	4/4 (100%)	24/24 (100%)
Brossart et al. 1995	Tyrosinase	–	–	–	50/50 (100%)
Foss et al. 1995	Tyrosinase	–	–	–	0/6
Battayani et al. 1995	Tyrosinase	2/10 (20%) (I+II)		22/51 (43%)	16/32 (50%)
Hoon et al. 1995	Tyrosinase, p97, MAGE3, MUC18	3/6 (50%)	10/11 (96%)	31/36 (86%)	63/66 (94%)
Mellado et al. 1996	Tyrosinase	4/17 (24%)	10/22 (45%)	7/17 (40%)	33/35 (94%)
Kunter et al. 1996	Tyrosinase	0/16 (I+II)		0/16	9/32 (28%)
Pittmann et al. 1996	Tyrosinase	–	–	–	3/24 (13%)
Reinhold et al. 1997	Tyrosinase	0/31 (I+II)		1/21 (5%)	5/13 (38%)
Gläser et al. 1997	Tyrosinase	1/43 (2%) (I+II)		0/15	12/44 (27%)
Jung et al. 1997	Tyrosinase	–	–	–	13/50 (26%)
Farthmann et al. 1998	Tyrosinase	6/46 (13%) (I+II)		7/41 (17%)	16/36 (44%)
Ghossein et al. 1998	Tyrosinase	–	2/16 (13%)	6/40 (15%)	1/17 (6%)
Curry et al. 1998	Tyrosinase, MelanA	1/5 (20%)	27/41 (66%)	58/77 (75%)	–
De Vries et al. 1999	Tyrosinase, MelanA	2/5 (40%)	0/1	8/27 (30%)	33/73 (45%)
Mellado et al. 1999	Tyrosinase	2/11 (18%) (I+II)		6/33 (19%)	2/13 (15%)
Palmieri et al. 1999	Tyrosinase, p97, MUC18, MelanA	20/87 (23%)	24/67 (36%)	27/49 (55%)	28/32 (87%)
Waldmann et al. 1999	Tyrosinase	–	–	–	7/20 (35%)
Schittek et al. 1999	Tyrosinase, MelanA	14/74 (19%)	14/45 (31%)	14/48 (29%)	30/58 (52%)
Berking et al. 1999	Tyrosinase, p97, MAGE-3, MelanA, gp100	1/8 (13%) (I+II)		5/21 (24%)	18/48 (38%)
Alao et al. 1999	Tyrosinase	–	–	1/4 (25%)	5/17 (29%)

tients, 20% were RT-PCR-positive and, in stages II and III, 40%, which is very similar to our results and those of Mellado et al. (1996).

Using RT-PCR for various markers (tyrosinase, p97, MUC18, and MelanA), Palmieri et al. (1999) demonstrated that each mRNA marker was significantly associated with disease stage. Each single marker and also the presence of all four PCR-positive markers remained statistically independent prognostic factors for tumour progression (Palmieri et al. 1999). In our study, a positive RT-PCR result was significantly associated with clinical stage ($\chi^2 = 16.8$, $p < 0.001$). Concerning tumour type, patients with ALM and LMM melanomas were more often RT-PCR-positive than those with type NM or SSM melanomas ($p < 0.009$).

Strikingly, PCR-positive patients showed significantly higher tumour thickness than PCR-negative patients (median 1.3 mm versus 2.4 mm). Most importantly, we could show that a positive PCR result correlated with tumour progression but that negative PCR results do not exclude further metastasis, especially in stage III (Schittek et al. 1999a). This implies that, in our patient group, a longer follow-up period is needed to analyse definitively the clinical impact of the RT-PCR, especially in earlier stages of the disease.

Conclusions

Several studies have demonstrated a statistically significant association between clinical stage of malignant melanoma and detection by RT-PCR of tumour-associated antigens in peripheral blood. The limited number of cases in most of the previous studies and the different methodologic approaches to sample preparation might be responsible for the contrasting results on the reliability of the RT-PCR assay to test tumour progression in malignant melanoma patients. Furthermore, tumour cells seem to be shed intermittently in the circulation, which will lead to sampling errors, as only a few millilitres of blood are analysed at any given time. In addition, the influence of PCR analysis protocol has to be analysed in more detail, i.e., concerning optimal blood volume and number of blood samples analysed, number of PCR analyses performed, and the correlation of these experimental conditions to the clinical outcome. The very high rate of PCR-positive patients in advanced melanoma reported in some studies could be explained in part by unrecognised contamination leading to false positive results. The development of more specific multiple-marker PCR assays would increase the sensitivity of this technique by overcoming the problem of tumour cell heterogeneity. Assessment of a subset of patients with a higher risk of recurrence needs longer follow-up and further studies to define the role of RT-PCR in monitoring malignant melanoma patients. Currently, increasing sensitivity for detection of circulating tumour cells to more than 50% of patients with disseminated melanoma seems to be unlikely. It is interesting that between 15% and 30% positive results have been obtained from patients with primary melanoma. So far, in melanoma patients with no detectable metastases (stages I, II), the significance of a positive RT-PCR result is not evident at the moment. Our presently limited experience shows that staging examinations in these patients revealed no proof of macrometastasis. Therefore, it is presently unclear as to whether these positive findings are related to long-term prognosis or if they merely reflect the rate of false positive findings in the highly sensitive RT-PCR technique. Further studies are necessary to define better the significance of the presence of these circulating antigens in tumour progression, early detection of relapse, and monitoring the effectiveness of systemic therapy in patients with melanoma.

ACKNOWLEDGEMENTS. This work was supported by a grant from the Deutsche Forschungsgemeinschaft (GA 446/2-1).

References

Adema GJ, de Boer AJ, Vogel AM, Loenen WA, Figdor CG (1994) Molecular characterization of the melanocyte lineage-specific antigen gp100. J Biol Chem 269:20126–20133

Alao JP, Mohammed MQ, Slade MJ, Retsas S (1999) Detection of tyrosinase mRNA by RT-PCR in the peripheral blood of patients with advanced metastatic melanoma. Melanoma Res 9:395–399

Battayani Z, Grob JJ, Xerri L, Noe C, Zarour H, Houvaeneghel G, Delpero JR, Birmbaum D, Hassoun J, Bonerandi JJ (1995) Polymerase chain reaction detection of circulating melanocytes as a prognostic marker in patients with melanoma. Arch Dermatol 131:443–447

Berking C, Schlupen EM, Schrader A, Atzpodien J, Volkenandt M (1999) Tumour markers in peripheral blood of patients with malignant melanoma: multimarker RT-PCR versus a luminometric assay for S-100. Arch Dermatol Res 291:479–484

Brossart P, Keilholz U, Scheibenbogen C, Mohler T, Willhauck M, Hunstein W (1994) Detection of residual tumour cells in patients with malignant melanoma responding to immunotherapy. J Immunother 15:38–41

Brossart P, Keilholz U, Willhauck M, Scheibenbogen C, Mohler T, Hunstein W (1993) Hematogenous spread of malignant melanoma cells in different stages of disease. J Invest Dermatol 101:887–889

Brossart P, Schmier JW, Kruger S, Willhauck M, Scheibenbogen C, Mohler T, Keilholz U (1995) A polymerase chain reaction-based semiquantitative assessment of malignant melanoma cells in peripheral blood. Cancer Res 55:4065–4068

Brouwenstijn N, Slager EH, Bakker ABH, Schreurs MWJ, VanderSpek CW, Adema GJ, Schrier PI, Figdor CG (1997) Transcription of the gene encoding melanoma-associated antigen gp100 in tissues and cell lines other than those of the melanocytic lineage. Brit J Cancer 76:1562–1566

Buzaid AC, Balch CM (1996) Polymerase chain reaction for detection of melanoma in peripheral blood: too early to assess clinical value. J Natl Cancer Inst 88:569–570

Chen YT, Stockert E, Jungbluth A, Tsang S, Coplan KA, Scanlan MJ, Old LJ (1996) Serological analysis of Melan-A(MART-1), a melanocyte-specific protein homogeneously expressed in human melanomas. Proc Natl Acad Sci USA 93:5915–5919

Coulie PG, Brichard V, Van Pel A, Wolfel T, Schneider J, Traversari C, Mattei S, De Plaen E, Lurquin C, Szikora JP et al (1994) A new gene coding for a differentiation antigen recognized by autologous cytolytic T lymphocytes on HLA-A2 melanomas. J Exp Med 180: 35–42

Curry BJ, Myers K, Hersey P (1998) Polymerase chain reaction detection of melanoma cells in the circulation: relation to clinical stage, surgical treatment, and recurrence from melanoma. J Clin Oncol 16:1760–1769

Curry BJ, Smith MJ, Hersey P (1996) Detection and quantitation of melanoma cells in the circulation of patients. Melanoma Res 6:45–54

Datta YH, Adams PT, Drobyski WR, Ethier SP, Terry VH, Roth MS (1994) Sensitive detection of occult breast cancer by the reverse-transcriptase polymerase chain reaction. J Clin Oncol 12:475–482

De-Vries TJ, Fourkour A, Punt CJA, van-de-Locht LTF, Wobbes T, van-den-Bosch S, de-Rooij MJM, Mensink EJBM, Ruiter DJ, and van-Muijen GNP (1999) Reproducibility of detection of tyrosinase and MART-1 transcripts in the peripheral blood of melanoma patients: a quality control study using real-time quantitative RT-PCR Brit J Cancer 80: 883–891

Farthmann B, Eberle J, Krasagakis K, Gstottner M, Wang NP, Bisson S, Orfanos CE (1998) RT-PCR for tyrosinase-mRNA-positive cells in peripheral blood: Evaluation strategy and correlation with known prognostic markers in 123 melanoma patients. J Invest Dermatol 110:263–267

Foss AJ, Guille MJ, Occleston NL, Hykin PG, Hungerford JL, Lightman S (1995) The detection of melanoma cells in peripheral blood by reverse transcription-polymerase chain reaction. Brit J Cancer 72:155–159

Gaugler B, Van den Eynde B, van der Bruggen P, Romero P, Gaforio JJ, De Plaen E, Lethe B, Brasseur F, Boon T (1994) Human gene MAGE-3 codes for an antigen recognized on a melanoma by autologous cytolytic T lymphocytes. J Exp Med 179:921–930

Gerhard M, Juhl H, Kalthoff H, Schreiber HW, Wagener C, Neumaier M (1994) Specific detection of carcinoembryonic antigen-expressing tumour cells in bone marrow aspirates by polymerase chain reaction. J Clin Oncol 12:725–729

Ghossein RA, Coit D, Brennan M, Zhang ZF, Wang Y, Bhattacharya S, Houghton A, Rosai J (1998) Prognostic significance of peripheral blood and bone marrow tyrosinase messenger RNA in malignant melanoma. Clin Cancer Res 4:419–428

Ghossein RA, Rosai J (1996) Polymerase chain reaction in the detection of micrometastases and circulating tumour cells. Cancer 78:10–16

Glaser R, Rass K, Seiter S, Hauschild A, Christophers E, Tilgen W (1997) Detection of circulating melanoma cells by specific amplification of tyrosinase complementary DNA is not a reliable tumour marker in melanoma patients: A clinical two-center study. J Clin Oncol 15:2818–2825

Hillaire S, Barbu V, Boucher E, Moukhtar M, Poupon R (1994) Albumin messenger RNA as a marker of circulating hepatocytes in hepatocellular carcinoma. Gastroenterology 106:239–242

Hoon DS, Wang Y, Dale PS, Conrad AJ, Schmid P, Garrison D, Kuo C, Foshag LJ, Nizze AJ, Morton DL (1995) Detection of occult melanoma cells in blood with a multiple-marker polymerase chain reaction assay. J Clin Oncol 13:2109–2116

Jimbow K, Hara H, Vinayagamoorthy T, Luo D, Dakour J, Yamada K, Dixon W, Chen H (1994a) Molecular control of melanogenesis in malignant melanoma: functional assessment of tyrosinase and lamp gene families by UV exposure and gene co-transfection, and cloning of a cDNA encoding calnexin, a possible melanogenesis "chaperone". J Dermatol 21:894–906

Jimbow K, Luo D, Chen H, Hara H, Lee MH (1994b) Coordinated mRNA and protein expression of human LAMP-1 in induction of melanogenesis after UV-B exposure and co-transfection of human tyrosinase and TRP-1 cDNAs. Pigment Cell Res 7:311–319

Jung FA, Buzaid AC, Ross MI, Woods KV, Lee JJ, Albitar M, Grimm EA (1997) Evaluation of tyrosinase mRNA as a tumour marker in the blood of melanoma patients. J Clin Oncol 15:2826–2831

Kawakami Y, Battles JK, Kobayashi T, Ennis W, Wang X, Tupesis JP, Marincola FM, Robbins PF, Hearing VJ, Gonda MA, Rosenberg SA (1997) Production of recombinant MART-1 proteins and specific antiMART-1 polyclonal and monoclonal antibodies: use in the characterization of the human melanoma antigen MART-1. J Immunol Methods 202:13–25

Kawakami Y, Eliyahu S, Delgado CH, Robbins PF, Rivoltini L, Topalian SL, Miki T, Rosenberg SA (1994) Cloning of the gene coding for a shared human melanoma antigen recognized by autologous T cells infiltrating into tumour. Proc Natl Acad Sci USA 91:3515–3519

Kunter U, Buer J, Probst M, Duensing S, Dallmann I, Grosse J, Kirchner H, Schluepen EM, Volkenandt M, Ganser A, Atzpodien J (1997) Peripheral Blood Tyrosinase Messenger RNA Detection and Survival in Malignant Melanoma. J Nat Cancer Inst 88:590–594

Kwon BS, Haq AK, Pomerantz SH, Halaban R (1987) Isolation and sequence of a cDNA clone for human tyrosinase that maps at the mouse c-albino locus [published erratum appears in Proc Natl Acad Sci USA 1988 Sep; 85(17):6352]. Proc Natl Acad Sci USA 84:7473–7477

Luca M, Hunt B, Bucana CD, Johnson JP, Fidler IJ, Bar Eli M (1993) Direct correlation between MUC18 expression and metastatic potential of human melanoma cells. Melanoma Res 3:35–41

Matsumura M, Niwa Y, Hikiba Y, Okano K, Kato N, Shiina S, Shiratori Y, Omata M (1995) Sensitive assay for detection of hepatocellular carcinoma associated gene transcription (alpha-fetoprotein mRNA) in blood. Biochem Biophys Res Commun 207:813–818

Mattano LA Jr, Moss TJ, Emerson SG (1992) Sensitive detection of rare circulating neuroblastoma cells by the reverse transcriptase-polymerase chain reaction. Cancer Res 52:4701–4705

Mellado B, Colomer D, Castel T, Munoz M, Carballo E, Galan M, Mascaro JM, Vives Corrons JL, Grau JJ, Estape J (1996) Detection of circulating neoplastic cells by reverse-transcriptase polymerase chain reaction in malignant melanoma: association with clinical stage and prognosis. J Clin Oncol 14:2091–2097

Mellado B, Gutierrez L, Castel T, Colomer D, Fontanillas M, Castro J, Estape J (1999) Prognostic significance of the detection of circulating malignant cells by reverse transcriptase-polymerase chain reaction in long-term clinically disease-free melanoma patients. Clin Cancer Res 5:1843–1848

Moreno JG, Croce CM, Fischer R, Monne M, Vihko P, Mulholland SG, Gomella LG (1992) Detection of hematogenous micrometastasis in patients with prostate cancer. Cancer Res 52:6110–6112

Muhlbauer M, Langenbach N, Stolz W, Hein R, Landthaler M, Buettner R, Bosserhoff AK (1999) Detection of melanoma cells in the blood of melanoma patients by melanoma-inhibitory activity (MIA) reverse transcription-PCR Clin Cancer Res 5:1099–1105

Naito H, Kuzumaki N, Uchino J, Kobayashi R, Shikano T, Ishikawa Y, Matsumoto S (1991) Detection of tyrosine hydroxylase mRNA and minimal neuroblastoma cells by the reverse transcription-polymerase chain reaction. Eur J Cancer 27:762–765

Palmieri G, Strazzullo M, Ascierto PA, Satriano SMR, Daponte A, Castello G (1999) Polymerase chain reaction-based detection of circulating melanoma cells as an effective marker of tumour progression. J Clin Oncol 17:304–311

Pickl WF, Majdic O, Fischer GF, Petzelbauer P, Fae I, Waclavicek M, Stöckl J, Scheinecker C, Vidicki T, Aschauer H, Johnson JP, Knapp W (1997) MUC18/MCAM (CD146), and activation antigen of human T lymphocytes. J Immunol 158:2107–2115

Pittman K, Burchill S, Smith B, Southgate J, Joffe J, Gore M, Selby P (1996) Reverse transcriptase-polymerase chain reaction for expression of tyrosinase to identify malignant melanoma cells in peripheral blood. Ann Oncol 7:297–301

Reinhold U, LudtkeHandjery HC, Schnautz S, Kreysel HW, Abken H (1997) The analysis of tyrosinase-specific mRNA in blood samples of melanoma patients by RT-PCR is not a useful test for metastatic tumour progression. J Invest Dermatol 108:166–169

Schittek B, Blaheta HJ, Florchinger G, Sauer B, Garbe C (1999b) Increased sensitivity for the detection of malignant melanoma cells in peripheral blood using an improved protocol for reverse transcription-polymerase chain reaction. Brit J Dermatol 141:37–43

Schittek B, Bodingbauer Y, Ellwanger U, Blaheta HJ, Garbe C (1999a) Amplification of MelanA messenger RNA in addition to tyrosinase increases sensitivity of melanoma cell detection in peripheral blood and is associated with the clinical stage and prognosis of malignant melanoma. Brit J Dermatol 141:30–36

Seiden MV, Kantoff PW, Krithivas K, Propert K, Bryant M, Haltom E, Gaynes L, Kaplan I, Bubley G, DeWolf W et al (1994) Detection of circulating tumour cells in men with localized prostate cancer. J Clin Oncol 12:2634–2639

Sers C, Riethmüller G, Johnson JP (1994) MUC18, a melanoma-progression associated molecule, and its potential role in tumour vascularization and hematogenous spread. Cancer Res 54:5689–5694

Shih IM, Elder DE, Hsu MY, Herlyn M (1994) Regulation of Mel-CAM/MUC18 expression on melanocytes of different stages of tumour progression by normal keratinocytes. Am J Pathol 145:837–845

Smith B, Selby P, Southgate J, Pittman K, Bradley C, Blair GE (1991) Detection of melanoma cells in peripheral blood by means of reverse transcriptase and polymerase chain reaction. Lancet 338:1227–1229

Van den Eynde B, Peeters O, De Backer O, Gaugler B, Lucas S, Boon T (1995) A new family of genes coding for an antigen recognized by autologous cytolytic T lymphocytes on a human melanoma. J Exp Med 182:689–698

Waldmann V, Deichmann M, Bock M, Jackel A, Naher H (1999) The detection of tyrosinase-specific mRNA in bone marrow is not more sensitive than in blood for the demonstration of micrometastatic melanoma. Brit J Dermatol 140:1060–1064

Zippelius A, Kufer P, Honold G, Kollermann MW, Oberneder R, Schlimok G, Riethmüller G, Pantel,K (1997) Limitations of reverse-transcriptase polymerase chain reaction analyses for detection of micrometastatic epithelial cancer cells in bone marrow. J Clin Oncol 15:2701–2708

Facts and Pitfalls in the Detection of Tyrosinase mRNA in the Blood of Melanoma Patients by RT-PCR

S. Seiter, G. Rappl, W. Tilgen, S. Ugurel, and U. Reinhold

Department of Dermatology, The Saarland University Hospital, 66421 Homburg/Saar, Germany

Abstract

Reverse transcription (RT) of tyrosinase mRNA and specific cDNA amplification to facilitate the early detection of circulating tumor cells in melanoma patients have been reported. The significance and practical value of these procedures for the diagnosis of tumor dissemination in melanoma patients is, however, still unclear. We analyzed peripheral blood samples of melanoma patients of different clinical stages for the presence of tyrosinase mRNA by reverse transcriptase polymerase chain reaction (RT-PCR). In addition to a nested RT-PCR-based system, we evaluated the new PCR enzyme-linked immunosorbent assay tyrosinase system for sensitivity and specificity in detecting circulating melanoma cells. Our results showed a high sensitivity and specificity for this system in detecting one melanoma cell in 1 ml of whole blood. Using different methods of detection, no tyrosinase mRNA was detectable in blood samples of patients with primary melanoma and regional lymph node metastases. In a small number of patients with visceral metastases (10–30%), we found tyrosinase mRNA-positive results. Analyses of different blood samples taken at 2-h intervals indicate that tumor cells persist only transiently in the peripheral blood. Successful establishment of melanoma cell growth from tyrosinase mRNA-positive samples indicates that viable tumor cells exist in melanoma patients' peripheral blood. Our results indicate a low amount of tyrosinase-specific transcripts in a small subset of stage IV patients and suggest that the analysis of tyrosinase mRNA in peripheral blood samples is not helpful as a prognostic marker or monitoring tool in melanoma patients.

Background

During the past two decades, the incidence of malignant melanoma has steadily increased. Although surgical treatment for localized melanoma is highly successful and new approaches have been tested, the available therapeutic options for patients with advanced disease have not resulted in improved survival. Therefore, early detection of disease progression resulting in early treatment may be an important factor in improving patient survival. At present, the clinical course of patients with melanoma is routinely monitored by physical examination, computerized tomography, magnetic resonance imaging, and radionuclide imaging. These modalities, although informative, do not detect micrometastases or circulating tumor cells posing a major risk of relapse. Ashworth first detected circulating tumor cells in the blood of patients in 1869, but only in 1934 did Pool and Dunlop make the first systematic attempts to demonstrate cancer cells in the blood of living patients, attributing their presence to a potential risk of metastasis formation. Based on the assumption that a growing tumor sheds viable tumor cells into the peripheral blood, it has been suggested that detection of circulating melanoma cells in the peripheral blood may function as a sensitive prognostic marker. Applying a molecular method in 1991, Smith et al. [1] demonstrated the presence of circulating tumor cells in the blood of melanoma patients. Using a nested reverse transcription polymerase chain reaction (RT-PCR) to detect tyrosinase mRNA, which is expressed in melanoma cells but not in normal peripheral blood cells, they could detect tyrosinase mRNA in the blood of three out of five melanoma patients. As this work suggested that tyrosinase mRNA might be useful as a marker in the early detection of micrometastases, numerous clinical centers started assays to test patients' blood for the presence of tyrosinase mRNA. Those efforts were further supported by a publication of Brossart et al. in 1993 [2]. Having tested a larger patient population in different stages of disease, they could demonstrate that all patients with stage IV melanoma had circulating tumor cells in their peripheral blood and 35% of the stage III patients were positive for tyrosinase mRNA. Furthermore, they also showed that 17% of the patients with stage II melanoma were positive for tyrosinase mRNA, suggesting that patients might have circulating tumor cells in their peripheral blood even in the early stages of disease. The "molecular marker" for melanoma seemed to be born. The second publication by Brossart et al. in 1994 [3] again demonstrated high numbers of patients positive for tyrosinase mRNA, particularly in stage IV patients.

Tyrosinase Testing Around the World, 1995–1999

Following the appearance of these publications, testing for tyrosinase mRNA was started in many centers around the world. However, in 1995, Foss et al. published a series of 42 stage IV patients, all of whom tested negative for tyrosinase mRNA [4]. Since 1995, more than 30 papers have been published on this topic (Table 1), with the numbers of patients testing positive for tyrosi-

Table 1. Publications on the detection of circulating melanoma cells by tyrosinase mRNA PCR

Year	No. of publications
1991	1
1993	2
1994	1
1995	4
1996	7
1998	6
1999	5
Total	33

nase mRNA varying greatly [1–20]. In stage IV melanoma, the percentage of positive patients varied from 0–100%. However, the vast majority of papers published demonstrated 20–30% positive patients in stage IV and 0–15% in stages I–III (Fig. 1). These publications resulted in extensive discussion on the validity and accuracy of the published data. Questions about specificity and sensitivity of the techniques used or contamination issues vary. Figure 1 shows the results of all papers on the use of tyrosinase mRNA detection in the peripheral blood of patients with melanoma using PCR. Looking at all published data, the question to answer first should be whether and, if so, in what percentage of patients in stage IV melanoma circulating tumor cells can be detected by performing molecular testing with RT-PCR for tyrosinase mRNA. The reason for answering this question first seems clear to most of us: if a patient with malignant melanoma presents with stage IV disease, in most cases he has lymphogenous and/or hematogenous metastatic spread, and if the data obtained by immunohistochemistry were valid, these patients should also have tumor cells in their peripheral blood. Assuming that the detection of tumor cells from peripheral blood works as well as demonstrated by Smith et al. in 1991 [1], one should be able to detect tyrosinase mRNA in the peripheral blood in a high percentage of patients. Spiking experiments performed by various groups demonstrated a sensitivity of one cell/1 ml of blood. However, with the exception of two groups, tyrosinase mRNA expression has been detected in only 0–44% of stage IV patients tested. In view of these discrepant data, many laboratories have stopped performing the test.

How Can We Explain the Conflicting Data?

For a number of years, PCR has been used in routine testing for various different clinical questions. Therefore, it is well-known that PCR methods can pose technical challenges to some laboratories, in particular concerning sensitivity and specificity. These major considerations are reflected by the vast number of papers published on the use of PCR and, in particular, on RT-PCR in routine testing. A major problem in PCR is the creation of false posi-

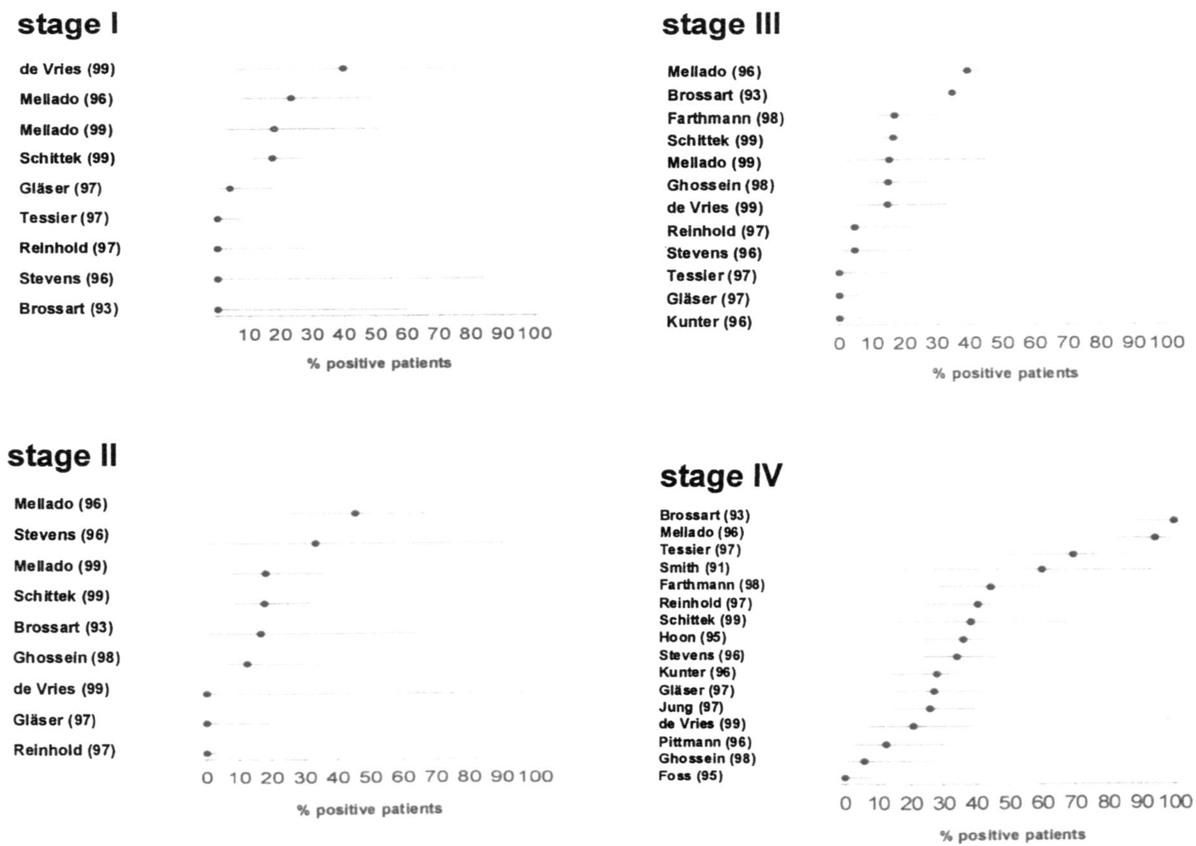

Fig. 1. Meta-analysis of different studies on the detection of tyrosinase mRNA in the peripheral blood of melanoma patients in different stages of disease performed by various laboratories since 1991. Stages are defined according to the American Joint Committee on Cancer (AJCC) system. *Dots* represent the percentage of patients tested positive for tyrosinase mRNA. *Lines* represent 95% confidence intervals

tive samples by contamination. Reading through the papers published on tyrosinase RT-PCR, we find the following statement by Foss et al. [4]: "We had significant technical problems with false positives which took 12 months to overcome." Therefore, the high percentages of positive samples detected in some laboratories may have to be carefully reanalyzed for the possibility of contamination.

Another serious problem limiting the general use of PCR-based techniques is the issue of false negative samples. Poor RNA quality could be one cause of false negative samples. However, as housekeeping gene controls are generally also run, poor quality RNA samples are easy to detect and can therefore be eliminated. Nonetheless, low numbers of amplifiable target mRNA as well as the absence of tyrosinase mRNA expression on melanoma cells or possible inhibition of reverse transcriptase activity by melanin could also account for false negative results. Taking into account the high sensitivity achieved when performing spiking experiments with, for example, SK-Mel-28 cells implies that in vivo testing might follow different rules. One possible explanation is that the cells circulating in a patient's blood are different from those used for sensitivity tests, and standard procedure with cultured cells might have changed over the years and therefore result in overexpression of tyrosinase or any other mRNA. Furthermore, the circulating tumor cells might lose the expression of certain antigens during metastatic progression, as demonstrated in several publications. These data would imply that our methods for detecting circulating tumor cells might not be sufficient to detect circulating tumor cells due to inadequate sensitivity. Another issue causing discrepant results may be the fact that the actual number of circulating tumor cells is below the sensitivity we can actually achieve by testing a defined volume of blood, usually 5 ml. We demonstrated that transiently circulating tumor cells in melanoma patients are capable of proliferating [17]. We cultured PBMC of melanoma patients and were able to establish growth of cells with melanocyte-like morphology in samples from two patients with visceral metastases which tested positive for tyrosinase mRNA using RT-PCR as well as for different melanoma-associated antigens using immunohistochemistry. These experiments further support the observation that circulating tumor cells really exist in patients and, furthermore, that they express well-known tumor cell markers. Moreover, the rare detection of melanoma cells may imply that tumor cells are also rare and possibly only transiently present in the blood of melanoma patients. Analysis of blood samples taken at 2-hour intervals from the same stage IV patients demonstrated tyrosinase mRNA-positive as well as -negative samples in follow-up.

In view of all these data, one could devise a simple model to explain the findings. If we agree that there are but few tumor cells circulating in the peripheral blood of melanoma patients, one can think of them as minute spheres floating freely. If we sample 5 ml of blood, we may or may not catch one of those spheres. If we take another 5 ml of the same blood, these statistics would apply again. Therefore, taking many samples and analyzing all of them should yield a higher percentage of positive results in the same patients.

Different methods of sample preparation (whole blood lysis, application of density gradient techniques, etc.) may also lead to discrepant results, as demonstrated by different groups. However, no consensus has been reached on the best method for creating comparable and reliable results in different laboratories. In view of these technical considerations, standardizing the methods among different laboratories is needed to be able to compare results.

Quality Assurance Testing Among Different Laboratories

Discrepant results published on the detection of tyrosinase mRNA in the peripheral blood of melanoma patients resulted in different approaches to validate all previously published data. In early 1997, members of the European Organization for Research and Treatment of Cancer (EORTC) Melanoma Cooperative Group met in Lausanne/Switzerland to discuss the use of tyrosinase mRNA and the varying numbers of positive samples in melanoma patients. As expected, all participating laboratories used different methods of sample preparation (whole blood or peripheral blood mononuclear cells, PBMC) and PCR protocols to detect tyrosinase mRNA. Therefore, the participants felt that the discrepancies observed may be due to the different techniques used. In order to test this hypothesis and further evaluate the possible clinical use of this method, a quality-assurance initiative of the Melanoma Cooperative Group was started. This study was designed to assess the reliability of the methods in use and determine the most common causes of disparities. Using a test panel of either blood samples from healthy donors spiked with defined numbers of melanoma cells or coded samples from patients, the testing was performed in nine different laboratories throughout Europe.

Strikingly, all laboratories reported correct results for all samples of the cDNA dilution series. None of the nine laboratories generated faultless results from whole blood samples, but four of them reported sufficient results, defined as missing only one of the two positive samples with the lowest concentration of melanoma cells. The remaining laboratories reported more false positive or false negative results. Extraction of amplifiable RNA from PBMC was successful in all laboratories. Four laboratories had sufficient results whereas three had more than one false negative result or missed a positive sample. Two laboratories reported false positive results which were, however, not reproducible. These data suggested that sample preparation, RNA extraction, and cDNA synthesis rather than PCR protocols may account for most of the heterogeneity in results with tyrosinase PCR assays. Internal and external standards controlling the whole process of sample preparation and PCR amplification should be developed to control the whole process and ensure sensitivity on a sample basis.

Problems seemed easy to overcome when the company Boehringer Mannheim (Germany) announced it had developed a highly sensitive PCR-based enzyme-linked immunosorbent assay (ELISA) as well as a standardized sample preparation kit for detecting tyrosinase mRNA in peripheral blood. Preliminary testing using blood from healthy donors spiked with defined numbers of melanoma cells in varying concentrations demonstrated a high sensitivity and specificity for this kit. Taking into account that this test represents a standardized highly reproducible method, its use could possibly solve problems in sensitivity and specificity in different laboratories due to discrepant techniques. However, before setting the testing kit to general use, members of the Dermatologic Cooperative Oncology Group (DeCOG) in Germany felt it had to be validated first on a large scale in different laboratories. Therefore, the DeCOG initiated an interlaboratory study: blood samples from healthy donors spiked with defined numbers of tumor cells as well as samples from patients with malignant melanoma in different stages of disease were prepared in a blinded fashion and sent to the seven participating laboratories in Germany (Departments of Dermatology, Universities of Kiel, Regensburg, Tuebingen, Ulm, Munich TU, Munich LMU, and Homburg/Saar). As analysis of all samples has still not been completed by all participants, no definite results are available on this test kit.

Spiking experiments performed in all participating laboratories using this kit demonstrated a high sensitivity (one tumor cell/ml whole blood) and specificity in SK-Mel-28-spiked samples; 7.4% of samples tested false positive and 1.4% (a single sample) tested false negative. However, the questions of whether this test can be used in the clinical setting to follow up patients or define those at risk of relapse and whether it can be used in different or even nonspecialized laboratories still remains open.

Should We Transfer the Tyrosinase-mRNA-Based Technology into a Clinical Setting?

In view of all published data on this technique and all conflicting results discussed previously, questions remain to be answered before the technique can be applied in a clinical setting. No consensus has yet been achieved on the best method of sample preparation, red cell lysis or isolation of white cell fractions. Furthermore, it is not clear whether total RNA extraction or poly-A-RNA isolation should be used. All these procedures should be standardized before allowing large scale clinical use. Furthermore, RNA-based assays can pose technical challenges to clinical laboratories. Most importantly, any test used in a clinical setting must have demonstrated its clinical value in long-term clinical outcome studies. No such study on the use of tyrosinase mRNA testing in the peripheral blood is yet available to support its routine clinical use and cost.

Although tumor cells could be detected at least in subgroups of melanoma patients by most of the groups working on that problem, the results indicate that analyzing tyrosinase mRNA in blood samples from melanoma patients is not suitable for the detection of early metastatic progression. Other diagnostic procedures such as sentinel node biopsy may possibly demonstrate better results for the detection of micrometastatic disease.

References

1. Smith B, Selby P, Southgate J, Pittman K, Bradley C, Blair GE (1991) Detection of melanoma cells in peripheral blood by means of reverse transcriptase and polymerase chain reaction. Lancet 338:1227–1229
2. Brossart P, Keilholz U, Willhauck M, Scheibenbogen C, Mohler T, Hunstein W (1993) Hematogenous spread of malignant melanoma cells in different stages of disease. J Invest Dermatol 101:887–889
3. Brossart P, Keilholz U, Scheibenbogen C, Mohler T, Willhauck M, Hunstein W (1994) Detection of residual tumor cells in patients with malignant melanoma responding to immunotherapy. J Immunother 15:38–41
4. Foss AJ, Guille MJ, Occleston NL, Hykin PG, Hungerford JL, Lightman S (1995) The detection of melanoma cells in peripheral blood by reverse transcription-polymerase chain reaction. Br J Cancer 72:155–159
5. de Vries TJ, Fourkour A, Punt CJ et al. (1999) Reproducibility of detection of tyrosinase and MART-1 transcripts in the peripheral blood of melanoma patients: a quality control study using real-time quantitative RT-PCR. Br J Cancer 80:883–891
6. Farthmann B, Eberle J, Krasagakis K et al. (1998) RT-PCR for tyrosinase-mRNA-positive cells in peripheral blood: evaluation strategy and correlation with known prognostic markers in 123 melanoma patients. J Invest Dermatol 110:263–267
7. Ghossein RA, Coit D, Brennan M et al. (1998) Prognostic significance of peripheral blood and bone marrow tyrosinase messenger RNA in malignant melanoma. Clin Cancer Res 4:419–428
8. Glaser R, Rass K, Seiter S, Hauschild A, Christophers E, Tilgen W (1997) Detection of circulating melanoma cells by specific amplification of tyrosinase complementary DNA is not a reliable tumor marker in melanoma patients: a clinical two-center study. J Clin Oncol 15:2818–2825
9. Hoon DS, Wang Y, Dale PS et al. (1995) Detection of occult melanoma cells in blood with a multiple-marker polymerase chain reaction assay. J Clin Oncol 13:2109–2116
10. Jung FA, Buzaid AC, Ross MI et al. (1997) Evaluation of tyrosinase mRNA as a tumor marker in the blood of melanoma patients. J Clin Oncol 15:2826–2831
11. Keilholz U, Willhauck M, Rimoldi D et al. (1998) Reliability of reverse transcription-polymerase chain reaction (RT-PCR)- based assays for the detection of circulating tumour cells: a quality-assurance initiative of the EORTC Melanoma Cooperative Group. Eur J Cancer 34:750–753
12. Kunter U, Buer J, Probst M et al. (1996) Peripheral blood tyrosinase messenger RNA detection and survival in malignant melanoma. J Natl Cancer Inst 88:590–594
13. Mellado B, Colomer D, Castel T et al. (1996) Detection of circulating neoplastic cells by reverse-transcriptase polymerase chain reaction in malignant melanoma: association with clinical stage and prognosis. J Clin Oncol 14:2091–2097
14. Mellado B, Gutierrez L, Castel T et al. (1999) Prognostic significance of the detection of circulating malignant cells by reverse transcriptase-polymerase chain reaction in long-term clinically disease-free melanoma patients. Clin Cancer Res 5:1843–1848
15. Palmieri G, Strazzullo M, Ascierto PA, Satriano SM, Daponte A, Castello G (1999) Polymerase chain reaction-based detection of circulating melanoma cells as an effective marker of tumor progression. Melanoma Cooperative Group. J Clin Oncol 17:304–311
16. Pittman K, Burchill S, Smith B et al. (1996) Reverse transcriptase-polymerase chain reaction for expression of tyrosinase to identify malignant melanoma cells in peripheral blood. Ann Oncol 7:297–301
17. Reinhold U, Ludtke-Handjery HC, Schnautz S, Kreysel HW, Abken H (1997) The analysis of tyrosinase-specific mRNA in blood samples of melanoma patients by RT-PCR is not a useful test for metastatic tumor progression. J Invest Dermatol 108:166–169
18. Schittek B, Blaheta HJ, Flärchinger G, Sauer B, Garbe C (1999) Increased sensitivity for the detection of malignant melanoma cells in peripheral blood using an improved protocol for reverse transcription-polymerase chain reaction. Br J Dermatol 141:37–43
19. Stevens GL, Scheer WD, Levine EA (1996) Detection of tyrosinase mRNA from the blood of melanoma patients. Cancer Epidemiol Biomarkers Prev 5:293–296
20. Tessier MH, Denis MG, Lustenberger P, Dreno B (1997) Detection of circulating neoplastic cells by reverse transcriptase and polymerase chain reaction in melanoma. Ann Dermatol Venereol 124:607–611

Morphologically Intact Melanoma Cells May Be Detected in Peripheral Blood of Melanoma Patients*

A. Benez, U. Schiebel, and G. Fierlbeck

Department of Dermatology, Eberhard-Karls-University Liebermeisterstr. 25, 72076 Tübingen, Germany

Abstract

The detection of circulating melanoma cells has been the subject of numerous investigations in recent years. We developed a cellular approach to identifying circulating melanoma cells in peripheral blood using immunomagnetic cell sorting. The examination covered 205 blood samples from 155 melanoma patients and 30 samples from healthy persons and nonmelanoma patients. After density gradient centrifugation, the interphase was incubated with the 9.2.27 antibody. Positive cells were labeled with magnetic microbeads and enriched by immunomagnetic cell sorting. Cells were stained using an alkaline phosphatase–anti-alkaline phosphatase assay and examined by light microscopy. In spiking experiments, melanoma cells seeded at a concentration of one melanoma cell per milliliter of whole blood could be detected reliably. Circulating melanoma cells were not found in 30 controls, nor were 9.2.27-positive cells found in 41 patients with primary malignant melanoma. In patients with regional lymph node metastases and disseminated disease, circulating 9.2.27-positive cells could be detected in 3 of 29 patients (10%) and 13 of 85 patients (15%) examined, respectively. We conclude that immunomagnetic cell sorting is a promising method with high sensitivity and specificity. The method is not suitable for early detection of metastases but is a valuable tool for further investigating the biological characteristics of circulating melanoma cells.

* Supported by a grant from the Federal Ministry of Education, Science, Research, and Technology (Fö. 01KS9602) and the Interdisciplinary Clinical Research Center (IKFZ), Tübingen, Germany.

Introduction

Detecting tumor cells in the bloodstream has been the object of numerous investigations with various solid tumors. The methods used are based either on cellular examination techniques or molecular biological methods. In malignant melanoma, recent investigations have concentrated on molecular biological methods to detect circulating melanoma cells [1–13]. The assay most often used is based on the detection of tyrosinase messenger RNA expression by reverse transcription polymerase chain reaction (RT-PCR). This method is considered to be extremely sensitive, however, detection rates vary considerably. In patients with distant metastases, previously published detection levels vary from 0% to 100% [9–12]. Most recent reports state that polymerase chain reaction-based detection of circulating melanoma cells is not suitable for early detection of metastasis [7, 8]. However, other investigators found that it might be an effective marker of tumor progression [3, 5, 13].

We developed a cellular approach to detect circulating melanoma cells using an immunocytologic assay with tumor cell enrichment by magnetic activated cell sorting.

Patients and Methods

The study included 205 50-ml blood samples from 155 consecutively selected melanoma patients (80 males, 75 females, mean age 51 years, range 17–84 years). An additional 30 healthy individuals and nonmelanoma patients were examined.

Leukocytes and tumor cells were separated from erythrocytes by density gradient centrifugation. The cell suspension was incubated with the murine monoclonal antibody 9.2.27 (kindly provided by Prof. Dr. R. A. Reisfeld, Department of Immunology, Scripps Research Institute, La Jolla, Calif., USA) and with goat antimouse microbeads (Miltenyi Biotec, Bergisch Gladbach, Germany). The cell suspension was passed over an LS+ separation column placed in the magnetic field of a Midi MACS separator (Miltenyi Biotec). Cells from the positive fraction were concentrated by centrifugation and attached to glass slides. The antibody reaction was developed with the indirect immunoenzyme alkaline phosphatase-anti-alkaline phosphatase (APAAP) technique (Dako, Hamburg, Germany).

Results

In spiking experiments, melanoma cells seeded at a concentration of one melanoma cell per ml whole blood could be detected reliably in five independent experiments. This corresponds to a sensitivity of one melanoma cell in more than 1×10^6 mononuclear cells. No positive cells were detectable in control samples. The recovery rate was consistently more than 10% of tumor cells seeded in the blood samples (mean 11.4%).

No positive staining was detected in the specimens from 30 healthy donors and nonmelanoma patients. Circulating melanoma cells could not be detected in 41 patients with AJCC clinical stage I/II disease independently of whether the blood samples were taken before or after surgical removal of the primary tumor. In patients with clinical stage III disease, 9.2.27-positive cells were found in three of 29 patients examined (10%), all of whom had clinically detectable metastases at the time of analysis. In patients with disseminated metastases (clinical stage IV), circulating cells were detected in 13 out of 85 patients (15%) examined.

Discussion

Recent investigations of malignant melanoma focused on molecular biological examination techniques for the detection of circulating melanoma cells using RT-PCR for detection of tyrosinase mRNA [1–13]. One of the main disadvantages of PCR is that it is an indirect method with no morphological correlate and cannot provide direct evidence for the actual presence of intact cancer cells in the blood containing these expressed mRNA sequences.

To overcome this limitation, we developed a new method for detecting circulating melanoma cells based on a cellular examination technique using an immunocytologic assay with immunomagnetic cell enrichment. As a marker for melanoma cells we chose the murine monoclonal antibody 9.2.27, which recognizes the core protein (250 kDa) of a human melanoma-associated chondroitin sulfate proteoglycan (MCSP) [14]. The antigen is uniformly expressed on >90% of human melanoma tissues and cultured cells [16, 17]. In our assay, tumor cells were enriched by magnetic activated cell sorting (MACS). Because the majority of mononuclear cells are eliminated by MACS, only a few slides must be analyzed after immunocytochemical staining.

In spiking experiments, we demonstrated that one melanoma cell per milliliter of whole blood can be reliably detected with this assay. The sensitivity reported for detection of tyrosinase mRNA in model experiments is in the same range [5, 8, 9] or slightly higher [6].

To our knowledge, this is the first report to demonstrate that 9.2.27-positive melanoma cells with typical morphological characteristics of malignant cells may be identified in a number of melanoma patients with advanced disease. Thus, 9.2.27-positive cells were found in three of 29 patients with stage III melanoma and in 13 of 85 patients with disseminated disease. Positive cells were not detected in patients with primary tumors, independently of whether blood samples were taken before or after surgery, nor in patients after surgical removal of regional lymph nodes and/or in-transit metastases.

Given the relatively low percentage in our study of positive cells in circulation, even in patients with advanced disease, a negative result certainly does not exclude the existence of metastases or micrometastatic disease. Consequently, this assay cannot be used as a diagnostic procedure for melanoma staging. The main advantage of our assay in comparison to PCR techniques is that not only mRNA sequences but whole melanoma cells may be identified. Although the method is not suitable for early detection of metastases, it is a valuable tool in further investigating phenotypic and biological characteristics of circulating melanoma cells.

References

1. Keilholz U, Willhauck M, Scheibenbogen C, de Vries TJ, Burchill S (1997) Polymerase chain reaction detection of circulating tumour cells. EORTC Melanoma Cooperative Group, Immunotherapy Subgroup. Melanoma Res 7 Suppl 2:S133–141
2. Curry BJ, Myers K, Hersey P (1998) Polymerase chain reaction detection of melanoma cells in the circulation: relation to clinical stage, surgical treatment, and recurrence from melanoma. J Clin Oncol 16:1760–1769
3. Farthmann B, Eberle J, Krasagakis K, Gstottner M, Wang N, Bisson S, Orfanos CE (1998) RT-PCR for tyrosinase-mRNA-positive cells in peripheral blood: evaluation strategy and correlation with known prognostic markers in 123 melanoma patients. J Invest Dermatol 110:263–267
4. Ghossein RA, Coit D, Brennan M, Zhang ZF, Wang Y, Bhattacharya S, Houghton A, Rosai J (1998) Prognostic significance of peripheral blood and bone marrow tyrosinase messenger RNA in malignant melanoma. Clin Cancer Res 4:419–428
5. Mellado B, Colomer D, Castel T, Munoz M, Carballo E, Galan M, Mascaro JM, Vives Corrons JL, Grau JJ, Estape J (1996) Detection of circulating neoplastic cells by reverse-transcriptase polymerase chain reaction in malignant melanoma: association with clinical stage and prognosis. J Clin Oncol 14:2091–2097
6. Curry BJ, Smith MJ, Hersey P (1996) Detection and quantitation of melanoma cells in the circulation of patients. Melanoma Res 6:45–654
7. Glaser R, Rass K, Seiter S, Hauschild A, Christophers E, Tilgen W (1997) Detection of circulating melanoma cells by specific amplification of tyrosinase complementary DNA is not a reliable tumor marker in melanoma patients: a clinical two-center study. J Clin Oncol 15:2818–2825
8. Reinhold U, Ludtke Handjery HC, Schnautz S, Kreysel HW, Abken H (1997) The analysis of tyrosinase-specific mRNA in blood samples of melanoma patients by RT-PCR is not a useful test for metastatic tumor progression. J Invest Dermatol 108:166–169
9. Brossart P, Schmier JW, Kruger S, Willhauck M, Scheibenbogen C, Mohler T, Keilholz U (1995) A polymerase chain reaction-based semiquantitative assessment of malignant melanoma cells in peripheral blood. Cancer Res 55:4065–4068
10. Brossart P, Keilholz U, Scheibenbogen C, Mohler T, Willhauck M, Hunstein W (1994) Detection of residual tumor cells in patients with malignant melanoma responding to immunotherapy. J Immunother 15:38–41
11. Brossart P, Keilholz U, Willhauck M, Scheibenbogen C, Mohler T, Hunstein W (1993) Hematogenous spread of malignant melanoma cells in different stages of disease. J Invest Dermatol 101:887–889
12. Foss AJ, Guille MJ, Occleston NL, Hykin PG, Hungerford JL, Lightman S (1995) The detection of melanoma cells in peripheral blood by reverse transcription-polymerase chain reaction. Br J Cancer 72:155–159
13. Palmieri G, Strazzullo M, Ascierto PA, Satriano SMR, Daponte A, Castello G (1999) Polymerase chain reaction-based detection of circulating melanoma cells as an effective marker of tumor progression. J Clin Oncol 17:304–311
14. Pluschke G, Vanek M, Evans A, Dittmar T, Schmid P, Itin P, Filardo EJ, Reisfeld RA (1996) Molecular cloning of a human melanoma-associated chondroitin sulfate proteoglycan. Proc Natl Acad Sci USA 93:9710–9715

15. Heyderman E, McCartney JC (1985) Epithelial membrane antigen and lymphoid cells. Lancet 1:109–110
16. Bumol TF, Reisfeld RA (1982) Unique glycoprotein-proteoglycan complex defined by monoclonal antibody on human melanoma cells. Proc Natl Acad Sci USA 79:1245–1249
17. Harper JR, Quaranta V, Reisfeld RA (1986) Ammonium chloride interferes with a distinct step in the biosynthesis and cell surface expression of human melanoma-type chondroitin sulfate proteoglycan. J Biol Chem 261:3600–3606
18. Oldham RK, Foon KA, Morgan AC, Woodhouse CS, Schroff RW, Abrams PG, Fer M, Schoenberger CS, Farrell M, Kimball E et al. (1984) Monoclonal antibody therapy of malignant melanoma: in vivo localization in cutaneous metastasis after intravenous administration. J Clin Oncol 2:1235–1244

Prognosis of Metastatic Melanoma: No Correlation of Tyrosinase mRNA in Bone Marrow and Survival Time

V. Waldmann, J. Wacker, M. Deichmann, A. Jäckel, M. Bock, and H. Näher

Department of Dermatology, University of Heidelberg, Voßstrasse 2, 69115 Heidelberg, Germany

Abstract

Recent publications suggest that tyrosinase mRNA in blood as well as in bone marrow is detectable only in a subgroup of patients with metastatic melanoma. This would imply that tyrosinase mRNA is of limited value as a tumor marker. We addressed the question of whether patients with metastatic melanoma and RT-PCR-detectable tyrosinase mRNA in blood or bone marrow have a different prognosis than tyrosinase mRNA-negative patients. Twenty melanoma patients with widespread clinical metastases were enrolled; the survival time after first diagnosis of visceral metastases was correlated to tyrosinase mRNA presence in blood and bone marrow samples. The time of survival of eight patients with metastatic melanoma and detectable tyrosinase mRNA in either blood or bone marrow was not different from the prognosis of 12 patients without detectable tyrosinase mRNA in either blood or bone marrow. Detection of tyrosinase mRNA in blood or bone marrow samples of melanoma patients with advanced disease seems to have no substantial relevance for survival time and outcome of disease. In this constellation, detection of tyrosinase mRNA by RT-PCR is not a valid tumor marker. Nevertheless, tyrosinase positivity in bone marrow in earlier tumor stages might indicate increased risk for the development of distant metastases. This should be addressed in further studies.

Introduction

The prognosis of patients suffering from metastatic malignant melanoma is still very poor. Therefore, elaboration and evaluation of adjuvant treatment protocols is of clinical importance. However, existing adjuvant treatment protocols have side effects, are expensive and therapy has to be continued for at least months. In this setting, it would be useful to have a marker of micrometastatic disease for early identification of patient subpopulations who

Recent Results in Cancer Research, Vol. 158

would possibly benefit most from adjuvant therapy. Detection of tyrosinase mRNA and thus of disseminated melanoma cells in blood, bone marrow, lymph nodes or subcutaneous fat surrounding the primary melanoma has been suggested as an indicator for early, clinically still latent, progression of melanoma disease (Smith et al. 1991; Rankin 1996; Farthmann et al. 1998; Waldmann et al. 2000). Tyrosinase is an enzyme in the melanin synthetic pathway and its expression is restricted to melanin-producing cells, which are normally not found in peripheral blood or bone marrow (Bennett 1991). Despite the high sensitivity of RT-PCR-based tyrosinase detection, with a detection limit of about one cell in 10^7 normal cells (Burchill et al. 1995; Curry et al. 1996), recent publications suggest a prevalence of tyrosinase mRNA in blood of patients with clinical diagnosed metastatic melanoma in the range of only 26–44% (for review see Waldmann et al. 2000). The prevalence of tyrosinase mRNA in bone marrow of patients with overt clinical metastases from melanoma does not exceed the prevalence in blood samples (Ghossein et al. 1998; Waldmann et al. 1999). Thus, detection of tyrosinase-specific mRNA in bone marrow does not contribute to a higher overall detection sensitivity of putatively tyrosinase-positive patients. In this respect, melanoma seems to be in marked contrast to solid epithelial tumors, in which bone marrow is a significant reservoir for micrometastatic tumor cells. However, this might not exclude that PCR-positivity defines a subgroup of patients with rapid, progressive metastatic disease. Therefore, we tested the hypothesis whether metastatic melanoma patients with RT-PCR-detectable tyrosinase mRNA in blood or bone marrow might have a different survival time and disease outcome than patients without detectable hematogenous spread of melanoma cells.

Material and Methods

Patient Selection

Blood and bone marrow samples from 20 patients with malignant melanoma were obtained with informed consent (Table 1). Of these, 14 patients had newly diagnosed visceral metastases and had not received prior systemic immunotherapy or chemotherapy. In addition, five patients with current treatment by chemo- and/or immunotherapy for multiple visceral metastases of melanoma were included. One patient suffered from huge, untreated locoregional and skin metastases, but had no systemic melanoma manifestation.

Reverse Transcription-Polymerase Chain Reaction for Tyrosinase mRNA

All blood and bone marrow samples were collected at the same time interval, between 9.00 and 10.00 h, and were examined microscopically for bone marrow depletion. The mononuclear cell fraction of peripheral blood and bone

Table 1. Histological parameters and results of tyrosinase mRNA RT-PCR from blood and bone marrow samples of patients with advanced melanoma disease

Patient	Histology	Sex	Stage	Therapy	Breslow	Clark	Blood	Marrow	Survival
1	NM	M	IV	DTIC	2.0	V	–	–	10
2	LMM	F	IV	DTIC/IFN/ DVP	?	IV	–	–	2
3	SSM	M	IV	–	2.0	IV	–	–	4
4	NM	M	IV	–	1.9	IV	–	–	6
5	NM	M	IV	–	4.0	III	–	–	8
6	SSM	F	IV	–	0.7	III	–	–	16+
7	NM	M	IV	–	6.0	IV	–	–	15+
8	UP	M	IV	–	–	–	–	–	18+
9	Mucosal	M	IV	DTIC/IFN	–	–	–	–	27+
10	Mucosal	F	IV	–	–	–	–	–	5
11	Uveal	F	IV	–	–	–	–	–	22+
12	Uveal	F	IV	–	–	–	–	–	5
13	SSM	F	IV	TEM	5.0	III	+	+	25+
14	LMM	M	IV	–	2.7	IV	+	+	21+
15	SSM	M	IV	–	3.2	IV	+	+	11
16	NM	F	III	–	6.1	IV	+	+	14+
17	SSM	M	IV	–	4.0	IV	+	+	9
18	UP	M	IV	DVP	–	-++	3		
19	UP	M	IV	–	–	–	–	+	5
20	UP	M	IV	–	–	–	+	–	3

Breslow index is given in millimeters; survival time is given in months from first diagnosis of visceral metastases to death from melanoma (adapted from Waldmann et al. 2000).
Abbreviations: *SSM*, superficial spreading melanoma; *NM*, nodular melanoma; *LMM*, lentigo maligna melanoma; *UP*, unknown primary; *III*, regional lymph node metastases, in this case with multiple untreated regional skin metastases; *IV*, visceral metastases; +, patient still alive; *DTIC*, dacarbazine; *DVP*, dacarbazine+cisplatin+vindesine; *TEM*, temozolamide; *IFN*, α-interferon.

marrow was isolated by Ficoll gradient, as described previously (Boyum 1968). For reverse transcription, approximately 1 µg of total isolated RNA was added to 25 µl of RT buffer containing 0.4 µg of random hexamers, 1 mmol dNTPs, 20 units of of AMV reverse transcriptase (Promega, Madison, Wisconsin, USA) and 40 units RNAsin (Promega). The reaction mixture was incubated at 65 °C for 5 min followed by incubation at 42 °C for 1 h. Then, 2 µl of the sample were resuspended in 50 µl of PCR buffer containing 40 pmol of the two outer primers (see below) and 2.5 units of Taq DNA polymerase. PCR was carried out in a thermal cycler for 1.5 min at 94 °C for denaturation, followed by 1.5 min at 60 °C for annealing and 1.5 min at 72 °C for extension for a total of 30 cycles. For the second round of PCR, a pair of inner primers was used (see below) and amplification was done with an identical temperature profile in a 1:10 dilution. The integrity of RNA from blood and bone marrow samples was confirmed by RT and amplification of a human β-actin probe, resulting in a DNA fragment of 630 bp. The procedure has been described in detail (Waldmann et al. 1999).

Synthetic Oligonucleotides

The DNA sequences of the primers used for PCR amplification were as according to Smith et al. (1991). The two outer primers used for the first round of PCR amplified a fragment of 284 bp of tyrosinase cDNA; amplification by the two inner primers used for the second round of PCR resulted in a product of 207 bp. Primers were obtained from Biometra (Göttingen, Germany).

Assessment of Sensitivity and Specificity

As a positive control, we used MM-I, a primary melanoma cell line which has been established in our laboratory. Cells of this line are tyrosinase-positive. Various amounts of MM-I cells were diluted in 10 ml of blood, total RNA was extracted, RT-PCR was performed and putative amplification products assessed on agarose gel electrophoresis, as for bone marrow and blood samples. Each amplification and gel electrophoresis included negative controls which contained no DNA. By this procedure ten or more MM-I cells per 10 ml of blood resulted in a positive tyrosinase amplification product upon conventional agarose gel electrophoresis (Fig. 1). This means a detection limit of one tyrosinase-positive cell per ml. The procedure has been described in detail (Waldmann et al. 1999).

Survival Time of Patients

Time of survival was calculated in months between first diagnosis of visceral metastases and death from melanoma disease. Five patients who tested nega-

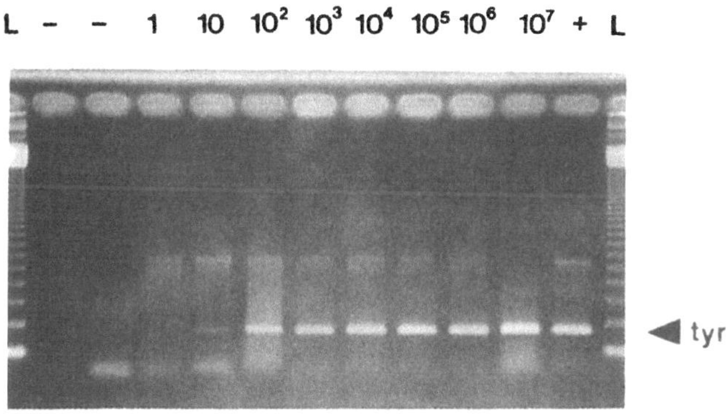

Fig. 1. Detection of tyrosinase-specific mRNA in normal blood mixed with MM-I cells, which are tyrosinase-positive. A different amount of MM-I cells (*top*, $1-10^7$) were mixed with 10 ml of normal human blood. Amplification of tyrosinase mRNA (*tyr*, amplification product 207 bp) and detection by ethidium bromide is successful down to 10 cells in 10 ml. *L*, length standard; – indicates negative controls for PCR; + is a positive control (MM-I cells). (From Waldmann et al. 1999)

tive for tyrosinase in blood and bone marrow are still alive as of this writing, as are three patients who tested positive in either blood or bone marrow. All other patients died from their melanoma disease.

Results

Blood and bone marrow samples from 20 patients with widespread clinical metastases of malignant melanoma were analysed for the presence of tyrosinase mRNA by RT and subsequent DNA amplification by PCR. Some 60% (12 of 20) were negative for tyrosinase in both blood and bone marrow. Of 15 patients with newly diagnosed clinical metastases and without previous systemic chemotherapy or immunotherapy, six were positive for tyrosinase mRNA in either blood or bone marrow; in these patients bone marrow depletion can be excluded. Of five patients who had received previous chemo- and/or immunotherapy, two were positive; microscopic examination of H&E-stained slides of the bone marrow aspirates showed the presence of bone marrow.

In the group of all 20 patients, of 19 stage IV patients and of all 15 patients in stage IV except those with mucosal and uveal melanomas, tyrosinase-negative patients had a mean (median) of survival between 9.9 and 11.5 months (9.0), compared to a mean of survival between 11.0 (9.0) and 11.4 (10.0) months for tyrosinase-positive patients (Table 2). Therefore, it can be concluded that eight patients with metastatic melanoma and detectable tyrosinase mRNA in either blood or bone marrow did not have a shorter survival and a worse prognosis than 12 patients without detectable tyrosinase mRNA in either blood or bone marrow. Interestingly, three of four patients with metastases from unknown primary melanoma were tyrosinase-positive and had a very poor prognosis, with 3, 3 and 5 months survival times after first diagnosis of metastases (Fig. 2), compared to the one tyrosinase-negative patient with a rather good outcome of 18 months of survival; this patient is still alive as of this writing.

Table 2. Mean (A) and median (M) of survival time for melanoma patients negative for tyrosinase mRNA in blood and bone marrow (negative) and for patients positive for tyrosinase mRNA in either blood or bone marrow (positive)

		Negative	Positive
$n=20$	A	11.5	11.4
	M	9.0	10.0
IV ($n=19$)	A	11.5	11.0
	M	9.0	9.0
Derm IV ($n=15$)	A	9.9	11.0
	M	9.0	9.0

Patient subgroups are as follows: $n=20$, all patients; IV, stage IV patients; Derm IV, all stage IV patients except mucosal and uveal melanomas.

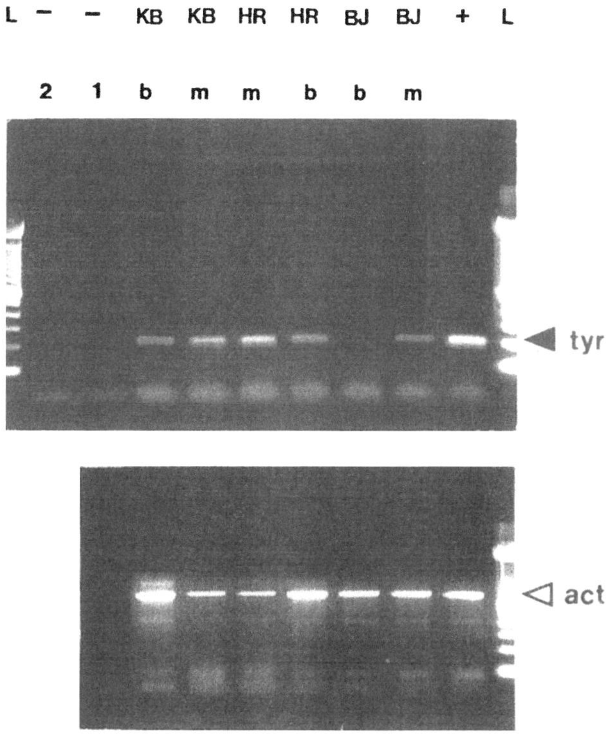

Fig. 2. *Top*: Analysis of tyrosinase mRNA expression in blood (*b*) and bone marrow (*m*) samples of three patients (KB, HR, BJ) with widespread clinical metastases of malignant melanoma by RT-PCR. *L*, length standard, – negative controls (*1* is negative control for the first PCR, *2* is negative control for the first and nested PCR); + is a positive control (MML I cells). The amplification product of tyrosinase RT-PCR is indicated (*tyr*). Whereas patients KB and HR are positive in blood and bone marrow, patient BJ is negative in blood but positive in bone marrow. *Bottom*: RNA integrity was controlled in all samples by RT-PCR with primers for human β-actin. The amplification product is indicated (*act*). (From Waldmann et al. 1999)

Discussion

In summary, 12 of 20 patients with metastatic melanoma were negative for tyrosinase in both blood and bone marrow. Two patients with metastatic uveal melanoma were both negative for tyrosinase in blood and bone marrow. Due to the low number of examined patients, statistical analysis is impossible; however, it can be concluded that the prevalence of tyrosinase mRNA positivity in bone marrow does not exceed the prevalence in blood samples from patients with metastatic melanoma. We and others therefore suggested that RT-PCR detection of tyrosinase-specific mRNA in bone marrow has no substantial advantage compared with that in blood and does not contribute to a higher overall detection sensitivity of putatively tyrosinase-positive patients (Ghossein et al. 1998; Waldmann et al. 1999). Evaluation of the follow-up of the present 20 patients does not demonstrate a substantial benefit in survival time for tyrosinase-negative patients. Thus, detection of tyrosinase mRNA does not define a subgroup of patients with rapidy progression of their metastatic melanoma disease compared to patients negative in RT-PCR for tyrosinase mRNA in blood and bone marrow. As tyrosinase positivity was not a predictor of short survival and the prevalence of tyrosinase-specific mRNA in stage IV patients is only 40%, this suggests that detection of tyrosinase-specific mRNA in blood as well as in bone marrow is only of limited use as a marker for micrometastatic melanoma and its progression (Waldmann et al. 1999, 2000).

The present data are in accordance with findings from tyrosinase mRNA RT-PCR studies on blood samples, which suggested that detection of tyrosinase mRNA-positive cells in peripheral blood is not an adequate marker either for identifying melanoma patients with distant metastases or for defining individual prognosis (Farthmann et al. 1998). However, tyrosinase positivity in bone marrow in earlier tumour stages might indicate increased risk for the development of overt distant metastases and may be of value as a progression marker not only in these patients but also for monitoring of chemotherapeutic success in patients with visceral metastases and positivity for tyrosinase prior to therapy. These questions should be addressed for in further studies.

This might also be the case for patients with metastases from unknown primary melanoma: of four patients examined, we found three to be tyrosinase-positive and having a poor prognosis, with a mean survival of 4 months after diagnosis of stage IV, compared to one tyrosinase-negative patient with more than 18 months of survival. For this subgroup of melanoma patients a larger study seems to be necessary for evaluating the usefulness of tyrosinase mRNA RT-PCR as a melanoma marker.

The finding that bone marrow is not a reservoir for micrometastatic disease in tumour progression of malignant melanoma is in marked contrast to solid tumours such as colon or breast cancer (Lindemann et al. 1992), in which micrometastasis in bone marrow can be found in progressive tumour disease. One explanation for this may be that these epithelial tumours have a completely different tumour biology than malignant melanoma. Indeed, the molecular steps that finally lead to colon cancer, for example, do not seem to play a significant role in melanoma initiation or progression (Waldmann et al. 1999). In melanoma, mutations of p16 (CDKN2), p53, *ras*, neurofibromatosis type I gene (NF-1), *bcl*-2 and the retinoblastoma gene have been described, however with low prevalence rates.

Another explanation for the failure of tyrosinase detection to act as a melanoma progression marker might be that continuous dissemination of melanoma cells does not occur and that, therefore, single sample preparation results in limited sensitivity. It is also possible that tyrosinase expression is not obligatory for melanoma cells during metastasis. The frequent coincidence of melanocytic and amelanocytic metastases in clinically advanced melanoma disease is in accordance with this contention. Therefore, as melanoma is heterogeneous for its melanoma-associated antigens, multiple-marker PCR assays to detect mRNA of different antigens have been developed to obtain a higher sensitivity for detection of melanoma cells in blood (Hoon et al. 1995; Sarantou et al. 1997; deVries et al. 1997). It remains to be determined whether these assays might be useful for detection of micrometastatic melanoma cells in bone marrow.

References

Bennet DJ. Colour genes, oncogenes and melanocytes differentiation (1991) J Cell Sci 98:135–139

Boyum A (1968) Separation of leukocytes from blood and bone marrow. Scand J Clin Invest 21:51–55

Burchill S, Bradbury M, Pittman K, Southgate J, Smith B, Selby P (1995) Detection of epithelial cancer cells in peripheral blood by reverse transcriptase-polymerase chain reaction. Br J Cancer 71:278–281

Curry B, Smith M, Hersey P (1996) Detection and quantitation of melanoma cells in the circulation of patients. Melanoma Res 6:45–54

Farthmann B, Eberle J, Krasagakis K, Gstöttner M, Wang N, Bisson S, Orfanos C (1998) RT-PCR for tyrosinase-mRNA-positive cells in peripheral blood: Evaluation strategy and correlation with known prognostic markers in 123 melanoma patients. J Invest Dermatol 110:263–267

Ghossein R, Coit D, Brennan M, Zhang Z, Wang Y, Bhattacharya S, Houghton A, Rosai J (1998) Prognostic significance of peripheral blood and bone marrow tyrosinase messenger RNA in malignant melanoma. Clin Cancer Res 4:419–428

Hoon DS, Wang Y, Dale PS et al. (1995) Detection of occult melanoma cells in blood with a multiple-marker polymerase chain reaction assay. J Clin Oncol 13:2109–2116

Lindemann F, Schlimok G, Dirschedl P et al. (1992) Prognostic significance of micrometastatic tumour cells in bone marrow of colorectal cancer patients. Lancet 340:685–689

Rankin E (1996) Detection of early micrometastases in malignant melanoma. Europ J Cancer 32 A:1627–1629

Sarantou T, Chi DD, Garrison DA et al. (1997) Melanoma-associated antigens as messenger RNA detection markers for melanoma. Cancer Res 57:1371–1376

Smith B, Selby P, Southgate J, Pittman K, Bradley C, Blair G (1991) Detection of melanoma cells in peripheral blood by means of reverse transcriptase and polymerase chain reaction. Lancet 338:1227–1229

de Vries TJ, Fourkour A, Wobbes T et al. (1997) Heterogeneous expression of immunotherapy candidate proteins gp100, MART-1 and tyrosinase in human melanoma cell lines and in human melanocytic lesions. Cancer Res 57:3223–3229

Waldmann V, Deichmann M, Jäckel A (2000) Minimal residual disease in metastatic melanoma and its detection by tumor marker candidates. Hautarzt (in press)

Waldmann V, Deichmann M, Bock M, Jäckel A, Näher H (1999) Tyrosinase-specific mRNA in bone marrow is not more sensitive than blood for the demonstration of micrometastatic melanoma. Br J Dermatol 140:1060–1064

Waldmann V, Wacker J, Deichmann M, Jäckel A, Bock M, Näher H (2000) No correlation of tyrosinase mRNA in bone marrow with prognosis of metastatic melanoma. Dermatol (in press)

III. Detection of Minimal Residual Disease in Sentinel Nodes

The Predictive Value of the Sentinel Lymph Node in Malignant Melanomas

D. Bachter[1], C. Michl[1], H. Büchels[2], H. Vogt[3], and B.R. Balda[1]

[1] Klinik für Dermatologie und Allergologie, Stenglinstrasse 2, 86156 Augsburg, Germany
[2] Department of Plastic Surgery, Augsburg, Germany
[3] Department of Nuclear Medicine, Augsburg, Germany

Abstract

At the beginning of a lymphogenous metastasizing process in malignant melanomas, the first tumor cells are found in the so-called sentinel lymph node (SLN), defined as the first tumor-draining lymph node. Its removal and histopathological examination enable us to discover metastases of malignant melanomas long before their possibility of detection by any other method. Since the beginning of 1995, we have performed more than 350 γ-probe-guided sentinel lymphonodectomies (γ-SLNE), without any clinical evidence of metastases as determined by lymphoscintigraphy. Using γ-SLNE, the detection and excision of the SLN succeeded in nearly all patients. The SLNs were fixed in formalin, completely cut into 1-mm thin slices and stained for routine H&E histology and with S-100 and HMB-45. In persons with melanomas thinner than 0.75 mm, we never found micrometastases. However, the SLNs were positive in melanomas from 0.76 to 1.50 mm in about 7% of patients, in melanomas from 1.51 to 4.00 mm in about 21% and in tumors thicker than 4 mm in about 44%. In primary melanomas with satellite or in-transit metastases, the SLNs contained metastases in 75% of patients. Normally, a radical lymph node dissection (RLND) follows, as it is considered to be the necessary consequence following detection of tumor cells. The lymph nodes of the RLNDs contained further metastases in about 30% of patients. The probability of the involvement of lymph nodes other than the SLN correlates with the extension of tumor cells in the SLN. During our 4-year-follow-up, we observed only a single lymph node recurrence in a patient with a negative SLN (false negative rate of about 0.4%). The development of systemic metastasis correlates not only with the Breslow tumor thickness, but also with the extent of the involvement of the melanoma metastasis in the SLN. Summarizing, it can be said that γ-SLNE has revolutionized melanoma surgery. Based on our data, it is absolutely necessary in the staging of malignant melanoma. In our opinion, the existing classification systems for staging lymph node involvement have to be revised in light of the results of SLNE.

Recent Results in Cancer Research, Vol. 158

Introduction

Malignant melanomas are known to spread most frequently to regional lymph nodes [7]. A considerable proportion of melanoma patients with clinical stage I and II (AICC/UICC) disease already show histological evidence of micrometastasis in regional lymph nodes [7]. Therefore, many centers perform regional lymphadenectomy in order to minimize the risk of tumor spread even in early clinical stages. However, the results of elective lymph node dissection (ELND) remain controversial, because a significant survival benefit has not been demonstrated yet [17, 21]. Since ELND is associated with considerable morbidity, there are as yet no commonly accepted recommendations for ELND.

A promising approach to solving the problem of appropriate patient selection for ELND is the sentinel lymphonodectomy (SLNE). The sentinel lymph node (SLN) is defined as the first lymph node draining the tumor. It has been assumed that the sentinel lymph node is an indicator representative of the whole lymph node region. According to the current hypothesis, tumor cells first spread to the SLN, thereby initiating lymphogenic metastasis. Thus a SLN free of tumor cells indicates a tumor-free lymph node region. In contrast, infiltration of tumor cells within the SLN corresponds to lymphogenic metastasis.

Preoperative Localization of the SLN

In order to visualize the lymphatic drainage and to identify the SLN, preoperative scintigraphic lymph node mapping is mandatory. Hereby technetium-labeled human albumin is injected intradermally around the tumor or the scar. Immediately images in at least two projections are made, pursuing the lymphatic channels until their ending in the first lymph node; this is the sentinel lymph node and is marked as such on the skin. There are two different methods to identify the SLN intraoperatively. These are discussed in the following sections.

Intraoperative Localization of the SLN

Lymphatic Mapping by the Vital Blue Dye Method

Morton et al. [14] first described the concept of SLN in malignant melanomas. In this report patent blue V (2,4-disulfo-5-hydroxy-4′,4″-bis (diethylamino)-triphenylcarbinol-monopotassium salt) dye is used for intraoperative localization of the SLN. About 0.5–1.0 ml of patent blue V is injected intradermally around the suspicious tumor, or on either side of the scar if the melanoma has already been excised. Subsequently, an incision is made over the lymph node basin, which has been detected lymphoscintigraphically and marked on the skin the day before. The blue-stained lymphatic channels and the SLN can now be identified. After ligation of the lymphatic channels, the SLN is removed completely and fixed in formalin. Finally, the wound is closed stepwise.

Lymphatic mapping, however, has some significant disadvantages. After injection of the dye, the SLN sometimes fails to stain, particularly if the tumor is located in the face, neck or trunk. The technique is time-consuming and requires extensive experience. Since the dye is washed out of the lymph node very rapidly, it sometimes has to be reinjected before the SLN has been identified. If the tumor is located in the patient's back, multiple intraoperative repositionings might be necessary. Rare complications include permanent tatooing of the skin with dye-rests. Also, in one case report, an allergic reaction to patent blue was described.

Intraoperative Localization of the SLN by γ-Probe Guidance

In 1993, Alex and Krag first described the γ-probe-guided intraoperative localization of lymph nodes [3], and the technique has been performed in our center since 1995 [4]. As a first step, one day before surgery, radioactively labeled human albumin or sulfur colloid is injected intradermally around the suspected tumor. The SLN is then localized scintigraphically and marked on the skin. If the amount of radiotracer was sufficient, the SLN can still be localized the next day without reinjection of the tracer. During surgery, the suspected tumor is excised with a margin of 1 cm on all sides (including the radioactively enhanced peritumoral tissue), immediately sent for frozen section and examined histologically. If malignancy is confirmed and the melanoma is thicker than 1 mm, the excision is widened with a resulting safety margin of 3 cm on all sides, and all tissue down to the fascia is removed. The defect is then closed.

As a next step, the SLN is localized externally using a 99 m Tc-collimated γ-probe (C-Trak-System, Care-Wise, Morgan Hill, CA). The mark on the skin from the day before makes orientation easier. A small incision is made exactly over the measured maximum of radioactivity. The lymph node is identified within the tissue by the γ-probe without causing significant tissue damage, and after careful ligation of draining lymphatic channels the SLN is removed. Afterwards it is important to measure radioactivity in the wound area in order to confirm whether the correct lymph node (SLN) has been removed and the excision has been performed completely. The defect is then closed stepwise. In most cases the SLN contains the highest amount of radioactivity of all the lymph nodes. Subsequent lymph nodes also containing radioactivity are not excised. Sometimes the SLN itself cannot be identified clearly and a conglomerate of lymph nodes has to be removed. In this case the radioactivity of each lymph node has to be measured, numbered and the SLN marked with a thread. Afterwards the lymph nodes are fixed in formalin.

Histological Examination of the SLN

After a 1-day fixation period in formalin, the lymph node is cut completely into 1-mm slices. Each slice is stained, both with HE and immunohistochemically with anti-S-100 and HMB-45. The immunohistochemical staining allows the differentiation between melanoma metastases and nevus cell nevi in lymph nodes. If there is evidence of micrometastases in the examined lymph node, a radical lymph node dissection (RLND) has to be performed. A careful histological examination of the stained specimen is required to identify small micrometastases. Frozen sections are not sufficient to visualize lymphatic metastasis.

Results

At the time of this analysis, 256 patients (132 women, 124 men, ages 15–87 years) without clinical evidence of lymphatic metastasis were examined. In 113 patients the melanoma was pre-excised. We diagnosed 165 superficial spreading, 57 nodal, 5 lentigo maligna-, 14 acral lentiginous and 15 non-classified malignant melanomas. The Breslow tumor thickness was between 0.20 and 17 mm, with a mean of 1.93 mm and a median of 1.20 mm. The main localizations were the trunk (104) and the lower limb (97).

According to the classification scheme of the German Dermatological Society, which is independent of the Clark level, we found 50 patients in stage Ia (≤0.75 mm), 101 in stage Ib (0.76–1.50 mm), 74 in stage IIa (1.51 mm–4.00 mm), 23 in stage IIb (>4 mm) and 8 in stage IIIa (melanomas with in-transit or satellite metastases).

The intraoperative localization of the SLN was first performed by γ-probe guidance ($n=176$) only, later in combination with the vital blue dye technique ($n=80$). The SLN stained blue in 75% of patients. In 223 patients there was one lymphatic drainage basin, while in 27 patients the melanoma drained into two and in three patients into three different lymph node regions.

In two patients with tumors in the cervical region in which the melanoma drained into two SLNs in two different lymph node regions, we could only localize one of them during the operation, because of its proximity to the injection site.

In clinical stage Ia we never found tumor cells in the SLN. In stage Ib we detected metastases in 7% of patients, in stage IIa in 21%, in stage IIb in 44% and in stage IIIa in 75%.

In 31 of 41 patients with melanoma-positive SLNs, a RLND was performed in a second operation after the SLNE. In about 30% we found further, non-sentinel, nodes involved. During our follow-up-period (mean 18 months, median 16 months, minimum 1 month, maximum 45 months), 15 patients developed melanoma metastases, from which three died. In only one patient with a negative SLN was there a regional lymph node recurrence, corresponding to a false-negative rate of 0.4%.

Conclusions

The removal of the SLN has nowadays become a standard approach in the primary therapy of malignant melanomas [4–6, 9, 10, 12, 13, 15, 16, 20]. The ELND showed no clear evidence of benefiting patients [17, 21]. In our opinion, this surgical procedure must be regarded as obsolete, as the SLNE delivers a minimally invasive surgical method that allows exact staging of the melanoma-draining lymph node region.

Although the complication rate is low, there is the question in which melanomas SLNE should be performed. As can be expected, the number of SLNs containing melanoma cells increases with tumor thickness, ranging between 14% and 36%, depending on the patient collective. The current literature does not differentiate according to tumor thickness, but to tumor stage. Most treatment centers remove the SLN only in tumors thicker than 1 mm. Clinical experience, however, shows that there is also lymphogenous metastasis in thin melanomas. Since there are only a few publications that address the issue of lymphogenous metastasis in melanomas less than 1 mm thick, we performed SLNE also in these patients. We never found a patient in clinical stage Ia whose SLN was harvesting tumor cells. The same results were obtained by Pijpers et al. [15]. Krag et al. [12] reported only one patient with a positive SLN in a group of 24 patients with melanomas less than 0.75 mm thick. That is why, in our opinion, SLNE is not necessary in patients with melanomas thinner than 0.75 mm. However, in thicker tumors (≥0.76 mm), the necessity of surgical removal of the SLN is evident. The percentage of positive SLNs in melanomas ranging between 0.75 and 1 mm corresponds to the distribution of the total collective in stage Ib and is about 6%.

Another reason for the different results could be the different methods used in histological examination of the SLN. As the micrometastases in the SLN mostly consist of very small tumor cell formations, we do not perform frozen sections. Following formalin fixation, the SLNs were cut parallel to the longitudinal axis into approximately 1 mm-thick slices. From each slice three consecutive paraffin sections were cut in a microtome. In this way, the total profile of the lymph node is as completely conserved as possible. All lymph nodes must be examined by immunohistochemistry (S-100, HMB-45), which improves the detection rate of micrometastases [8.18].

The biological significance of submicroscopic proof of metastases using special techniques should be regarded critically. The cultivation of melanoma cells of histologically negative SLNs and the use of reverse transcriptase-polymerase chain reaction (RT-PCR) [23] lead obviously to an upstaging (31–44%). There is nothing known about the false-positive rate, as especially benign nevus cell nevi, which are found in the lymph nodes in a non-negligible percentage of patients, can cause false-positive results [18]. When we removed additional lymph nodes during the SLNE, which were either nearby or had low counts of radioactivity, we never found tumor-cell-harvesting ones. The metastases always were in the SLN only.

Another question is whether SLNE can be regarded as a therapeutic measure. In patients who underwent RLND after finding a positive SLN, we found that, in about 30%, further lymph nodes, besides the SLN, were involved. In the literature, the percentages range from 13 to 50% [9, 12, 15, 16]. Our examinations revealed a clear correlation between the amount of involvement of the SLN and the probability of finding metastases in further lymph nodes. Since no adjuvant therapies for the eradication of melanoma cells currently exist, a radical lymph node section must follow the identification of tumor cells in a SLN.

The preoperative lymphoscintigraphy is very important regarding the sensitivity of this procedure, with the radiotracer having a decisive influence. Technetium-labeled human albumin seems to be the best defined substance concerning particle size (1.15). Immediately after injection of the radiotracer, early images in at least two projections should be performed [22]. These reveal the lymphatic flow to the SLNs. Imaging should be repeated as long as the lymphatic pathway leads into the first lymph node; this is the sentinel node and is marked as such on the skin. In some cases drainages leading into one or several different lymph nodes can be seen; these so-called interval lymph nodes can cause difficulties in the interpretation. They occur especially in patients with pre-excised melanomas and may not have any filter function, or are only lacunae of lymph vessels. On the one hand, interval lymph nodes are hot spots that cannot be detected after a short period of time. On the other hand, these are lymph nodes that lie in between the primary tumor and the regional lymph node station and thus have true sentinel characteristics.

Intraoperative localization of the SLN by γ-probe guidance, facilitated by use of patent blue V dye, is the method of choice [2–6, 9, 12, 13, 20]. In the facial and cervical regions, we do not use dye injection, as the operation site becomes unclear due to diffusion of the dye into deeper layers and the risk of a permanent blue dye tattoo in these sites. However, these complications are rare – we have seen them only twice, but they have also been described by other authors [14]. Obligate is the blue/green coloring of the urine, in one case we observed a blue coloring of the whole body in a slender patient.

The use of blue dye only for detection of the SLN is, in our opinion, not acceptable. The SLN is not always stained blue, and the intraoperative localization does not always succeed, even when performed by very experienced surgeons [2, 5, 14]. Especially when the SLN is located in the axillary or cervical region, the blue dye method often fails. Other disadvantages are the higher complication rate caused by the necessity of lifting greater skin flaps, and a longer learning curve for the surgeon. In our collective, all sentinels that were stained blue also harvested the radiotracer. Additional blue but not radioactively labeled lymph nodes never occurred. Other groups reported the same results [2, 15]. The γ-probe-guided technique, however, is much easier to learn and simpler to perform. By the exact spatial resolution of the γ-probe, the SLN can be localized also in difficult anatomic regions, so that a tissue-sparing removal is possible. Very small incisions can be performed leading to good cosmetic results. Moreover, this procedure can, in many cases, be performed under local anesthesia. We could detect all SLNs without any problems, except for two in patients with primary tumors on the neck and a second SLN in the supraclavicular region. Here the radioactive background was so high that no differentiation of the SLN was possible. The supraclavicular region often leads to problems because of infiltration of the radiotracer into deep tissue [1, 15].

Our complication rate is negligible. We never observed late complications; some patients developed small seromas or hematomas after the SLNE that could be cured by current therapeutic modalities.

Often we hear questions about radiation exposure for the surgeons; however, we never registered any significant radiation exposure on our ring dosimeters.

Although the follow-up period is relatively short, a positive tendency can be seen. Local recurrences after SLNE are rare (0–1.5%) [5, 14]. We observed only one such incident in a group of 214 patients. This was a lymph node recurrence in the groin after SLNE with negative SLN. A possible explanation could be that the patient's melanoma was pre-excised with a large safety margin. This operation could have changed the drainage conditions, so that the lymphatic drainage led to another lymph node that we falsely regarded as the sentinel.

Summarizing, it can be said that the SLNE is a milestone in the surgery of melanomas. This technique allows an exact staging and spares early removal of the regional lymph nodes in patients with proven lymph node metastases. Nonetheless, the value of this method concerning survival time has yet to be evaluated.

References

1. Alazraki N, Eshima D, Eshima L et al. (1997) Lymphoscintigraphy, the sentinel node concept, and the intraoperative gamma probe in melanoma, breast cancer and other potential cancers. Sem Nucl Med 27:55–67
2. Albertini JJ, Cruse CW, Rapaport D et al. (1996) Intraoperative radio-lympho-scintigraphy improves sentinel lymph node identification for patients with melanoma. Ann Surg 223:217–224
3. Alex JC, Krag DN (1993) Gamma-probe-guided localization of lymph nodes. Surg Oncol 2:137–144
4. Bachter D, Balda BR, Vogt H, Büchels H Die "sentinel"-Lymphonodektomie mittels Szintillationsdetektor. Hautarzt 1996; 47:754–58
5. Bachter D, Balda BR, Vogt H, Büchels H (1998) Primary therapy of malignant melanomas: sentinel lymphadenectomy. Int J Derm 37:101–105
6. Büchels H, Vogt H, Bachter D (1997) Szintillationsgesteuerte Sentinel-Lymphadenektomie beim malignen Melanom. Chirurg 68:45–50
7. Balch CM (1988) The role of elective lymph node dissection in melanoma: rationale, results and controversies. J Clin Oncol 6:163–172
8. Cochran AJ, Wen DR, Morton DL (1998 Occult tumor cells in the lymph nodes of patients with pathological stage I malignant mela- noma: an immunohistochemical study. Am J Surg Path) 12:612–618

9. Glass FL, Messina JL, Cruse W et al. (1996) The use of intraoperative radiolymphoscintigraphy for sentinel node biopsy in patients with malignant melanoma. Dermatol Surg 22:715–720
10. Godellas CV, Berman CG, Lyman G et al. (1995) The identification and mapping of melanoma regional nodal metastases: Minimal invasive surgery for the diagnosis of nodal metastases. Am Surg 61:97–101
11. Heller R, Becker J, Waselle J et al. Detection of submicroscopic lymph node metastases in patients with melanoma. Arch Surg 1991; 126:1455–1460
12. Krag DN, Meijer SJ, Weaver DL (1995) Minimal-access surgery for staging of malignant melanoma. Arch Surg 130:654–658
13. Leong SPL, Steinmetz I, Habib FA et al. (1997) Optimal selective sentinel lymph node dissection in primary malignant melanoma. Arch Surg 132:666–673
14. Morton DL, Wen DR, Wong JH (1992) et al. Technical details of intraoperative lymphatic mapping for early stage melanoma. Arch Surg 127:392–399
15. Pijpers R, Borgstein PJ, Meijer S et al. (1997) Sentinel node biopsy in melanoma patients: Dynamic lymphoscintigraphy followed by intraoperative gamma probe and vital dye guidance. World J Surg 21:788–793
16. Reintgen D, Cruse CW, Wells K et al. (1994) The orderly progression of melanoma nodal metastases. Ann Surg 220:759–767
17. Sim FH, Taylor WF, Pritchard DJ, Soule E (1986) Lympadenectomy in the management of stage I malignant melanoma: a prospective randomized study. Mayo Clin Proc 61:697–705
18. Starz H, Balda BR, Büchels H (1998) Sentinel-Lymphonodektomie bei malignen Melanomen. Eine vorläufige Bilanz aus histomorphologischer Sicht. In: Garbe C, Rassner G (eds) Dermatologie. Leitlinien und Qualitätssicherunng für Diagnostik und Therapie. Springer, Berlin Heidelberg New York, pp 274–277
19. Uren RF, Howman-Giles RB, Shaw HM, Thompson JF, Mc Carthy WH (1993) Lymphoscintigraphy in high-risk melanoma of the trunk: predicting draining node groups, defining lymphatic channels and locating the sentinel node. J Nucl Med 34:1435–1440
20. Veen van der H, Hoekstra OS, Paul MA, Cuesta MA, Meijer S (1994) Gamma probe-guided sentinel node biopsy to select patients with melanoma for lymphadenectomy. Br J Surg 81:1769–1770
21. Veronesi U, Adamus J, Bandiera DC et al. (1997) Inefficacy of immediate node dissection in stage I melanoma of the limbs. N Engl J Med 297:627–630
22. Vogt H, Bachter D, Büchels H et al. (1999) Nachweis des Sentinel-Lymphknotens mittels präoperativer Lymphszintigraphie und intraoperativer Gammasondenmessung bei malignem Melanom. Nuklearmedizin 38:95–100
23. Wang X, Heller R, VanVoorhis N et al. (1994) Detection of submicroscopic lymph node metastases with polymerase chain reaction in patients with malignant melanoma. Ann Surg 220:768–774

Detection of Micrometastasis in Sentinel Lymph Nodes of Patients with Primary Cutaneous Melanoma

H.-J. Blaheta, B. Schittek, H. Breuninger, and C. Garbe

Department of Dermatology, Section of Dermatological Oncology, Eberhard-Karls-University, Liebermeister Strasse 25, 72076 Tübingen, Germany

Abstract

The technique of sentinel lymph node (SLN) biopsy has been demonstrated to be highly predictive for the detection of melanoma micrometastases in the regional lymph node basin. Therefore, the SLN was proposed to accurately reflect the lymph node status of patients with primary cutaneous melanoma. As the regional lymph node status is one of the most powerful predictors of survival in patients with primary melanoma, the histopathologic assessment is critically important for accurate staging. In approximately 20% (ranging from 9% to 42%) of patients with primary melanoma, the SLN was found to be tumor-positive by histopathology or immunohistochemistry. However, the true incidence of metastatic melanoma cells in (sentinel) lymph nodes is underestimated by histopathologic examination. Recently, the method of reverse transcription-polymerase chain reaction (RT-PCR) for tyrosinase mRNA has been used as a molecular marker for the presence of melanoma cells. Tyrosinase RT-PCR was demonstrated to significantly increase the detection of melanoma cells in SLNs as compared to histopathology. All lymph nodes positive by histopathology were shown to express tyrosinase by RT-PCR. Furthermore, tyrosinase transcripts were also detected in 36–52% of stage I and II melanoma patients with SLNs negative by histopathology. Importantly, the recurrence rate was significantly higher in patients with histologically negative SLNs who were found to be positive by RT-PCR than in patients with negative results by both techniques. These findings indicate that RT-PCR status of the SLN is more sensitive for detection of minimal melanoma disease than histopathology. Therefore, the RT-PCR status of the SLN may be suitable to improve melanoma staging and may serve as a prognostic factor in patients with primary cutaneous melanoma.

Recent Results in Cancer Research, Vol. 158

Introduction

The most powerful prognostic factor for patients with primary cutaneous melanoma is Breslow's tumor thickness (Breslow 1970). However, once patients develop regional lymph node metastasis, histopathologic features of the primary melanoma no longer contribute significantly to survival prediction. In this tumor stage, the extent of nodal involvement and the number of metastatic lymph nodes are strongly associated with unfavorable survival rates (Balch 1996; Buzaid 1995). Therefore, the regional lymph node status is one of the most powerful predictors of survival and prognosis for patients with melanoma (Balch 1996; Balch 1992).

The technique of sentinel lymph node (SLN) biopsy was developed as a minimally invasive technique of nodal tumor staging for melanoma patients with clinically negative regional lymph nodes (Morton 1992). The SLN is defined as the first lymph node in the regional lymph node basin that drains the site of the primary tumor. Previous studies have shown that the histologic status of the SLN reflects the status of the entire nodal basin, especially if the SLN is tumor-negative (Morton 1992, 1993; Reintgen 1994; Thompson 1995). As nodal tumor staging and therapeutic decisions are based on the SLN examination, the detection of melanoma cells is of critical importance.

More detailed histopathologic analysis of (sentinel) lymph nodes by immunohistochemistry has been demonstrated to improve the detection of occult melanoma cells. Approximately 10% of patients negative by routine histopathology using H&E staining are found positive after immunohistochemical examinations and serial sectioning (Cochran 1988; Yu 1999). However, the true incidence of occult melanoma micrometastases will be frequently underestimated. More recently, the technique of reverse transcription-polymerase chain reaction (RT-PCR) of tyrosinase mRNA was applied to the detection of micrometastatic melanoma in (sentinel) lymph nodes (Wang 1994; Van der Velde-Zimmermann 1996). The clinical relevance, however, of detecting minimal residual disease by RT-PCR in SLNs of patients with primary cutaneous melanoma has not been clearly established.

Examination of Sentinel Lymph Nodes by Histopathology and Immunohistochemistry

Standard pathologic assessment of (sentinel) lymph nodes usually consists of examining one to two H&E-stained sections of the central cut surface. Using this limited examination of (sentinel) lymph node specimens, the number of patients with microscopic disease will be frequently underestimated. In fact, in up to 12–14% of patients with (sentinel) lymph nodes found negative by routine H&E staining, occult microscopic metastases were identified immunohistochemically (Table 1). Up to now, a large number of studies has been performed, mostly using standard H&E staining in combination with immunohistochemistry for SLN analysis. Approximately 20% of stage I and II mel-

Table 1. Detection of melanoma micrometastasis (not identified by H&E) in (sentinel) lymph nodes by immunohistochemical examination in stage I and II melanoma patients

Reference	Markers	No. of patients	No. of positive patients
Cochran et al. 1988	S-100	100	14/100 (14%)
Yu et al. 1999	S-100, HMB-45, NK1C3, MART-1	94	11/94 (12%)

Table 2. Detection of melanoma micrometastasis in sentinel lymph nodes by histopathology in stage I and II melanoma patients

Reference	Markers	No. of patients	No. of positive patients
Morton et al. 1992	H&E, S-100, NKIC3	194	40/194 (21%)
Reintgen et al. 1994	H&E, S-100[a], HMB-45[a]	42	8/42 (19%)
Krag et al. 1995	H&E	118	15/118 (13%)
Pijpers et al. 1995	H&E, S-100, HMB-45	41	8/41 (20%)
Thompson et al. 1995	H&E	105	22/105 (21%)
Albertini et al. 1996	H&E, S-100, HMB-45	106	16/106 (15%)
Glass et al. 1996	H&E	132	31/132 (23%)
Leong et al. 1997	H&E, S-100[a]	160	30/160 (66%)
Gogel et al. 1998	H&E, S-100[a], HMB-45[a]	68	6/68 (9%)
Mraz-Gernhardt et al. 1998	H&E, S-100, HMB-45	215	64/215 (21%)
Shivers et al. 1998	H&E	114	23/114 (20%)
Blaheta et al. 1999	H&E, S-100, HMB-45	73	13/73 (18%)
Bostick et al. 1999	H&E, S-100, HMB-45	72	17/72 (24%)
Gershenwald et al. 1999	H&E, S-100, HMB-45	580	85/580 (15%)
Lukowsky et al. 1999	H&E, S-100	24	10/24 (42%)

[a] Not routinely performed.

anoma patients (ranging from 9% to 42%) were found to have microscopic metastases in the SLNs (Table 2). However, different immunohistochemical markers were used in these studies to detect melanoma.

The HMB-45 antibody, as one of the most commonly used markers, has been shown to be highly specific for melanocytic differentiation, improving the detection of melanoma (Gown 1986; Colombari 1988). Therefore, the HMB-45 antibody has long been considered as the "gold standard" for immunohistochemical detection of melanoma cells. However, the HMB-45 antibody is less sensitive for melanoma detection than S-100 protein.

The antibody for S-100 protein is frequently used as a second marker. This antibody is considered to be the most sensitive immunohistochemical marker for cells of melanocytic differentiation (Cochran 1988). However, S-100 protein may stain resident cells in lymph nodes, in particular dendritic reticulum cells, but may also stain some sinus macrophages, and occasionally Schwann cells in node-associated nerves (Cochran 1988). Due to this low specificity, interpretation of positive S-100 staining is difficult. This is especially a problem if only small deposits of tumor cells are present without suspicious cytological characteristics.

More recently, the monoclonal antibody to Melan-A/MART-1 (melanoma antigen recognized by T cells), a melanocytic specific transmembrane protein, has been added for the detection of micrometastatic melanoma cells (Busam 1998; Jungbluth 1998; Fetsch 1999). The expression of MART-1 and HMB-45 has been evaluated in metastatic melanoma lesions (Fetsch 1999). In lesions that stained for both markers (82%), immunoreactivity was demonstrated for MART-1 in 92% of lesions and for HMB-45 in 84% of lesions. Furthermore, the intensity and the percentage of stained cells were stronger and higher using MART-1 as compared to HMB-45. MART-1 expression was not observed in control samples of normal tissue, except melanocytes in normal skin that stained positively for MART-1. Therefore, the Melan-A/MART-1 antibody appears to have a sensitivity and specificity for metastatic melanoma superior to that of HMB-45 (Kageshita 1997; Fetsch 1999; Yu 1999).

Examination of Sentinel Lymph Nodes by Molecular Analysis

Using RT-PCR-based methods, specific tumor markers are identified with a significantly higher sensitivity as compared to histopathology. Tyrosinase, a key enzyme in melanin biosynthesis, is apparently a specific marker for cells derived from the melanocytic lineage (Kwon 1987). Therefore, tyrosinase RT-PCR has been used for the detection of lymph node micrometastasis in patients with primary cutaneous melanoma (Wang 1994; Van der Velde-Zimmermann 1996; Blaheta 1998, 1999; Shivers 1998; Bostick 1999).

Using this extremely sensitive RT-PCR technique, 49–66% of patients with primary cutaneous melanoma were identified with (sentinel) lymph nodes positive for tyrosinase or other melanoma-specific markers (Table 3). Except one study, all (sentinel) lymph nodes positive by histopathology or immunohistochemistry were demonstrated to express tyrosinase. Bostick and co-

Table 3. Detection of melanoma micrometastasis in (sentinel) lymph nodes by RT-PCR in stage I and II melanoma patients

Reference	Markers	No. of patients	No. of positive patients	No. of positive patients detected exclusively by RT-PCR
Wang et al. 1994	Tyrosinase	29	19/29 (66%)	8/18 (44%)
Velde-Zimmermann et al. 1996	Tyrosinase	16	10/16 (62%)	6/12 (50%)
Blaheta et al. 1998	Tyrosinase	79	52/79 (66%)	21/48 (44%)
Shivers et al. 1998	Tyrosinase	114	70/114 (61%)	47/91 (52%)
Blaheta et al. 1999	Tyrosinase	73	44/73 (66%)	23/60 (38%)
Bostick et al. 1999	Tyrosinase, MAGE-3, MART-1	72	35/72 (49%)	20/55 (36%)

workers showed expression of melanoma markers by RT-PCR in 16 of 17 patients (94%) with SLNs positive by histopathology (Bostick 1999). Moreover, tyrosinase transcripts were still detected in 36–52% of patients with (sentinel) lymph nodes negative by histopathology (Table 3). These results demonstrate that tyrosinase RT-PCR is able to detect cells of melanocytic origin with a sensitivity significantly higher than that achieved by histopathology and immunohistochemistry.

The specificity of tyrosinase RT-PCR was tested by analyzing lymph nodes and lymph node aspirates obtained from patients without melanoma (Blaheta 1998; Van der Velde-Zimmermann 1996; Schwuerzer-Voit 1996; Hatta 1998, 1999; Bostick 1999). Summarizing the results of these studies, a total of 120 control lymph nodes and six control lymph node aspirates were demonstrated negative for tyrosinase expression, documenting the specificity of this assay.

Advantages and Disadvantages of the Molecular Analysis in Addition to Histopathologic Examination

It has been demonstrated that metastatic melanoma cells are preferentially located in the subcapsular sinus at the hilum of the lymph node (Cochran 1988; Yu 1999). Further lymph node analysis by serial sectioning was demonstrated to be only of minor diagnostic value for detecting occult melanoma (Cochran 1988; Morton 1992). Due to the focal nature of melanoma micrometastases, it is of major importance to analyze especially the hilus region of the sentinel lymph node for metastatic melanoma cells. Examination of this central region of the sentinel lymph node by both diagnostic methods will lead to the highest concordance in comparing histopathology to RT-PCR. Accordingly, most of the previous studies have bisected the lymph nodes along the long axis, with special emphasis given to each cut surface that was analyzed separately (Wang 1994; Shivers 1998; Blaheta 1999). In addition, this lymph node preparation is the most practical technique for a routinely performed melanoma staging procedure like the SLN biopsy.

However, in principle, the same lymph node tissue cannot be analyzed simultaneously by histopathology and RT-PCR for detection of metastatic melanoma. Therefore, sampling error may occur when the lymph node is bisected for separate histopathologic and RT-PCR analysis. However, a high concordance of histopathology and RT-PCR was shown by detection of tyrosinase mRNA in all (sentinel) lymph nodes found positive by histopathology (Wang 1994; Blaheta 1998, 1999; Shivers 1998). In addition, tyrosinase transcripts were also detected in 36–52% of stage I and II melanoma patients with (sentinel) lymph nodes negative by histopathology (Table 3).

However, one cannot expect that all of the patients with positive RT-PCR findings suggesting the presence of minimal residual disease will subsequently develop melanoma progression. In fact, metastases will be expected (only) in about 25–30% of patients with primary cutaneous melanoma (Breslow's tumor thickness >1 mm; Garbe 1995; Buttner 1995). What is the reason for the discrepancy between the (high) rate of positive RT-PCR findings and the (low) rate of patients who are expected to develop melanoma progression? Is the extreme sensitivity of RT-PCR a reason for false-positive results, and may therefore occult melanoma be overdiagnosed?

One source for false-positive detection of tyrosinase mRNA might be the presence of benign capsular melanocytic nevi in tumor-draining lymph nodes. Nodal nevocytes have been described in approximately 10% of patients (Bautista 1994; Shivers 1998; Blaheta 1999). SLNs with benign nevus cells found in the half assessed for histopathology were classified negative for metastatic disease regardless of the RT-PCR findings. However, the presence of nodal nevocytes does not exclude minimal residual disease in the part of the lymph node used for RT-PCR. On the other hand, the absence of nodal nevi in the half examined by histopathology does not exclude nevocytes in the part of the lymph node used for RT-PCR. Nonetheless, this approach will reduce false-positive tyrosinase RT-PCR results. Interestingly, not all lymph nodes with capsular nevi were found positive for tyrosinase (unpublished data).

Finally, the presence of melanoma-specific markers identified by RT-PCR only appears to detect minimal tumor burden and does not necessary indicate autonomous tumor cell proliferation. Determination of the tumor burden by quantitative RT-PCR may become a helpful technique to further classify melanoma patients with positive findings by RT-PCR only.

Different reports have demonstrated that sentinel lymph node analysis by RT-PCR in combination with histopathology is able to improve the detection of occult melanoma cells. Therefore, the benefit of RT-PCR analysis obtaining a more accurate nodal staging may justify that (a small part) of lymph node tissue is not available for histopathologic examinations.

Clinical Impact of the Detection of Micrometastases in Regional Lymph Nodes

The prognostic significance of micrometastases in regional lymph nodes of patients with early stage melanoma (AJCC stages I and II) is well established and is associated with a dramatic decrease of the 5-year survival rate to 50% (Balch 1992). Therefore, it has long been known that the regional lymph node status is one of the most powerful predictors of survival and prognosis for patients with cutaneous melanoma (Buzaid 1995; Balch 1996). Accordingly, the sensitive detection of melanoma cells in the SLNs is of major importance to obtain an accurate staging and for selecting patients for adjuvant therapy and clinical follow-up procedures. Performing more extensive analysis of SLNs by immunohistochemistry and RT-PCR can enhance the detection of melanoma cells as compared to standard histopathology (Wang 1994; Shivers 1998). However, the question of whether the presence of melanoma cells exclusively detected by RT-PCR reliably indicates subsequent tumor recurrence has not been clearly answered. Recently, a significant decrease in disease-free survival and overall survival was demonstrated for patients with histologically negative SLNs who were upstaged by positive RT-PCR as compared to those with negative findings by both methods (Shivers 1998). We were able to confirm the clinical relevance of RT-PCR detection of melanoma cells in SLNs of patients with primary cutaneous melanoma (unpublished data). In our study, we found that recurrence rates were significantly higher in patients with submicroscopic tumor cells than in patients with negative RT-PCR examination ($P=0.01$). Therefore, tyrosinase RT-PCR, in addition to histopathology, for SLN analysis identifies clinically relevant, minimal residual disease in patients with primary melanoma. More recently, another study was able to demonstrate that patients with histopathologically negative SLNs who were positive by a multiple-marker RT-PCR were at increased risk of tumor recurrence (Bostick 1999). These data indicate that the staging procedure of SLN biopsy combined with the highly sensitive RT-PCR assay is a promising approach to improve tumor staging and prognostication of patients with primary cutaneous melanoma.

Conclusions

It has been well established that the histologic detection of lymph node micrometastases is the most important prognostic factor in patients with primary melanoma. However, even a more detailed, histopathologic lymph node examination by immunohistochemistry will underestimate the true incidence of occult metastatic disease. Previous studies have shown that tyrosinase RT-PCR is able to detect melanoma cells in lymph nodes with a significantly higher sensitivity than that achieved by histopathology. Determination of the clinical impact of minimal residual disease in SLNs detected exclusively by RT-PCR requires long-term follow-up of these patients. In our own study, we found that, after a median follow-up period of 19 months, tumor relapse was significantly higher in patients with histologically negative SLNs who were positive by RT-PCR than in patients with negative results by both techniques (unpublished data). These data are in concordance with a recent study of Shivers et al. (1998), demonstrating the clinical significance of RT-PCR detection of melanoma cells in SLNs after a similar follow-up time. These early findings indicate that RT-PCR analysis of the SLN more accurately reflects the outcome of patients with primary melanoma than does the histopathologic examination. Therefore, the RT-PCR status of the SLN may be suitable to improve melanoma staging and may serve as powerful prognostic factor in patients with primary cutaneous melanoma.

Acknowledgements. This study was supported in part by a grant from the Fortune program of the University of Tuebingen, Germany (no. 1260065).

References

Albertini JJ, Cruse CW, Rapaport D, Wells K, Ross M, DeConti R, Berman CG, Jared K, Messina J, Lyman G, Glass F, Fenske N, Reintgen DS (1996) Intraoperative radiolymphoscintigraphy improves sentinel lymph node identification for patients with melanoma. Ann Surgery 223:217–224

Balch CM, Soong S, Shaw HM, Urist MM, and McCarthy SW (1992) An analysis of prognostic factors in 8500 patients with cutaneous melanoma. In: Balch C (ed) ed 2. JB Lippincott, Philadelphia, Cutaneous melanoma 165–187

Balch CM, Soong SJ, Bartolucci AA, Urist MM, Karakousis CP, Smith TJ, Temple WJ, Ross MI, Jewell WR, Mihm MC, Barnhill RL, Wanebo HJ (1996) Efficacy of an elective regional lymph node dissection of 1 to 4 mm thick melanomas for patients 60 years of age and younger. Ann Surg 224:255–263

Bautista NC, Cohen S, Anders KH (1994) Benign melanocytic nevus cells in axillary lymph nodes. A prospective incidence and immunohistochemical study with literature review. Am J Clin Pathol 102:102–108

Blaheta H-J, Schittek B, Breuninger H, Maczey E, Kroeber S, Sotlar K, Ellwanger U, Thelen MH, Rassner G, Bultmann B, Garbe C (1998) Lymph node micrometastases of cutaneous melanoma: Increased sensitivity of molecular diagnosis in comparison to immunohistochemistry. Int J Cancer 79:318–323

Blaheta H-J, Schittek B, Breuninger H, Sotlar K, Ellwanger U, Thelen MH, Mazcey E, Rassner G, Bueltmann B, Garbe C (1999) Detection of melanoma micrometastasis in sentinel nodes by RT-PCR correlates with tumor thickness and is predictive for micrometastatic disease in the lymph node basin. Am J Surg Pathol 23:822–828

Bostick PJ, Morton DL, Turner RR, Huynh KT, Wang HJ, Elashoff R, Essner R, Hoon DSB (1999) Prognostic significance of occult metastases detected by sentinel lymphadenectomy and reverse transcriptase-polymerase chain reaction in early-stage melanoma patients. J Clin Oncol 17:3238–3244

Breslow A (1970) Thickness, cross-sectional areas and depth of invasion in the prognosis of cutaneous melanoma. Ann Surg 172:902–908

Busam KJ, Chen YT, Old LJ, Stockert E, Iversen K, Coplan KA, Rosai J, Barnhill RL, Jungbluth AA (1998) Expression of Melan-A (MART1) in benign melanocytic nevi and primary cutaneous malignant melanoma. Am J Surg Pathol 22:976–982

Buettner P, Garbe C, Bertz J, Burg G, d'Hoedt B, Drepper H, Guggenmoos Holzmann I, Lechner W, Lippold A, Orfanos CE et al. (1995) Primary cutaneous melanoma. Optimized cutoff points of tumor thickness and importance of Clark's level for prognostic classification. Cancer 75:2499–2506

Buzaid AC, Tinoco L, Ross MI, Legha SS, Benjamin RS (1995) Role of computed tomography in the staging of patients with local-regional metastases of melanoma. J Clin Oncol 13:2104–2108

Cochran AJ, Wen DR, Morton DL (1988) Occult tumor cells in the lymph nodes of patients with pathological stage I malignant melanoma. An immunohistological study. Am J Surg Pathol 12:612–618

Colombari R, Bonetti F, Zamboni G, Scarpa A, Marino F, Tomezzoli A, Capelli P, Menestrina F, Chilosi M, Fiore DL (1988) Distribution of melanoma specific antibody (HMB-45) in benign and malignant melanocytic tumours. An immunohistochemical study on paraffin sections. Virchows Arch A Pathol Anat Histopathol 413:17–24

Fetsch PA, Marincola FM, Filie A, Hijazi YM, Kleiner DE, Abati A (1999) Melanoma-associated antigen recognized by T cells (MART-1) – The advent of a preferred immunocytochemical antibody for the diagnosis of metastatic malignant melanoma with fine-needle aspiration. Cancer Cytopathol 87:37–42

Garbe C, Buettner P, Bertz J, Burg G, d'Hoedt B, Drepper H, Guggenmoos-Holzmann I, Lechner W, Lippold A, Orfanos CE (1995) Primary cutaneous melanoma. Identification of prognostic groups and estimation of individual prognosis for 5093 patients. Cancer 75:2484–2491

Gershenwald JE, Thompson W, Mansfield PF, Lee JE, Colome MI, Tseng CH, Lee JJ, Balch CM, Reintgen DS, Ross MI (1999) Multi-institutional melanoma lymphatic mapping experience: The prognostic value of sentinel lymph node status in 612 stage I or II melanoma patients. J Clin Oncol 17:976–983

Glass LF, Messina JL, Cruse W, Wells K, Rapaport D, Miliotes G, Berman C, Reintgen D, Fenske NA (1996) The use of intraoperative radiolymphoscintigraphy for sentinel node biopsy in patients with malignant melanoma. Dermatol Surg 22:715–720

Gogel BM, Kuhn JA, Ferry KM, Fisher TL, Preskitt JT, O' Brien JC, Lieberman ZH, Stephens JS, Krag DN (1998) Sentinel lymph node biopsy for melanoma. Am J Surg 176:544–547

Gown AM, Vogel AM, Hoak D, Gough F, McNutt MA (1986) Monoclonal antibodies specific for melanocytic tumors distinguish subpopulations of melanocytes. Am J Pathol 123:195–203

Hatta N, Fujimoto A, Takehara K, Takata M (1999) Mapping of occult melanoma micrometastases in the inguinal lymph node basin by immunohistochemistry and RT-PCR. Melanoma Res 9:401–406

Hatta N, Takata M, Takehara K, Ohara K (1998) Polymerase chain reaction and immunohistochemistry frequently detect occult melanoma cells in regional lymph nodes of melanoma patients. J Clin Pathol 51:597–601

Jungbluth AA, Busam KJ, Gerald WL, Stockert E, Coplan KA, Iversen K, MacGregor DP, Old LJ, Chen YT (1998) A103: An anti-Melan-A monoclonal antibody for the detection of malignant melanoma in paraffin-embedded tissues. Am J Surg Pathol 22:595–602

Kageshita T, Kawakami Y, Hirai S, Ono T (1997) Differential expression of MART-1 in primary and metastatic melanoma lesions. J Immunother 20:460–465

Krag DN, Meijer SJ, Weaver DL, Loggie BW, Harlow SP, Tanabe KK, Laughlin EH, Alex JC (1995) Minimal-access surgery for staging of malignant melanoma. Arch Surg 130:654–658

Kwon BS, Haq AK, Pomerantz SH, Halaban R (1987) Isolation and sequence of a cDNA clone for human tyrosinase that maps at the mouse c-albino locus. Proc Natl Acad Sci USA 84:7473–7477

Leong SPL, Steinmetz I, Habib FA, McMillan A, Gans JZ, Allen RE, Morita ET, ElKadi M, Epstein HD, KashaniSabet M, Sagebiel RW (1997) Optimal selective sentinel lymph node dissection in primary malignant melanoma. Arch Surg 132:666–673

Lukowsky A, Bellmann B, Ringk A, Winter H, Audring H, Fenske S, Sterry W (1999) Detection of melanoma micrometastases in the sentinel lymph node and in nonsentinel nodes by tyrosinase polymerase chain reaction. J Invest Dermatol 113:554–559

Morton DL, Wen DR, Foshag LJ, Essner R, Cochran A (1993) Intraoperative lymphatic mapping and selective cervical lymphadenectomy for early-stage melanomas of the head and neck. J Clin Oncol 11:1751–1756

Morton DL, Wen DR, Wong JH, Economou JS, Cagle LA, Storm FK, Foshag LJ, Cochran AJ (1992) Technical details of intraoperative lymphatic mapping for early stage melanoma. Arch Surg 127:392–399

MrazGernhard S, Sagebiel RW, KashaniSabet M, Miller JR, Leong SPL (1998) Prediction of sentinel lymph node micrometastasis by histological features in primary cutaneous malignant melanoma. Arch Dermatol 134:983–987

Pijpers R, Collet GJ, Meijer S, Hoekstra OS (1995) The impact of dynamic lymphoscintigraphy and gamma probe guidance on sentinel node biopsy in melanoma. Eur J Nucl Med 22:1238–1241

Reintgen D, Cruse CW, Wells K, Berman C, Fenske N, Glass F, Schroer K, Heller R, Ross M, Lyman G et al. (1994) The orderly progression of melanoma nodal metastases. Ann Surg 220:759–767

Schwuerzer-Voit M, Proebstle TM, Sterry W (1996) Identification of lymph node metastases by use of polymerase chain reaction (PCR) in melanoma patients. Eur J Cancer 32 A:264–268

Shivers SC, Wang XN, Li WG, Joseph E, Messina J, Glass LF, DeConti R, Cruse CW, Berman C, Fenske NA, Lyman GH, Reintgen DS (1998) Molecular staging of malignant melanoma: Correlation with clinical outcome. JAMA 280:1410–1415

Thompson JF, McCarthy WH, Bosch CM, O'Brien CJ, Quinn MJ, Paramaesvaran S, Crotty K, McCarthy SW, Uren RF, Howman Giles R (1995) Sentinel lymph node status as an indicator of the presence of metastatic melanoma in regional lymph nodes. Melanoma Res 5:255–260

Van der Velde-Zimmermann D, Roijers JF, Bouwens Rombouts A, De Weger RA, De Graaf PW, Tilanus MG, Van den Tweel JG (1996) Molecular test for the detection of tumor cells in blood and sentinel nodes of melanoma patients. Am J Pathol 149:759–764

Wang X, Heller R, VanVoorhis N, Cruse CW, Glass F, Fenske N, Berman C, Leo Messina J, Rappaport D, Wells K et al. (1994) Detection of submicroscopic lymph node metastases with polymerase chain reaction in patients with malignant melanoma. Ann Surg 220:768–774

Yu LL, Flotte TJ, Tanabe KK, Gadd MA, Cosimi AB, Sober AJ, Mihm MC, Duncan LM (1999) Detection of microscopic melanoma metastases in sentinel lymph nodes. Cancer 86:617–627

IV. Early Recognition and Monitoring by Serological Markers

Monitoring Malignant Melanoma with the S-100B Tumour Marker

J.M.G. Bonfrer and C.M. Korse

The Netherlands Cancer Institute (Antoni van Leeuwenhoek Huis), Amsterdam, The Netherlands

Abstract

To assess the usefulness of the S-100B tumour marker in monitoring therapy and during follow-up we measured S-100B serum concentration in 31 patients participating in a phase I trial studying the effect of vaccination with GM-CSF gene-transduced autologous tumour cells. The S-100B serum concentration before treatment is a strong independent prognostic factor for survival, as in this study the 11 patients with low (<0.16 μg/l) S-100B levels were at considerably lower risk for death. All patients alive at the end of the study ($n=8$) had a S-100B level within the reference range at the start of the study. At a level of 0.16 μg/l the presence of disease could be predicted with 99% certainty for 63% of the patients. Nine patients became progressive after a stable disease. In four of them S-100 increased over 50% before clinical observation of progression, giving a lead time of more than a month in 44% of cases. In patients who acquired a status of no clinical evidence of disease after treatment, the S-100B concentration invariably decreased by more than 100%.

Introduction

Malignant melanoma shows a rapidly increasing incidence in the western world. The affected age group is relatively young and the prognosis is poor when tumour thickness is more than 4 mm (Lee and Carter 1970). In fact, patients with lesions more than 2 mm and those with histologically involved regional lymph nodes are at risk of developing disseminated disease (Balch et al. 1979). For patients with metastatic disease, the prognosis is generally poor because responses to systemic therapy have been disappointingly low (Ahmann et al. 1989).

Standard chemotherapy has been dacarbazine (DTIC) as a single-agent regimen, with response rates of 20–25%, but a 6-month survival after the start of therapy occurs in only 5% of the cases (Lee et al. 1995). A different approach is to provide the host with antigens to develop an autoimmune response to melanoma cells. This active specific immunotherapy may be enhanced by vaccination of the patient. Transfection of autologous tumour with genes encoding cytokines may protect against challenge with wild-type tumour (McIllmurray et al. 1977). Routine clinical follow-up of the response to therapy is usually done following patient complaints and includes inspection of the treated regions. Additionally, a yearly or half-yearly CT scan may be done.

The S-100 protein was demonstrated to be expressed in cultured melanoma cells (Gaynor et al. 1980), and this opened the way for investigation into the presence of S-100 in a variety of tissues. As the protein was originally extracted from brain tissue, it was not surprising that the molecule was detected in tissues other than melanotic cells (Hakajima et al. 1982). The function of S-100 is not exactly known, but its biochemical properties strongly suggest that it activates cell processes along the Ca^{2+} signal-transduction pathway (Schäfer and Heizmann 1996). The availability of a sensitive test for the determination of S-100B protein in serum has resulted in several publications describing the relation between S-100B and the stage of the disease (Schoultz et al. 1996; Bei Guo et al. 1995). Later data showed that the S-100B serum concentration before treatment is a strong independent prognostic factor for survival (Bonfrer et al. 1998; Hansson et al. 1997). We have measured the S-100B concentration in serum from patients participating in a study performed at the Netherlands Cancer Institute to assess the usefulness of this tumour marker in monitoring the disease status during the follow-up period of this trial.

Materials and Methods

A dose-finding phase I trial to study the effect of vaccination with autologous tumour cells transduced with the GM-CSF gene was performed at the Netherlands Cancer Institute (Rankin et al. 1995). This study was carried out in cooperation with the Somatix Therapy Corporation (Alameda, Ca, USA). Patients were eligible to enter the study when their disease was not potentially curable. Renal and hepatic function had to be adequate and life expectancy had to be more than 3 months. Patients were to be followed at fixed times by physical examinations, laboratory tests, chest X-ray, ECG and CT scan, when this was clinically indicated. Clinical evaluation was performed according to WHO criteria. For our study, data from each patient who had undergone five or more S-100B determinations after the start of this trial were used in evaluation of the S-100B assay. As a result, we could include 31 patients (14 female) with a mean age of 49 years (27–70 years). The average follow-up period was 17 months with a range of 5–60 months. The total number of samples that was assayed for the S-100B concentration was 257 (range 6–25 per patient). All samples were analysed without knowledge of the clinical status of the patient.

S-100B Assay

The Sangtec S-100 luminescence immunoassay (LIA) is a two-site immunoluminometric test based on three monoclonal antibodies which specifically bind to the βb subunit of the S-100B protein. The assay detects the βbβb and αaβb dimer in serum (Nyberg et al. 1996). The standard range is 0.1–20 μg/l and a lower detection limit of 0.02 μg/l was established. Day to day variation was found to be 5% at the level of 1.0 μg/l as well as at 10 μg/l. The normal range for this assay was established in our laboratory as 0.16 μg/l (Bonfrer et al. 1998). Byk Sangtec advises a reference value of 0.12 μg/l (package insert).

Statistical Methods

Survival curves were performed using the procedure of Kaplan and Meier (1958).

Receiver operating characteristic (ROC) curves were plotted to show the sensitivity vs the specificity for a range of S-100B levels (Robertson and Zweig 1981).

Results

Of 31 patients monitored in this study, 23 (74%) died of their disease within the follow-up period. At the end of the study, four patients (13%) were still alive with no clinical evidence of disease (NED) and four (13%) were alive with tumour. The initial S-100B serum concentration before the start of the trial was above the reference level of 0.16 μg/l in 11 cases (35%), with a maximum of 159.3 μg/l. Twenty patients (65%) did not have an elevated S-100B serum level. If the cut-off level is set at the advised value of 0.12 μg/l, this number was 14 (45%), respectively 17 (55%). We investigated the prognostic power of an initially raised marker level in this group of patients with disseminated disease at the start of the study. The Kaplan-Meier survival curve of the S-100B serum level showed that patients with S-100B levels <0.16 μg/l at the start of the trial were at a considerably lower risk for death (Fig. 1). This curve is comparable to the curve using 0.12 μg/l as a dividing line. Life expectancy of patients entering the trial with an elevated S-100B level (≥ 0.16 μg/l) is a median 14 months, but with levels below this cut-off it is about 2 years. Moreover, all eight (26%) patients still alive at the end the follow-up period had a S-100B concentration within the reference range at the start of the study. Of this group four patients were alive with NED. In this

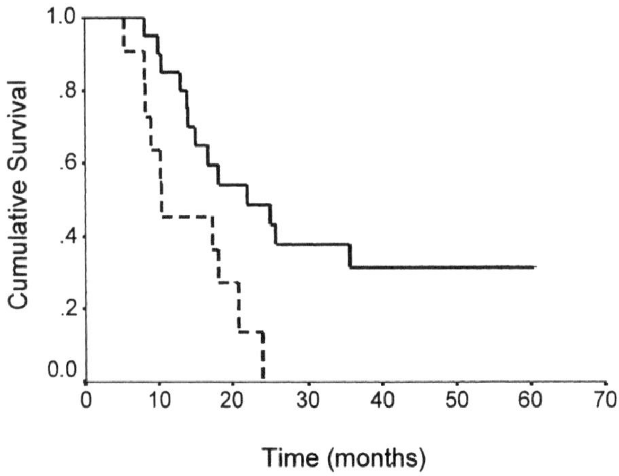

Fig. 1. Survival curve of all patients ($n=31$) according to the S-100B level before vaccination. A positive level (>0.16) was found in 11 patients. Difference is significant ($p=0.01$)

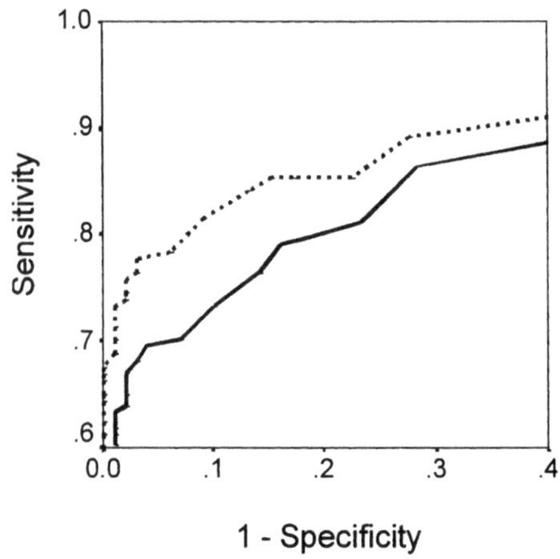

Fig. 2. Receiver operating characteristic (ROC) curves for S-100B in predicting disease progression (PD, *dotted line*) or presence of tumour (PR/SD/PD, *solid line*) compared to the group of patients with no evidence of disease

group, no elevated S-100B serum levels occurred during the follow-up period. The specificity/sensitivity ratio is shown in the ROC curve comparing S-100 levels indifferent subsets of the patient group (Fig. 2). To make a distinction between patients with NED or patients with clinically detectable tumour, the ROC curve shows that at a level of 0.10 µg/l it is possible to predict the presence of melanoma in 70% of the cases with a specificity of 95%. The ROC curve showing the patient group with NED and progression of disease (PD) only demonstrates an expected clearer disparity. To predict the clinically proven presence of disease with 99% certainty, 63% of the patients will then be identified by a serum S-100B level of 0.16 µg/l (Table 1). If this level is decreased to 0.12 µg/l the sensitivity is increased to 68% with a marginal loss of 2% specificity.

Table 1. Sensitivity and specificity ratio of S-100B at the indicated concentration for NED vs PD, NED vs PR/SD/PD and NED/PR/SD vs PD

	S-100B (µg/l)	Sensitivity (%)	Specificity (%)
NED vs PD	0.10	78	96
	0.12	76	94
	0.16	74	99
NED vs PR/SD/PD	0.10	70	99
	0.12	68	99
	0.16	63	99
NED/PR/SD vs PD	0.10	78	88
	0.12	77	90
	0.16	74	95

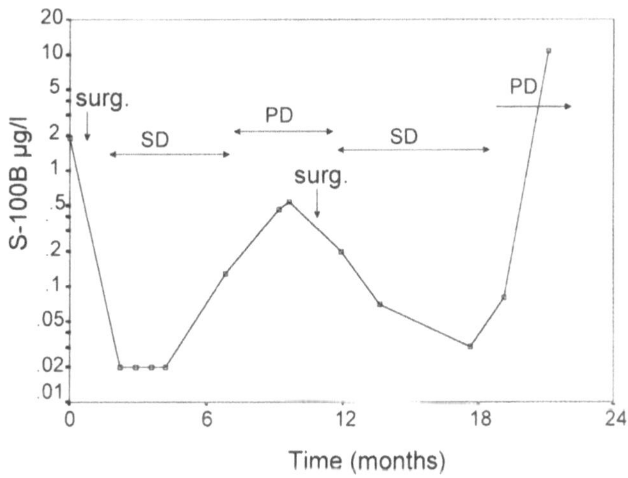

Fig. 3. Course of the S-100B serum levels in a patient with two biochemical remissions, clinically assessed as stable disease (*SD*). *PD*, progression of disease

In 20 patients (65%), the course of the disease remained unchanged during the period of monitoring. After the operation to obtain tumour tissue, four patients acquired a status of NED, which did not change during the study. The highest level of S-100B in this group was 0.07 µg/l. The median was <0.02 µg/l. All but one of the patients with continuous progression had overall increasing serum S-100B levels. In this single patient the S-100B protein was never detectable. In three patients (19%) with invariable PD, the S-100B concentration started to rise between 6 and 9 months after the clinically proven progression. In the remaining 12 patients (75%), the S-100B increase was sometimes irregular because palliative treatment caused intermittent decreases of the S-100B level. Eleven patients (35%) had a clinically demonstrable change in their disease status during the follow-up period. In two patients progression occurred again after a short partial remission (Fig. 3).

In four cases, newly detected melanoma was removed by surgery or treated with DTIC. In all four cases the S-100B level decreased by more than 100%. Of the nine patients who went into progression from a state of stable disease, six had serum S-100B concentrations that increased by 100% or more. An increase of S-100B of more than 50% was seen in four cases before the clinical observation of progression. This means that a positive lead time was seen in 4/9 (44%) of the cases. In two cases the S-100B concentration did not rise above 0.12 μg/l (3 in the case of 0.16 μg/l; Fig. 4). The last S-100B result of each individual patient in the given period of observation is given in Fig. 5.

Discussion

The introduction of the S-100B protein in the diagnostic procedures for patients with malignant melanoma was based on the demonstration of its presence in tumour tissue by immunohistochemical procedures using polyclonal antibodies (Cochran et al. 1982). The availability of monoclonal antibodies to S-100 subtypes provided a promising tool for implementing a more specific antibody. Cho proved the importance of measuring the S-100βb fraction as a parameter for the invasiveness of the tumour (Cho et al. 1990). The use of serum assays was initially restricted, since the tests were difficult to use in routine biochemistry, but as they were able to diagnose advanced cases of melanoma, the outlook for their use became promising (Fagnart et al. 1988; Missler and Wiesmann 1995). The first available commercial assay to detect S-100B was a rather insensitive immunoradiometric method (Bei Guo et al. 1995), but a sensitivity of 41% in stage IV malignant melanoma did confirm

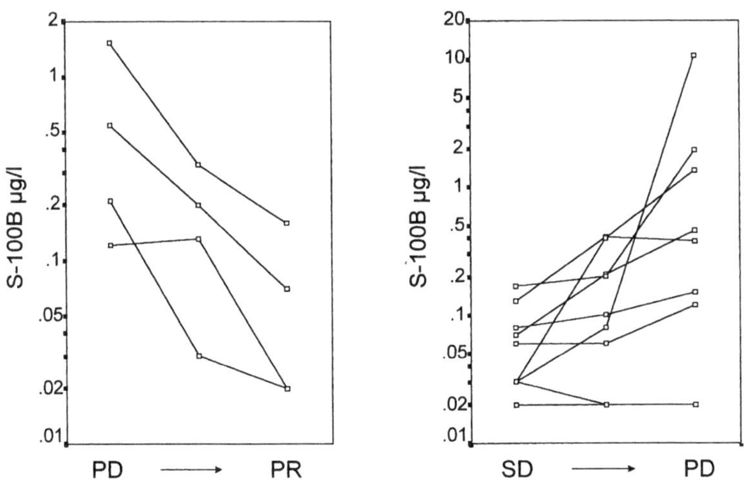

Fig. 4. Three consecutive determinations of S-100B in 13 patients during follow-up. Each measurement was done between 2 and 4 weeks after the previous test. *PD*, progression of disease; *PR*, partial response; *SD*, stable disease

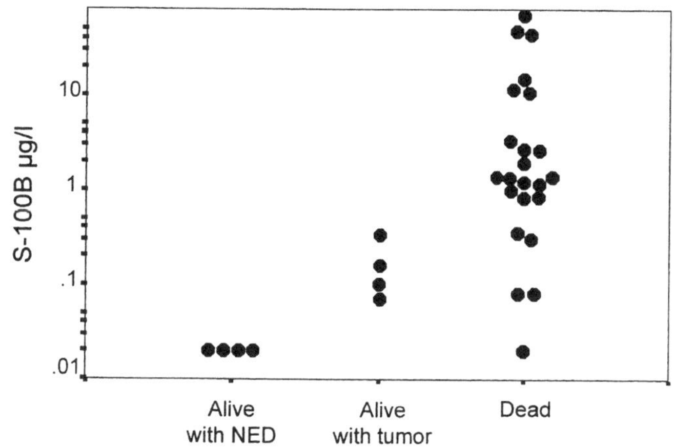

Fig. 5. The last available S-100B result of each patient ($n=31$) at the end of the follow-up period. *NED,* no evidence of disease

its possible use. Because healthy people invariably had S-100 levels below the detection level, it was necessary to improve the suitability of the assay. This study has been performed with a sensitive automated test with a detection limit of 0.02 µg/l, which is far below the reference level of 0.16 µg/l used in our laboratory (Bonfrer et al. 1998) or the 0.12 µg/l recommended by the manufacturer. This study confirms the earlier published finding that a positive serum S-100B concentration is a prognostic sign for poor longer survival (Bonfrer et al. 1998; Hansson et al. 1997). The availability of prognostic signs is an important factor in the decision to participate in various treatment programs or clinical trials. In this study, it was shown that also patients who are entering a phase I/II trial after previous treatment may be divided into subgroups with a good or bad prognosis, depending on their S-100B serum concentration. Thus, in future trials a certain level of S-100B should be included as inclusion or exclusion criterion. In many clinical trials assessing treatment of prostate cancer, the PSA level is now used as one of the biochemical endpoints of the study (Ellis et al. 1997). As noted above, the cut-off level in this study is somewhat higher than the level currently recommended by the manufacturer (0.12 µg/l). In our study, we showed that this difference has only a small impact on the results in terms of sensitivity and specificity in our group of patients. As expected, using 0.16 µg/l leads to a higher specificity if one compares patients with clinically detectable tumour and those with NED, but the significance of the difference between both levels is difficult to assess in this relatively small group with only a few patients in the latter group. The most important feature of tumour markers is their use in monitoring disease activity after treatment. Measuring S-100B levels after primary local surgical therapy may allow detection of early disease progression, and the failure of S-100B to decline to normal levels may be an early indication of persistent melanoma activity. Although the sensitivity of S-100B for low-stage disease seems rather low, this application is important in the follow-up of new surgical strategies, like lymphatic mapping and selective lymphadenectomy (Morton et al. 1992). An increasing S-100B level can be followed by a positive emission tomography (PET) scan to detect the presence of minimal residual disease, thereby leading to surgical dissection of the tumour and a subsequent increase in the life expectancy of melanoma patients (Böni et al. 1995). The search for an effective treatment to improve survival time has been the subject of many studies. Until now, the standard chemotherapy has been dacarbizine as a single agent, which gives response rates of 10–20% but without a proven prolongation of the median survival (Lee et al. 1998). An important new field of treatment is immunotherapy or a combination of immunotherapy with chemotherapy. The Somatix study (Rankin et al. 1995) was a phase I trial to try to generate a potent anti-tumour response. The clinical evaluation of this study is currently being carried out. The use of S-100B measurements does not seem to be hampered by the introduction of biological therapies. At least in this study, the administered biological therapy did not effect the use of the tumour marker. Our data show that S-100B levels have a high sensitivity and specificity in predicting failure of treatment. The exact relation of this biochemical reaction to clinical progression has yet to be shown. For clinical trials, guidelines about the increase of S-100B as a definition of biochemical failure are necessary. The introduction of a routine immunological assay for the determination of S-100B protein concentration in serum in the early 1990s resulted in its gradual clinical implementation. The availability of a more sensitive assay since 1995 may have an important impact on the staging and monitoring of malignant melanoma. The biological role of the S-100 molecule in malignant melanoma is not yet understood but will be an important key in the further contribution of the S-100 assay to the management of this disease.

References

Ahmann DL, Creagan ET, Hahn RG et al. (1989) Complete responses and long-term survivals after systemic chemotherapy for patients with advanced malignant melanoma. Cancer 63:224–227

Balch CM, Soong SJ, Murad TM et al. (1979) A multifactorial analysis of melanoma. II. Prognostic factors in patients with stage I (localized) melanoma. Surgery 86:343

Bei Guo H, Stoffel-Wagner B, Bierwirth T, Mezger J, Klingmüller D (1995) Clinical significance of serum S-100 in metastatic malignant melanoma. Eur J Cancer 31 A:1898–1902

Bonfrer JMG, Korse CM, Nieweg OE, Rankin EM (1998) The luminescence immunoassay S-100: a sensitive test to measure circulating S-100B: its prognostic value in malignant melanoma. Br J Cancer 77(12):2210–2214

Böni R, Böni RA, Steinert H, Burg G, Buck A, Marincek B, Berthold T, Dummer R, Voellmy D, Ballmer B (1995) Staging of metastatic melanoma by whole-body positron emission tomography using 2-fluorine-18-fluoro-2-desoxy-D-glucose. Br J Dermatol 132:556–562

Cho KH, Hashimoto K, Taniguchi Y, Pietruk T, Zarbo RJ, An T (1990) Immunohisto-chemical study of melanocytic naevus and malignant melanoma with monoclonal antibodies against S-100 subunits. Cancer 66:765–771

Cochran AJ, Wen DR, Herschman HR, Gaynor RB (1982) Detection of S-100 protein as an aid to the identification of melanocytic tumors. Int J Cancer 30:295–297

Ellis WJ, Vessella RL, Noteboom JL, Lange PH, Wolfert RL, Rittenhouse HG (1997) Early detection of recurrent prostate cancer with an ultrasensitive chemiluminescent prostate-specific antigen assay. Urology 50:573

Fagnart OC, Sindic CJ, Laterre C (1988) Particle counting immuno-assay of S-100 protein in serum. Possible relevance in tumors and ischemic disorders of the central nervous system. Clin Chem 34:1387–1391

Gaynor R, Irie R, Morton DL, Herschmann HR (1980) S-100 protein in cultured human malignant melanoma. Nature 286:400–401

Green RJ, Schuchter LM (1998) Systemic treatment of metastatic melanoma with chemotherapy. In: Koh HK (ed) Hematology/oncology clinics of North America. WB Saunders Company, Orlando, FL, vol 12(4), pp 863–875

Hakajima T, Kameya T, Watanabe S, Hirota T, Sato Y, Shimosato Y (1982) An immunoperoxidase study of S-100 protein distribution in normal and neoplastic tissues. Am J Surg Pathol 6:715–727

Hansson LO, Schoulz E von, Djureen E, Hansson J, Nilsson B, Ringborg U (1997) Prognostic value of serum analyses of S-100 protein βb in malignant melanoma. Anticancer Res 17:3071–3074

Kaplan EL, Meier P (1958) Nonparametric estimation from incomplete observations, J Am Stat Assoc 53:457–481

Lee JAH, Carter AP (1970) Secular trendsin mortality from malignant melanoma. J Natl Cancer Inst 45:91–97

Lee SM, Betticher DC, Thatcher N (1995) Melanoma: Chemotherapy. Br Med Bull 51:609–630

McIllmurray MB, Embleton MJ, Reeves WG et al. (1977) Controlled trial of active immunotherapy in management of stage IIB malignant melanoma. Br Med J 1:540

Missler U, Wiesmann (1995) Measurement of S-100 protein in human blood and cerebrospinal fluid: analytical method and preliminary clinical results. Eur J Clin Chem Clin Biochem 33:743 748

Morton DL, Wen DR, Wong JH et al. (1992) Technical details of intraoperative lymphatic mapping and selective lymphadenectomy or "wait and watch"'. Surg Oncol Clin North Am 1:247

Nyberg L, Kroon R, Ullén A, Brundell J, Haglid KG, Stigbrand T (1996) Sangtec 100 LIA a new sensitive monoclonal assay for measuring protein S-100 in patients with malignant melanoma. In Final Program and Abstract Book of the XXIV Meeting of the ISOBM, The Interdependence of Tumour Biology and Clinical Oncology p. 108. San Diego, CA

Rankin EM, Spits H, Orsini D, Gallee, M, Nooijen WJ, Batchelor D, Kroon B, Israels SP, Clift S, Parry G, Rokovich J, Berns A, Gerritsen WR (1995) A phase I study of vaccination with autologous, GM-CSF-transduced and irradiated tumour cells in patients with advanced melanoma. In: Proceedings of ASCO vol 14, p 226

Robertson EA, Zweig MH (1981) Use of receiver operating characteristic curves to evaluate the clinical performance of analytical systems. Clin Chem 27:1569–1574

Schäfer BW, Heizmann CW (1996) The S-100 family of EF-hand calciumbinding proteins: functions and pathology. TIBS 21:134–140

Schoultz E von, Hansson LO, Djureen E, et al. (1996) Prognostic value of serum analyses of S-100βb protein in malignant melanoma. Melanoma Res 6:133–137

Melanoma Inhibitory Activity (MIA), a Serological Marker of Malignant Melanoma

A.K. Bosserhoff[1], D. Dreau[4], R. Hein[3], M. Landthaler[2], W.D. Holder[4], and R. Buettner[1]

[1] Institute of Pathology, RWTH-Aachen, Germany
[2] Department of Dermatology, University of Regensburg, Regensburg, Germany
[3] Department of Dermatology, TU Munich, Germany
[4] Department of General Surgery Research, Charlotte, North Carolina, USA

Abstract

Melanoma inhibitory activity (MIA) was originally identified as an 11 kDa protein secreted from malignant melanoma cells. We have shown that MIA is strongly expressed in melanoma and melanoma cell lines but not in melanocytes and normal skin. We also observed that MIA mRNA expression correlates with progressive malignancy of melanocytic tumors.

Measuring MIA in serum or plasma by a sensitive and quantitative ELISA and investigating the potential of MIA serum levels as a novel marker for malignant melanomas showed that the protein can be used to monitor therapy and follow-up. The present study measured the variations in blood concentrations of MIA in 84 patients with stage II–IV melanoma by ELISA. Patients treated with repeated injections of a polyvalent melanoma vaccine (PMV), interferon-α-2b (IFN-α2b) or interleukin-2 (IL-2) were followed during treatment duration. Before treatment, patients treated with PMV or IFN-α2b had comparable low MIA concentrations, whereas most IL-2-treated patients had higher MIA levels. At the end of treatment, MIA concentrations were higher in patients with progressive disease (PD) than in patients with no clinical evidence of melanoma (NPD) for PMV, IFN-α2b or IL-2 therapy (3.7 ± 0.2 vs 11.5 ± 5.4 ng/ml, 3.8 ± 0.2 vs 8.3 ± 1.7 ng/ml, and 2.3 ± 0.7 vs 20.2 ± 7.4 ng/ml, respectively, $p < 0.05$). In contrast to the stable MIA concentrations measured in NPD patients, significant increase in MIA levels were observed in PD patients over time regardless of treatment. For PMV- and IFN-α2b-treated patients, a rise in MIA levels occurred significantly earlier than clinical diagnosis of melanoma recurrence.

In conclusion, our data suggest that quantitation of MIA serum levels may be used for detection of both clinically apparent and non-apparent metastatic melanoma disease and for monitoring therapy.

Recent Results in Cancer Research, Vol. 158

Introduction

The incidence of cutaneous melanoma is rising worldwide. The treatment of early stage melanoma consists primarily of surgical removal of the tumor. As in many cancers, early diagnosis is the key to improving patient survival. The overall 5-year survival rate for malignant melanoma is 81%, but survival depends on the depth of invasion, anatomic location, presence of ulceration, the patient's age and sex, histological factors, and clinical subtype of the tumor. Regrettably, the diagnosis of metastatic or recurrent melanoma is frequently delayed by the absence of early diagnostic tools.

In the absence of useful diagnostic methods, physicians rely primarily on patient history, as well as physical and radiological examinations to detect melanoma progression. However, detection of clinical disease by the latter approaches requires significant tumor volume. Unlike prostate-specific antigen (PSA) in patients with prostate cancer, there is no similar marker in melanoma. Several potential markers including S-100 (Seregni et al. 1998; Kroiss et al. 1998; Bonfrer et al. 1998; von Schoultz et al. 1996), tyrosinase (Glaser et al. 1997; Reinhold et al. 1997; Sarantou et al. 1997), and lipid-associated sialic acid (Miliotes et al. 1996; Reintgen et al. 1992) have been tested in melanoma patients with conflicting results.

Recently, an 11 kDa protein, melanoma-inhibitory activity protein (MIA), was isolated from the cell culture supernatant of a melanoma cell line and expression was shown to correlate with clinical stage (Bosserhoff et al. 1997a; Bogdahn et al. 1989; Apfel et al. 1992). Elevated MIA serum levels were found in approx. 70% of patients with stage III and 95% of patients with stage IV melanoma but rarely in patients with other cancers. Plasma concentrations of MIA measured in these patients were related to the clinical stage of melanoma.

Material and Methods

Quantification of MIA Serum or Plasma Levels

MIA was measured by a one-step ELISA as described previously (Bosserhoff et al. 1997a). Briefly, two monoclonal antibodies, directed against 14-meric N-terminal and C-terminal peptides (MAB 1A12 and MAB 2F7; Roche, Germany), were raised and conjugated to horseradish-peroxidase (POD) and biotin, respectively. Then, 20 µl serum was coincubated with biotinylated MAB 2F7 and POD-conjugated MAB 1A12 antibodies in streptavidin-coated 96-well plates for 45 min. After washing three times with PBS, 200 µl ABTS-solution (2,2′-azino-di-[3-ethylbenz-thiazolinesulfonate]; Roche, Germany) was incubated in the wells for 30 min and measured colorimetrically at 405 nm. Using standard concentrations of recombinant MIA purified from stably transfected CHO cells, we measured linear signals at MIA concentrations between 0.1 and 50 ng/ml. Reproducibility of test results was confirmed by measuring repeatedly eight standard sera using different ELISA lots (mean SD=9.4%).

Patients and Treatments

Eighty-four patients with AJCC stage II to IV melanoma treated at Carolinas Medical Center were analyzed prospectively for plasma MIA concentrations. Patients who were treated by either a polyvalent melanoma vaccine (PMV; $n=52$), repeated injections of interferon-α-2b (IFN-α2b; $n=22$), or intravenous interleukin-2 (IL-2; $n=10$), were studied during the period of treatment.

Both PMV and IFN-α2b treatments were offered after surgical resection of all clinical disease to patients who had no evidence of other metastatic disease but a high risk of melanoma recurrence (>50% at 5 years). The PMV treatment is an experimental protocol derived from previous vaccine studies (Morton et al. 1992; Morton and Barth 1996). The treatment consisted of repeated injections of an irradiated cocktail of three allogenic melanoma cell lines grown in vitro (Dreau et al. 1997). Each patient received subcutaneous injections of 10^7 cells once a month for 12 months. For at least the first two injections, BCG was added to the immunization cocktail. Adjuvant IFN-α2b treatment consisted of 20 mIU/m^2 of recombinant IFN-α2b (IntronA, Schering, Kenilworth, NJ) given intravenously for 4 weeks (5 days/week) followed by 10 mIU/m^2 of recombinant IFN-α2b given subcutaneously for 11 months (three times/week). The patients with stage IV metastatic disease were treated with an intravenous IL-2 regimen. Patients received three large doses of intravenous IL-2 (720000 IU/kg every 8 h) followed by up to 12 smaller doses of intravenous IL-2 (72000 IU/kg every 8 h) over a 5-day period. This treatment was repeated 7–10 days later. Patients were evaluated for response to treatment 1 month later. Patients with regression or stable melanoma repeated the treatment.

For all treatment groups, recurrence or progression of melanoma determined by clinical and radiological examinations defined the end of treatment.

Clinical Follow-up and Diagnosis of Melanoma Recurrence

Patients were followed monthly (patients treated with IFN-α2b or IL-2) or every 3 months (patients treated with PMV) by physical examination and routine laboratory tests including complete blood count and liver function tests. Radiological examinations including chest X-rays, computed tomography, magnetic resonance imaging, and positron-emission tomography were also performed at various intervals. Suspected melanoma recurrence was confirmed by histopathological diagnosis of biopsies or fine-needle aspiration specimens, except in the case of liver or brain metastases.

Patients were evaluated for recurrent melanoma before, during, and after the treatment. Two categories of patients were defined based solely on the presence or absence of clinical disease at the end of the follow-up period: patients with no evidence of disease by physical examination and radiological evaluation (NPD) and patients with clinically identifiable disease (PD). At the beginning of treatment, patients with no evidence of disease (with one exception) received adjuvant therapy (PMV and IFN-α2b), whereas all patients treated with IL-2 had clinical evidence of disease.

Plasma Collection

After obtaining informed consent, blood samples were collected from each patient enrolled in the three immunotherapy protocols for the treatment duration. Samples were drawn before treatment and every 3 months thereafter for patients treated with PMV. For melanoma patients treated with IFN-α2b, blood samples were obtained before treatment, after 1 month, and every 3 months thereafter. For melanoma patients with unresectable metastases and treated with IL-2, blood samples were obtained before treatment and with each follow-up examination thereafter. The blood samples were centrifuged and the plasma stored at –70 °C until used.

Results

Patient Characteristics

MIA concentrations were measured over time in 84 treated patients. There were no significant differences in the patients' age (54 ± 1.3 years) or sex ratio (male/female, 2/1) concerning the kind of treatment. Sixteen, 29, and 39 patients were AJCC stage II, III, and IV, respectively. Most of the stage II and III patients (36/45) were treated with the PMV; 59% (13/22) of the patients treated with IFN-α2b were stage IV with no evidence of disease at the start of treatment. All patients treated with IL-2 were stage IV and had evidence of disease at the start of treatment. Only one patient with evidence of melanoma (a solitary, stable non-resectable tumor) was treated with PMV.

MIA Concentrations

Before treatment, MIA concentrations in patients were similar in the PMV and IFN-α2b treatment groups (4.5 ± 0.8 and 4.4 ± 0.4 ng/ml, respectively, $p > 0.5$, Fig. 1). Significantly higher MIA values were observed in IL-2-treated patients than in PMV- and IFN-α2b-treated patients (13.9 ± 3.2 vs 4.5 ± 0.8 and 4.4 ± 0.4 ng/ml, $p < 0.001$, Fig. 1).

Of the 84 patients treated with PMV, IFN-α2b, or IL-2, 13 (25%), six (27%), and eight (80%) patients, respectively, developed melanoma recur-

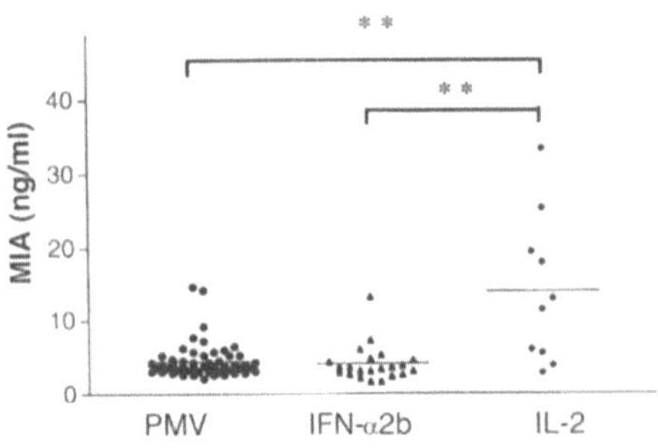

Fig. 1. MIA concentrations before treatment in melanoma patients treated with PMV, IFN-α2b, or IL-2. MIA values measured in PMV and IFN-α2b treated patients were significantly lower than MIA values in IL-2 patients before treatment (**$p<0.001$, ANOVA). A similar difference was measured between PD and NPD melanoma patients considered for immunotherapy regimens (**$p<0.001$, ANOVA)

rence or progression as defined solely by radiological and physical examination during or after treatment (PD patients, Table 1). This included one patient with a solitary melanoma tumor treated with PMV. Most of the patients treated with PMV or IFN-α2b remained free of melanoma for the duration of the follow-up (NPD patients, Table 1).

Before treatment, MIA concentrations were low in NPD patients treated with PMV ($n=39$) or IFN-α2b ($n=16$) (4.2±0.2 and 3.5±0.3 ng/ml, respectively, Table 1) and similar to MIA levels measured in PD patients following PMV or IFN-α2b therapy ($p>0.3$, Table 1). Prior to IL-2 treatment, MIA concentrations in the two patients who underwent surgical resection or had a complete response to IL-2 treatment were lower than in the patients with stage IV metastatic disease treated with IL-2 who progressed (3.4±0.4 vs 16.5±3.3 ng/ml, $p<0.05$, Table 1).

MIA concentrations were also measured over the treatment duration for each therapy, i.e., 12 months for PMV and IFN-α2b, and up to 2 months for IL-2 (Table 1). Over time, MIA levels were stable and below 4.5 ng/ml in most NPD patients regardless of therapy (Table 1). By contrast, MIA levels increased significantly over time in PD patients treated with PMV ($p<0.05$, Table 1). Similar trends were observed in PD patients treated with IFN-α2b or IL-2 (Table 1). MIA concentrations obtained at treatment end were higher than before therapy in PMV- (5.2±1.1 vs 11.5±5.4 ng/ml), IFN-α2b- (5.8±1.6 vs 8.3±1.7 ng/ml), and IL-2- (16.5±3.3 vs 20.2±7.4 ng/ml) treated PD patients (Table 1). This was not observed in NPD patients.

MIA Concentrations and Clinical Diagnosis

After treatment, 74% (20/27) of the patients with melanoma recurrence or progression had MIA concentrations higher than 4.5 ng/ml (Table 2). All the

Table 1. Plasma MIA concentrations (mean±SEM, [range], ng/ml) in melanoma patients treated with repeated injections of PMV, IFN-α2b or IL-2 measured over the treatment duration

Treatment	Group	n[a]	Time (months)							After treatment[c]
			0[b]	1	2	3	6	9	12	
PMV (n=52)	NPD[d]	39	4.2±0.2 [2.4–7.7]	–[e]	–	4.3±0.3 [2.1–6.6]	4.1±0.2 [2.6–5.7]	4.7±0.3 [2.3–6.8]	3.5±0.2 [1.2–6.9]	3.7±0.2 [1.2–6.9]
	PD[d*]	13	5.2±1.1 [2.4–14.6]	–	–	7.8±3.4 [2.7–52.5]	8.1±2.9** [2.4–33.3]	7.8±3.1 [2.9–35.5]	13.3±9.1** [2.6–77.1]	11.5±5.4** [2.6–77.1]
IFN-α2b (n=22)	NPD[d]	16	3.5±0.3 [1.6–6.2]	3.0±0.2 [1.9–3.7]	–	3.7±0.4 [1.5–5.6]	3.7±0.2 [2.3–4.8]	3.9±0.3 [2.2–4.9]	4.4±0.2 [3.6–5.0]	3.8±0.2 [1.9–5.1]
	PD[d]	6	5.8±1.6 [2.2–13.2]	6.8±2.0* [2.4–10.8]	–	6.9±2.2(**) [3.2–15.4]	4.7±0.8 [2.6–6.6]	6.1±1.1** [3.4–8.9]	–	8.3±1.7*** [3.4–15.4]
IL-2 (n=10)	NPD[d]	2	3.4±0.4 [3.0–3.8]	2.3±0.1 [2.3–2.4]	–	–	–	–	2.3±0.7 [2.3–2.4]	
	PD[d]	8	16.5±3.3** [5.6–33.3]	13.2±6.2 [3.8–31.5]	27.3±13.6 [9.1–67.7]	– –	– –	– –	20.2±7.4(**) [3.8–67.7]	

$p<0.05$: significant difference over time within treatment and patient groups (paired t-test). (**)$p=0.06$, $p<0.05$, and ***$p<0.01$: significant differences between NPD and PD groups within treatment (ANOVA)

[a] Patient number per treatment and group. Effective (n) remained constant in NPD groups, but since recurrence or progression defined treatment end, n decreased in PD groups, i.e., from 13 to 8 (0–12 months), 6 to 4 (0–9 months) and 8 to 4 (0–2 months) for PMV, IFN-α2b, and IL-2 treatment, respectively.

[b] MIA concentrations before treatment.

[c] MIA concentrations obtained in treated patients at treatment end regardless of treatment duration.

[d] Patient status determined by clinical examination at the end of treatment or during the follow-up period defined two patients groups based on the absence (NPD) or presence (PD) of evidence of melanoma recurrence or progression.

[e] No samples.

Table 2. Number of melanoma patients treated by PMV, IFN-a2b, or IL-2 immunotherapy diagnosed with recurrence or progression by clinical examination and MIA concentration

Therapy	*n*	Clinical recurrence[a]	MIA>4.5 ng/ml
PMV	52	13	8
IFN-α2b	22	6	4
IL-2	10	8	8
Overall	84	27	20

[a] Clinical recurrence determined by physical and radiological examination (see Materials and Methods for details).

melanoma progressions observed after IL-2 treatment were associated with an increase in MIA concentration. However, 5/13 and 2/6 patients treated with PMV or IFN-α2b, respectively, who developed melanoma recurrences did not have MIA concentrations higher than 4.5 ng/ml (Table 2). Using MIA values ranging from 4.0 to 5.0 ng/ml, the best MIA threshold value to discriminate between NPD and PD melanoma patients was 4.5 ng/ml. This threshold was associated with a sensitivity of $9/11 \times 100 = 82\%$ and a specificity of $52/73 \times 100 = 71\%$ before treatment. After treatment, MIA concentrations were associated with a sensitivity of $18/27 \times 100 = 67\%$ and a specificity of $45/57 \times 100 = 79\%$. However, confidence intervals (99.9% CI) for MIA concentrations obtained after treatment were significantly different from the 4.5 ng/ml threshold value for NPD and PD melanoma patients (2.96 to 4.14 ng/ml and 3.99 to 15.52 ng/ml, respectively, $p < 0.001$).

For most of the patients treated with IL-2, disease progression was observed at the same time an increase in MIA was detected (time difference of 0.37 ± 1.06 months, Table 3). For both IFN-α2b and PMV therapies, MIA concentrations higher than 4.5 ng/ml were detected earlier than the clinical diagnosis of melanoma recurrence (0.75 ± 0.75 vs 4.25 ± 1.97 months and 3.37 ± 1.54 vs 12.37 ± 4.01 months, respectively, Table 3). Regardless of the treatment, in 20 of 27 (74%) melanoma patients with increased MIA concentrations, clinical diagnosis was associated with MIA concentrations higher than 4.5 ng/ml, and the rise of MIA was detectable on average 5.9 ± 6.2 months earlier than the time of the clinical diagnosis ($p < 0.001$, Table 3).

Discussion

The present study measured MIA levels in the plasma of melanoma patients during treatment. The results obtained here suggest that: (1) MIA concentrations were higher in patients with evidence of disease than in patients without evidence of disease; (2) MIA concentrations were stable over time in melanoma patients with no evidence of disease, whereas a rise in MIA was observed in patients who developed or progressed with metastatic disease; and (3) in 74% of patients, an increase in MIA concentrations was observed before recurrence was detected by physical and radiological examination.

Table 3. Time to recurrence or progression in melanoma patients treated by PMV, IFN-a2b, or IL-2 immunotherapy determined by clinical examination and MIA concentration >4.5 ng/ml

Treatment	*n*	Clinical recurrence[a] (months)	MIA>4.5 ng/ml[b] (months)	Time difference[c] (months)	Range
PMV	8	12.37±4.01	3.37±1.54***	6.8±7.3	1–23
IFN-a2b	4	4.25±1.97	0.75±0.75	4.6±4.7	0–10
IL-2	8	1.87±0.47	0.37±0.37**	0.37±1.06	0–3
Overall	20	6.55±1.94	1.65±0.70**	5.9±6.2	0–23

** $p<0.01$ and ***$p<0.001$ significant difference between the time to melanoma recurrence or progression determined by clinical examination and MIA concentration >4.5 ng/ml (paired t test)
[a] Time between the start of treatment and diagnosis of progression by clinical examination.
[b] Time between the start of treatment and detection of MIA concentration higher than 4.5 ng/ml.
[c] Time between the detection of MIA concentration higher than 4.5 ng/ml and the diagnosis of progression by clinical examination.

The treatment of melanoma patients at high risk for recurrence or with progressive disease is different from that of patients with primary melanoma (Fusi et al. 1993). The most effective treatment available for primary tumors is surgical resection, which results in an overall 5-year survival rate of 81% (Rossi et al. 1997). However, recurrent malignant melanoma has been shown to behave distinctly different from primary disease (Fusi et al. 1993). Local recurrence, in-transit metastasis, and regional nodal metastasis are all associated with a 20–25% 5-year survival (Fusi et al. 1993); the survival of patients with distant organ disease is limited (Fusi et al. 1993). An early diagnosis of initial recurrent melanoma can contribute to longer survival if the disease can be surgically resected or if the metastases respond to specific therapies (Miliotes et al. 1996). Therefore, much research is directed toward the identification of a reliable marker for melanoma occurrence or recurrence.

Identification of a marker specific for melanoma similar to PSA in prostate cancer has been the focus of much research. The most commonly used diagnostic marker for melanoma remains S-100 protein (Cochran et al. 1993). The concentration of S-100 protein measured in the blood of melanoma patients showed significant correlations to both time to recurrence and survival (Miliotes et al. 1996). However, while S-100 protein is highly expressed in melanoma, it is also expressed in numerous other cell types including T lymphocytes, chondrocytes, and adipocytes (Cochran and Wen 1985). Moreover, S-100 protein expression appears to be extremely heterogeneous within melanoma tumors, as observed in immunohistochemistry studies. Additionally, the specificity of the antibodies against S-100 used in these assays, whether monoclonal or polyclonal, gave conflicting results, as suggested by flow cytometry analyses of melanoma cell lines (Dréau et al. unpublished). In fact, to conclusively diagnose melanoma, the use of a panel of antibodies rather than one has been suggested, especially to distinguish metastatic amelanotic malignant melanoma from other metastatic neoplasms. Our results suggest that MIA has a sensitivity and specificity comparable to S-100 measurement (Bosserhoff et al. 1997a). Whether MIA concentrations are more reflective than S-100 protein concentrations of melanoma evolution in patients treated by immunotherapy remains to be determined.

The increase in MIA concentrations in the blood of most (74%) of the patients with melanoma recurrence or progression, compared with values observed in non-recurring patients' blood, was consistent with the enhanced MIA serum levels observed previously in 100% ($n=49$) of melanoma patients with AJCC stage III or IV disease (Bosserhoff et al. 1997a). Moreover, MIA mRNA can be detected in the blood (Muhlbauer et al. 1999; La Valle GJ et al. 1998) and tumor specimens (Bosserhoff et al. 1996) of patients with advanced melanoma. Unlike S-100 protein, the MIA expression was restricted to cartilage, chondrosarcoma, and melanoma (Bosserhoff et al. 1997b) and was higher in metastatic melanoma than in primary melanoma.

Some patients with a clinical diagnosis of melanoma recurrence (26%) had low MIA levels, challenging the use of MIA blood concentrations as a clinical diagnostic test. Many factors may have contributed to the discrepancy observed here. In four of the seven patients, the clinical diagnosis of metastatic melanoma was made after standard melanoma diagnosis, using histopathological examination of lymph nodes (3) or spleen (1) biopsy specimens. However, all seven patients had multiple metastasis sites, i.e., liver (4), lymph nodes (4), bowel (2), brain (2), bone (1), breast (1), and lung (1), suggesting that metastatic sites were unlikely to affect MIA levels. Since the MIA ELISA test was shown both here and previously (Bosserhoff et al. 1997a) to be sensitive and reliable, the absence of detectable levels of MIA in the blood of seven patients with progressive metastatic melanoma may be indicative of the absence of expression or release of MIA protein, or of MIA protein alterations in some melanoma tumors. Although the reproducibility of the MIA measurements presented here was in keeping with previous analyses (Bosserhoff et al. 1996), MIA detection difficulties in the plasma of these patients cannot be entirely ruled out. Further analyses are needed to explain the absence of MIA increase in the blood of some patients with clinical progressive melanoma disease.

Nevertheless, increases in MIA concentrations, observed in 74% of patients with progressive melanoma disease, were detected, on average, 6 months before the diagnosis of melanoma recurrence or progression was made. This suggests that MIA measurement may allow an earlier diagnosis of melanoma progression or recurrence. More than 350 healthy control patients had a MIA blood concentration below the threshold value of 4.5 ng/ml (Bosserhoff et al, unpublished) selected here suggesting that this threshold may be used to screen not only patients monitored during immunotherapy but also the general population. Whether the measurement of blood MIA concentrations can detect early stages of melanoma development is currently under investigation.

Acknowledgements The authors wish to thank Ute Holtzapfel for her technical assistance, Pam Pitman, LPN and Paula Muehlbauer, RN, for providing detailed clinical records, and H. James Norton, Ph.D. for his advice on statistical evaluation of the data.

References

Apfel R, Lottspeich F, Hoppe J, Behl C, Durr G, Bogdahn U (1992) Purification and analysis of growth regulating proteins secreted by a human melanoma cell line. Melanoma. Res 2:327–336

Bogdahn U, Apfel R, Hahn M, Gerlach M, Behl C, Hoppe J, Martin R (1989) Autocrine tumor cell growth-inhibiting activities from human malignant melanoma. Cancer Res 49:5358–5363

Bonfrer JM, Korse CM, Nieweg OE, Rankin EM (1998) The luminescence immunoassay S-100: a sensitive test to measure circulating S-100B: its prognostic value in malignant melanoma. Br J Cancer 77:2210–2214

Bosserhoff AK, Hein R, Bogdahn U, Buettner R (1996) Structure and promoter analysis of the gene encoding the human melanoma-inhibiting protein MIA. J Biol Chem 271:490–495

Bosserhoff AK, Kaufmann M, Kaluza B, Bartke I, Zirngibl H, Hein R, Stolz W, Buettner R (1997a) Melanoma-inhibiting activity, a novel serum marker for progression of malignant melanoma. Cancer Res 57:3149–3153

Bosserhoff AK, Kondo S, Moser M, Dietz UH, Copeland NG, Gilbert DJ, Jenkins NA, Buettner R, Sandell LJ (1997b) Mouse CD-RAP/MIA gene: structure, chromosomal localization, and expression in cartilage and chondrosarcoma. Dev Dyn 208:516–525

Cochran AJ, Lu HF, Li PX, Saxton R, Wen DR (1993) S-100 protein remains a practical marker for melanocytic and other tumours. Melanoma Res 3:325–330

Cochran AJ, Wen DR (1985) S-100 protein as a marker for melanocytic and other tumours. Pathology 17:340–345

Dreau D, Foster M, Culberson C, Holder WDJ (1997) Specific IgG immune responses in melanoma patients treated with cell-vaccine. Proc Am Assoc Cancer Res 38:396

Fusi S, Ariyan S, Sternlicht A (1993) Data on first recurrence after treatment for malignant melanoma in a large patient population. Plast Reconstr Surg 91:94–98

Glaser R, Rass K, Seiter S, Hauschild A, Christophers E, Tilgen W (1997) Detection of circulating melanoma cells by specific amplification of tyrosinase complementary DNA is not a reliable tumor marker in melanoma patients: a clinical two-center study. J Clin Oncol 15:2818–2825

Kroiss MM, Bosserhoff AK, Vogt T, Buettner R, Bogenrieder T, Landthaler M, Stolz W (1998) Loss of expression or mutations in the p73 tumour suppressor gene are not involved in the pathogenesis of malignant melanomas. Melanoma Res 8:504–509

La Valle GJ, Williams NY, Walker MJ, Triozzi PL, Barbera-Guillem E (1998) Expression of melanoma inhibitory activitya in the peripheral blood of melanoma patients by the reverse transcriptase-polymerase chain reaction (RT-PCR). Proc Am Assoc Cancer Res 39:229

Miliotes G, Lyman GH, Cruse CW, Puleo C, Albertini PA, Rapaport D, Glass F, Fenske N, Soriano T, Cuny C, Van Voorhis N, Reintgen D (1996) Evaluation of new putative tumor markers for melanoma. Ann Surg Oncol 3:558–563

Morton DL, Barth A (1996) Vaccine therapy for malignant melanoma. CA. Cancer J Clin 46:225–244

Morton DL, Foshag LJ, Hoon DS, Nizze JA, Famatiga E, Wanek LA, Chang C, Davtyan DG, Gupta RK, Elashoff R (1992) Prolongation of survival in metastatic melanoma after active specific immunotherapy with a new polyvalent melanoma vaccine [published erratum appears in Ann Surg 1993 Mar; 217(3):309]. Ann Surg 216:463–482

Muhlbauer M, Langenbach N, Stolz W, Hein R, Landthaler M, Buettner R, Bosserhoff AK (1999) Detection of melanoma cells in the blood of melanoma patients by melanoma-inhibitory activity (MIA) reverse transcription-PCR [In Process Citation]. Clin Cancer Res 5:1099–1105

Reinhold U, Ludtke-Handjery HC, Schnautz S, Kreysel HW, Abken H (1997) The analysis of tyrosinase-specific mRNA in blood samples of melanoma patients by RT-PCR is not a useful test for metastatic tumor progression. J Invest Dermatol 108:166–169

Reintgen DS, Cruse CW, Wells KE, Saba HI, Fabri PJ (1992) The evaluation of putative tumor markers for malignant melanoma. Ann Plast Surg 28:55–59

Rossi CR, Foletto M, Vecchiato A, Alessio S, Menin N, Lise M (1997) Management of cutaneous melanoma M0: state of the art and trends [see comments]. Eur J Cancer 33:2302–2312

Sarantou T, Chi DD, Garrison DA, Conrad AJ, Schmid P, Morton DL, Hoon DS (1997) Melanoma-associated antigens as messenger RNA detection markers for melanoma. Cancer Res 57:1371–1376

Seregni E, Massaron S, Martinetti A, Illeni MT, Rovini D, Belli F, Agresti R, Greco M, Cascinelli N, Bombardieri E (1998) S-100 protein serum levels in cutaneous malignant melanoma. Oncol Rep 5:601–604

von Schoultz E, Hansson LO, Djureen E, Hansson J, Karnell R, Nilsson B, Stigbrand T, Ringborg U (1996) Prognostic value of serum analyses of S-100 beta protein in malignant melanoma. Melanoma Res 6:133–137

Quantification of Melanoma-Associated Molecules in Plasma/Serum of Melanoma Patients

A. Hauschild, R. Gläser, and E. Christophers

Department of Dermatology, University of Kiel, Schittenhelmstrasse 7, 24105 Kiel, Germany

Abstract

Tumor markers for metastatic melanoma have, so far, been infrequently used. Although there is good evidence from several studies that protein S-100B serum measurement could serve as a valid marker for micro- and/or macrometastasis, the S-100B-LIAmat test has not been established as part of national and international recommendations for the care of melanoma patients. Future studies should focus on early detection of metastatic disease with S-100B compared to routine clinical, laboratory and technical evaluations. Furthermore, preliminary, interesting results on the predictive value of S-100B for the monitoring of metastatic patients during treatment should be verified in multicenter trials. The same considerations are true for melanoma-inhibitory activity (MIA), a new and interesting tool for the detection of metastatic melanoma. However, available data on the clinical use of on the MIA-ELISA are too limited to speculate on an even higher sensitivity and specificity than reported for S-100B.

Melanin metabolites are candidates for valid melanoma markers, too. Quantification of 5-S-cysteinyldopa from blood or urine of melanoma patients has not been transferred from the laboratory to daily routine due to several technical problems in the assessment of this particular molecule.

Cytokines, adhesion molecules and metalloproteinases are shed from melanoma cells into the serum, but these cells are not the only source of elevated serum levels. Several inflammatory conditions are responsible for high serum concentrations of these molecules. In general, they are not sensitive and specific enough to serve as "melanoma markers."

Introduction

Tumor markers are substances that are detectable by different types of methods and potentially of value in the screening and/or differential diagnosis,

Recent Results in Cancer Research, Vol. 158

Table 1. Clinical value of potential melanoma markers. A meta-analysis of published studies

Group	Marker	Prognostic relevance shown in number of studies [a]	Number of patients
Melanin metabolites	α-MSH	0/1	37
	Tyrosinase	1/1	10
	Tyrosinase-RT-PCR	8/19	967
	5-S-CD	4/6	203
	6H5M12 C	1/2	75
Adhesion molecules	ICAM-1	4/8	633
	PECAM-1	0/1	119
	CD44	0/2	153
Cytokines	IL-2R	0/2	63
	IL-8	1/1	56
	IL-10	1/1	104
Melanoma-associated antigens	NSE	3/6	841
	LSA	3/4	618
	S-100	13/14	2454
	MIA	1/1	112

[a] In the personal/subjective opinion of the publishing author(s).

staging, follow-up and treatment monitoring of patients with malignant diseases (Table 1). In an overview of the value of tumor markers in clinical oncology (without special consideration of malignant melanoma), Hossfeld [1] recently questioned the use of expensive measurements of tumor markers without asking whether it benefits the patient. For example, it is known that a healthy person who undergoes 13 tumor marker tests has, by chance alone, a probability of only 51% of being classified as being disease-free [1, 2].

In the international guidelines for the care of melanoma patients, so far no serological tumor marker has reached an approved stage of relevance. In principal, a broad variety of molecules synthesized, secreted or shed into the blood, either directly by melanoma cells or as an indirect response by the patient's immune system, could serve as markers of tumor progression. These substances can be grouped as follows: melanin-related metabolites, melanoma-associated antigens, adhesion molecules and cytokines [3]. In the following sections we will critically comment on the sensitivity and specificity of particular markers. Furthermore, we will attempt to address the question whether such markers are useful in the routine care of melanoma patients.

Melanin-Related Metabolites

Melanin pigment formation is a metabolic pathway that is unique to the melanocytic lineage. Since pigment production is highly enhanced in metastatic melanoma, theoretically, a simple serum test evaluating melanin metabolites would be an ideal tool to monitor metastatic disease. Several attempts have been made to quantify different melanin metabolites either in blood (plasma/serum) or urine with varying success.

5-S-Cysteinyldopa (5-S-CD)

A group from Japan carefully examined four melanin-related metabolites for their predictive value in malignant melanoma [4]. Horokoshi et al. summarized that 5-S-CD appeared to be the best biochemical marker for detection of progressive melanoma. Serum 5-S-CD elevations significantly preceded the detection of metastatic sites by conventional procedures such as physical, laboratory and radiological examinations [4].

Despite these encouraging results, several questions remain unclear: Is high-performance liquid chromatography (HPLC) really useful as a daily routine analysis procedure? What is the relevant 5-S-CD cut-off value of Caucasian patients (seasonal and ethnic serum level variations during sun exposure)? A comparison of the results with those from simple routine assays (S-100B-LIAmat) should be taken in account before 5-S-CD can reach clinical significance in the daily routine.

Tyrosinase

Since Smith et al. [5] described the molecular detection of melanoma cells in peripheral blood using reverse transcription polymerase chain reaction (RT-PCR), a number of publications have focused on this new approach [6–15]. The detection of tyrosinase mRNA functions as an highly specific indicator of circulating melanoma cells in the peripheral blood. With respect to the sensitivity of tyrosinase RT-PCR, the results from different groups have varied from 0% to 100% in patients with distant melanoma metastases (stage IV; UICC classification).

In a clinical two-center study [12], we optimized and standardized a technique allowing detection of a single melanoma cell in 10 ml of blood. With this, at least in vitro, sensitive assay, a total of 153 blood samples was investigated. Interestingly, only 12/44 advanced melanoma patients (27.3%) were tyrosinase RT-PCR-positive, indicating that this type of molecular staging is not suitable for routine use [12]. Our data are supported by several other groups [8, 9, 14, 15], who reported sensitivities between 13% and 50%; but the results are in clear contrast to those of others, which described a sensitivity of 100% and 94% [6, 7, 11]. So far, tyrosinase RT-PCR cannot serve as a reliable tumor marker, even multimarker assays [13], as time- and cost-intensive alternatives, need confirmation and validation from comparable trials.

Melanoma-Associated Antigens

Earlier studies, in particular those from the United States, focused on two molecules that are shed from the surface of melanoma cells as well from other cell entities into the blood: neuron-specific enolase (NSE) and lipid-bound sialic acid (LASA). In addition, in recent years, two other melanoma-associated molecules, melanoma-inhibiting activity (MIA) and protein S-100B (S-100B), have generated great interest regarding their use in clinical studies. Both markers are now available on the market as serum test kits for use in daily practice.

Neuron-Specific Enolase

This enzyme was considered as a useful marker of endocrine tumors such as small-cell lung cancer and neuroblastoma. Studies in melanoma produced discrepant results. Whereas Hornef et al. [16] reported elevated NSE serum levels exclusively in stage IV melanoma patients, other clinicians found no statistically relevant correlation between NSE levels and the clinical course of disease [17, 18]. Interestingly, Wibe et al. [19] determined that NSE-positive patients had a median survival time of only 3 months compared with 12 months for NSE-negative metastatic melanoma patients. These data are comparable with results from our laboratory. In a large clinical investigation, 40 out of 84 stage IV patients became NSE-positive in the course of metastatic disease, but in the majority of cases the elevation of the NSE levels appeared shortly before the patients died. Thus, the clinical relevance of NSE remains questionable, in particular with respect to the low specificity.

Lipid-Bound Sialic Acid

Reintgen et al. carried out a clinical study on the use of plasma levels of LASA, a sialoglycolipid bound to membranes of a variety of tumor cells [20]. The authors compared NSE detection with that of LASA-P in a large cohort of melanoma patients with a follow-up of at least 2 years. Whereas NSE was found to be neither sensitive (27%) nor specific (77%), increased LASA-P served as an indicator of active malignant melanoma in about 65% of involved patients. Moreover, in 13 patients elevated LASA-P levels preceded recurrences by at least 9 months. However, it should be mentioned that the specificity of LASA-P appears to be in the same range (76%) as NSE [20]. A commercially available test system for LASA-P does not exist. The same group published a comparison of LASA-P and serum S-100B [21]. In this analysis LASA-P levels – in contrast to S-100B – was not associated with the time to recurrence or survival of melanoma patients.

Melanoma-Inhibitory Activity

Early experiments suggest that MIA, a small 11 kDa protein, is secreted from melanoma cells, but not from benign melanocytes, into the blood. In one monocenter study, all patients suffering from metastatic melanoma (either locoregional, stage III or advanced metastasis, stage IV) demonstrated elevated serum levels of MIA. Only a small proportion of healthy controls and patients with other benign or malignant diseases showed serum concentrations above the cut-off level, set at 6.5 μg/l in this particular study [22]. Thus, MIA represents an encouraging tumor marker with high sensitivity and reliable specificity for detecting metastatic melanoma. Final conclusions will be drawn after results of a multicenter trial on an extended number of melanoma patients in all stages of disease, as well as a representative variety of control patients, are available.

S-100B

The name "S-100" was coined by Moore [23] and describes an acidic calcium-binding protein derived from bovine brain extract that is soluble at neutral pH in 100% (saturated) ammonium sulfate. Using an immunoradiometric assay (IRMA), several studies have revealed the clinical significance of the quantification of S-100B subunit in serum. Both German [24] and Swiss [25] groups collected serum samples from 126 and 73 melanoma patients, respectively, and were able to detect elevated levels in a stage-dependent fashion (stage I/II: 1.3% vs 4.0%; stage III: 8.7% vs 21.4%; stage IV: 73.9% vs 79.4%). These results are supported by a large analysis involving 643 melanoma patients from Sweden [26], which demonstrated, for the first time, a highly statistically significant impact on the individual survival time. S-100B in serum was proposed as an independent prognostic factor for melanoma patients.

Our own study on 1339 serum samples from 412 melanoma patients and 107 control patients with cutaneous diseases was able to support these earlier results [27]. Using a cut-off level of 0.2 μg/l S-100B, 5/286 patients (1.7%) with primary tumors (stage I/II), 14/73 (19.2%) patients with locoregional metastasis (stage III) and 57/84 (67.9%) patients with advanced disease (stage IV) were S-100B positive (statistically significant differences for stage I/II vs III, I/II vs IV, and III vs IV, $p<0.001$). The estimated overall survival time was significantly longer ($p<0.001$) for patients with S-100B values below 0.2 μg/l than for patients with elevated S-100B levels (≥0.2 μg/l), independent of the stage of disease (I–IV). Regarding prognosis, we were furthermore able to distinguish different subgroups among stage III and IV patients using S-100B serum levels ($p<0.01$) [27].

Furthermore, in an additional investigation, treatment monitoring in 64 stage IV melanoma patients during chemo- and/or immunotherapy was evaluated [28]. S-100B IRMA tests were performed before, during and after treatment at scheduled time points. In the interim analysis at 4 weeks, 29/37

(78%) of patients with tumor progression during treatment showed a raised S-100B level. In the final analysis at 8 weeks, 31 of these 37 patients (84%) demonstrated rising S-100B values ($p<0.001$). Patients who were responding to treatment (stable or regressing metastatic disease) showed constant or declining S-100B levels in 38 of 40 patients (95%) in the interim analysis; at 8 weeks this increased further to 39 of 40 patients (98%; $p<0.001$) [28]. Thus, the use of S-100B adequately predicts treatment outcome in the majority of cases. Our observations are of great interest for therapeutic trials in the adjuvant and palliative setting, as the increase in S-100B levels might indicate that restaging and/or changes in therapy strategies are needed.

Recently, we evaluated 489 serum samples from 64 patients suffering from advanced melanoma (UICC/AJCC stage IV) to compare the sensitivity of a S-100B IRMA with both measurement of conventional blood parameters as well as other known clinical prognostic factors [29]. In a univariate statistical analysis, gender, bone metastasis, LDH and S-100B levels in serum samples were found to be significant prognostic markers ($p<0.05$), but S-100B represented the only relevant independent prognostic marker in a multivariate analysis ($p=0.016$). Furthermore, we could demonstrate that S-100B is of relevance independent of the specific sites of metastatic involvement. The other laboratory parameters could not approximate the sensitivity rate of S-100B. The overall survival rate was strongly associated with S-100B serum values [29]. The results of our study suggest that S-100B is a useful tool as a melanoma marker and an independent prognostic factor in advanced metastatic melanoma.

Since 1998, a S-100B luminoimmunometric assay (LIA) has been available. Bonfrer et al. reported on an enhanced sensitivity for S-100B-positive melanoma patients with metastatic disease and a sensitivity rate of about 80% for advanced metastatic melanoma patients [30]. Further studies are currently in the final phase of evaluation. These studies are aimed at answering the question whether the new test system is able to detect even micrometastatic disease in melanoma patients and at determining the practical value of S-100B in routine follow-up.

Adhesion Molecules

Controversial results have been reported regarding the ELISA detection of soluble intercellular adhesion molecule-1 (ICAM-1) in the serum. Whereas Altomonte et al. [31] found that 95% of melanoma patients showed increased ICAM-1 concentrations in a stage-dependent fashion, another group [32] could not measure statistical differences between ICAM-1 levels in primary melanomas and advanced metastatic disease.

Schaider et al. analyzed different adhesion molecules to clarify whether they could distinguish metastatic melanoma from primary melanoma and benign melanocytic diseases [33]. The authors concluded that adhesion molecule concentrations do not reflect the stage of disease or indicate the prognosis of individual patients.

Because adhesion molecules are elevated generally during several inflammatory processes, results should be interpreted with caution, unless prospective evaluations of the prognostic value are available. Disease monitoring by ICAM-1 is not feasible in melanoma patients who are also being treated with cytokines (interferon-α, interleukin-2), because these treatment modalities are capable of inducing secondary cytokines, which can enhance ICAM-1 levels in the serum. This conclusion is supported by our own unpublished results that evaluated ICAM-1 for routine follow-up of melanoma patients.

Cytokines

Interleukin-8

It has been shown that IL-8 is produced by several cell types including melanoma cells. Scheibenbogen and colleagues [34] could demonstrate elevated serum levels of IL-8 in 21 out of 56 patients with advanced metastatic melanoma using an ELISA assay. There was a significant correlation to tumor burden but not to particular metastatic sites [34]. Because IL-8 is expressed and released under several inflammatory conditions, the clinical value of these findings in terms of specificity and sensitivity remains unclear.

Interleukin-10

Another report on elevated cytokine levels in blood revealed elevated IL-10 levels in a stage-dependent manner in 104 untreated melanoma patients. Twenty-nine of 40 stage IV patients were positive in an IL-10 ELISA [35]. Again, these data should be considered as preliminary, because only a univariate analysis was performed and the specificity of IL-10 as a melanoma marker is, in general, low.

ACKNOWLEDGEMENTS. We thank Mrs. Frauke Ruser for typewriting this manuscript.

References

1. Hossfeld DK (1996) Tumor marker terrorism. Educational Book; 21. Congress European Society of Medical Oncology (ESMO); Wien, pp 191–192
2. Pohl AL (1992) Multiple testing with cancer markers. In: Sell S (ed): Serological Cancer Markers. Totowa, Humana Press, pp 473–494
3. Hauschild A (1997) The use of serological tumor markers for malignant melanoma. Onkologie 20:462–465
4. Horikoshi T, Ito S, Wakamatsu K, Onodera H, Eguchi H (1994) Evaluation of melanin-related metabolites as markers of melanoma progression. Cancer 73:629–636

5. Smith B, Selby P, Southgate J, Pittman K, Bradley C, Blair GE (1991) Detection of melanoma cells in peripheral blood by means of reverse transcriptase and polymerase chain reaction. Lancet 338:1227–1229
6. Brossart P, Keilholz U, Willhauck M, Scheibenbogen C, Möhler T, Hunstein W (1993) Hematogenous spread of malignant melanoma cells in different stages of disease. J Invest Dermatol 10:887–889
7. Brossart P, Schmier JW, Krüger S, Willhauck M, Scheibenbogen C, Möhler T, Keilholz U (1995) A polymerase chain reaction-based semiquantitative assessment of malignant melanoma cells in peripheral blood. Cancer Res 55:4065–4068
8. Battayani Z, Grob JJ, Xerri L, Noe C, Zarour H, Houvaeneghel G, Delpero JR, Birmbaum D, Hassoun J, Bonerandi JJ (1995) Polymerase chain reaction detection of circulating melanocytes as a prognostic marker in patients with melanoma. Arch Dermatol 131:443–447
9. Kunter U, Buer J, Probst M, Duensing S, Dallmann I, Grosse J, Kirchner H, Schluepen EM, Volkenandt M, Ganser A, Atzpodien J (1996) Peripheral blood tyrosinase messenger RNA detection and survival in malignant melanoma. J Nat Cancer Inst 88:590–594
10. Tobal K, Sherman LS, Foss AJ, Lightman SL (1993) Detection of melanocytes from uveal melanoma in peripheral blood using the polymerasse chain reaction. Invest Ophthal Vis Sci 34:2622–2625
11. Mellado B, Colomer D, Castel T, Munoz M, Carballo E, Galan M, Mascaro JM, Vives-Corrons JL, Grau JJ, Estape J (1996) Detection of circulating neoplastic cells by reverse-transcriptase polymerase chain reaction in malignant melanoma: association with clinical stage and prognosis. J Clin Oncol 14:2091–2097
12. Gläser R, Rass K, Seiter S, Hauschild A, Christophers E, Tilgen W (1997) Detection of circulating melanoma cells by specific amplification of tyrosinase complementary DNA is not a reliable tumor marker in melanoma patients: a clinical two-center study. J Clin Oncol 15:2818–2825
13. Hoon DSB, Wang Y, Dale PS, Conrad AJ, Schmid P, Garrison D, Kuo C, Foshag LJ, Nizze AJ, Morton DL (1995) Detection of occult melanoma cells in blood with a multiple-marker polymerase chain reaction assay. J Clin Oncol 13:2109–2116
14. Pittman K, Burchill S, Smith B, Southgate J, Joffe J, Gore M, Selby P (1996) Reverse transcriptase-polymerase chain reaction for expression of tyrosinase to identify malignant melanoma cells in peripheral blood. Ann Oncol 7:297–301
15. Reinhold U, Lüdtke-Handjery HC, Schnautz S, Kreysel HW, Abken H (1997) The analysis of tyrosinase-specific mRNA in blood samples of melanoma patients by RT-PCR is not a useful test for metastatic tumor progression. J Invest Dermatol 108:166–169
16. Hornef S, Lux J, Rassner G (1992) Neuronen-spezifsche Enolase (NSE) – ein geeigneter Tumormarker des malignen Melanoms? Hautarzt 43:77–80
17. Buzaid AC, Sandler AB, Hayden CL, Scinto J, Poo WJ, Clark MB, Hotchkiss S (1994) Neuron-specific enolase as a tumor marker in metastatic melanoma. Am J Clin Oncol 17:430–431
18. Couvreur R, Joos G, Geerts ML, Lambert J, Naeyaert JM (1993) Neuron-specific enolase as serum marker for malignant melanoma. Lancet 342:985
19. Wibe E, Hannisdal E, Paus E, Aamdal S (1992) Neuron-specific enolase as a prognostic factor in metastatic malignant melanoma. Eur J Cancer 28:1692–1695
20. Reintgen DS, Cruse CW, Wells KE, Saba HL, Fabri PJ (1992) The evaluation of putative tumor markers for malignant melanoma. Ann Plast Surg 28:55–59
21. Miliotes G, Lyman GH, Cruse CW, Puleo C, Albertini PA, Rapaport D, Glass F, Fenske N, Soriano T, Cuny C, van Voorhis N, Reintgen D (1996) Evaluation of new putative tumor markers for melanoma. Am Surg Oncol 3:558–563
22. Bosserhoff AK, Kaufmann M, Kaluza B, Bartke I, Zirngibl H, Hein R, Stolz W, Buettner R (1997) Melanoma inhibiting activity, a novel serum marker for progression of malignant melanoma. Cancer Res 57:3149–3153
23. Moore BW (19665) A soluble protein characteristic of the nervous system. Biochem Biophys Res Comm 19:739–744

24. Guo HB, Stoffel-Wagner B, Bierwirth T, Mezger J, Klingmüller D (1996) Clinical significance of serum S-100 in metastatic malignant melanoma. Eur J Cancer 31:924–928
25. Henze G, Dummer R, Joller-Jemelka HI, Böni R, Burg G (1997) Serum S-100 – a marker for disease monitoring in metastatic melanoma. Dermatology 194:208–212
26. von Schoultz E, Hansson LO, Djureen E, Hansson J, Kärnell R, Nilsson B, Stigbrand T, Ringborg U (1996) Prognostic value of serum analyses of S-100 beta protein in malignant melanoma. Melanoma Res 6:133–137
27. Hauschild A, Engel G, Brenner W, Gläser R, Mönig H, Henze E, Christophers E (1999) S-100B protein detection in serum is a significant prognostic factor in metastatic melanoma. Oncology 56:338–344
28. Hauschild A, Engel G, Brenner W, Gläser R, Mönig H, Henze E, Christophers E (1999) Predictive value of serum S-100B for monitoring patients with metastatic melanoma during chemotherapy and/or immunotherapy. Br J Dermatol 140:1065–1071
29. Hauschild A, Michaelsen J, Brenner W, Rudolph P, Gläser R, Henze E, Christophers E (1999) Prognostic significance of serum S-100B detection compared with routine blood parameters in advanced metastatic melanoma patients. Melanoma Res 9:155–161
30. Bonfrer JM, Korse CM, Nieweg OE, Rankin EM (1998) The luminescence immunoassay S-100: a sensitive test to measure circulating S-100B: its prognostic value in malignant melanoma. Br J Cancer 77:2210–2214
31. Altomonte M, Colizzi F, Esposito G, Maio M (1992) Circulating intercellular adhesion molecule 1 as a marker of disease progression in cutaneous melanoma. N Engl J Med 327:959
32. Viac J, Misery L, Schmitt D, Claudy A (1996) Follow-up of circulating ICAM-1 in malignant melanoma: correlation with the clinical course of the disease. Br J Dermatol 34:604–605
33. Schaider H, Rech-Weichselbraun I, Richtig E, Seidl H, Soyer HP, Smolle J, Kerl H (1997) Circulating adhesion molecules as prognostic factors for cutaneous melanoma. J Am Acad Dermatol 36:209–213
34. Scheibenbogen C, Möhler T, Haefele J, Hunstein W, Keilholz U (1995) Serum interleukin-8 (IL-8) is elevated in patients with metastatic melanoma and correlates with tumor load. Melanoma Res 5:179–181
35. Dummer W, Becker JC, Schwaaf A, Leverkus M, Moll T, Bröcker EB (1995) Elevated serum levels of interleukin-10 in patients with metastatic malignant melanoma. Melanoma Res 5:67–68

V. Clinical Relevance of Micrometastases Detection

Molecular Tools in the Detection of Micrometastatic Cancer Cells – Technical Aspects and Clinical Relevance

M. von Knebel Doeberitz, J. Weitz, M. Koch, J. Lacroix, A. Schrödel, and C. Herfarth

Division for Molecular Diagnostics and Therapy, Department of Surgery, University of Heidelberg, Im Neuenheimer Feld 110, 69120 Heidelberg, Germany

Abstract

The frequent failure to reduce the mortality due to epithelial cancers by common medical intervention results primarily from early dissemination of cancer cells, which is missed by conventional diagnostic procedures used for tumor staging. Individual carcinoma cells present in regional lymph nodes, blood or distant organs (e.g., bone marrow) can be detected by sensitive immunologic or molecular methods. Here, we review recently developed molecular assays for the detection of individual micrometastatic cancer cells and their clinical application in patients with epithelial tumors.

Introduction

Solid epithelial cancers are the most common cause of tumor-related death worldwide. Despite considerable progress in surgical treatment, a significant decrease in cancer-related mortality rates of patients with solid cancers has not been achieved. This is, at least in part, due to the early dissemination of tumor cells, which is generally occult at the time of primary diagnosis and treatment. Thus, it is reasonable to assume that the identification of disseminated cancer cells (DCC) using highly sensitive and specific techniques will allow better therapeutic management of the individual cancer patient. Over the past decade, various new and highly sensitive molecular assays have been developed that permit the identification of DCC in organs remote from the primary tumor. These assays are increasingly being used to develop early cancer detection methods as well as to establish new molecular staging assays. Here, recent molecular tools used for the detection of DCC in bone marrow, peripheral blood, and regional lymph nodes will be discussed.

In principle, either DNA- or RNA-based markers can be used, both with specific advantages but also critical limitations for the detection of rare residual cancer cells (von Knebel and Lacroix 1999). Specific mutations of defined DNA sequences, for example in proto-oncogenes (k-*ras*) and tumor suppressor genes (p53) (Sanchez-Cespedes et al. 1999a; Hayashi et al. 1994; Hayashi et al. 1995), changes in the methylation status of defined genes (for example p16; Belinsky et al. 1998), microsatellite instability (Mao et al. 1996) or even sequences of carcinogenic viruses (Kobayashi et al. 1998) have been used as markers. Since these alterations are not present in normal, non-transformed human tissues, they permit the identification of tumor-specific changes within the DNA of tumor cells or their precursors. One limitation of this approach is, however, the fact that DNA fragments might be released from decaying tumor cells in any tissues of the body. Since DNA molecules are relatively stable in human tissues, detection of the mutant or altered sequences does not per se point to the presence of *vital* cancer cells in the sample of investigation. Instead, these assays indicate, on a highly sensitive level, the presence of tumor cells that might have released DNA fragments with tumor-specific alterations (Goessl et al. 1998; Nawroz et al. 1996; Sanchez-Cespedes et al. 1998; Chen et al. 1996; Hibi et al. 1998). DNA-based assays, consequently, seem to be the most suitable to monitor the tumor burden (Fujiwara et al. 1999) or to detect cancers early (Chen et al. 1999). In some reports DNA-based markers have been used to detect residual tumor cells in lymph nodes (Sanchez-Cespedes et al. 1999b) or even at resection margins (Brennan et al. 1995), in both cases being clearly associated with a worse prognostic outcome for the respective patients. Overall, these assays are very promising; however, their true clinical relevance still awaits confirmation in large prospective studies (Sidransky 1997).

Another approach to detect DCC in clinical samples is the reverse transcriptase polymerase chain reaction (RT-PCR). In this method specific mRNA molecules are amplified which are only expressed in the tumor cells but not in surrounding tissues or other clinical samples under investigation (Raj et al. 1998; Ghossein et al. 1999a). One major advantage of using mRNA as a target for the detection assays instead of DNA is the reduced viability of RNA molecules in clinical samples once they are released from decaying cells. Thus, the detection of specific RNA transcripts points to the presence of vital tumor cells under investigation. For some cancers, specific transcripts which are selectively expressed in the tumor cells but not in normal non-neoplastic cells have been described, for example, mRNAs transcribed from specific fusion genes in various soft tissue sarcomas (Willeke et al. 1998a, b). Likewise, transcripts encoded by specific human papillomaviruses have been used to detect residual tumor cells of anogenital cancers, in particular cervical carcinoma (Czegledy et al. 1995). However, for most cancers such *true* tumor-specific mRNA molecules have not yet been characterized. Thus, transcripts of genes encoding tumor-associated proteins (CEA, MAGE, GAGE, β-HCG) or tissue-specific differentiation markers (e.g., cytokeratins, PSA, or tyrosinase) have been extensively used to detect DCC in bone marrow, lymph node or peripheral blood (Raj et al. 1998; Ghossein et al. 1999b). Although these mRNA-based assays can detect one cancer cell in about 10 ml of blood, corresponding to 10^7 normal non-transformed cells, the sensitivity and specificity of each assay largely depends on various technical factors. The precise amplification conditions, including temperature, choice of amplification primers, use of appropriate "nested" PCR primers, and the defined conditions of amplification reagents, are of particular importance. In addition inherent biological factors, for example the presence of pseudogenes or the expression of even the slightest amount of the target transcript in normal, non-transformed cells (illegitimate transcription), strongly influence the rate of false-positive test results (Zippelius et al. 1997; Bostick et al. 1998). Various pathophysiological conditions, such as the level of specific cytokines, may also markedly affect the expression levels of the target genes used for the RT-PCR-based detection of DCCs (Jung et al. 1998).

The perioperative analysis of blood samples taken from cancer patients who underwent surgery by molecular methods clearly points to a temporary intraoperative dissemination of tumor cells (Denis et al. 1997; Weitz et al. 1998). Whether these cells might reach and survive in secondary organs and form manifest metastases there is still unknown.

Recent reports from several clinical laboratories suggest that the detection of DCC in blood or bone marrow using RNA amplification assays has a strong prognostic impact on the survival of patients with cancers of the gastrointestinal tract (CK20; Soeth et al. 1997), prostate (PSA; Ghossein et al. 1997) and in melanoma (GAGE, tyrosinase; Cheung et al. 1999; Ghossein et al. 1998; Mellado et al. 1996, 1999; Keilholz 1998). However, there are also reports in which such a prognostic impact could not be confirmed (Millon et al. 1999; Oefelein et al. 1999). Additional prospective trials with more patients and, in particular, standardized amplification protocols are essentially needed before the clinical utility of these assays has been defined (De la Taille et al. 1999; Jung et al. 1997).

Molecular markers to identify single DCC may improve the diagnostic analysis of tumor-draining lymph nodes. Various publications have shown that a detailed immunohistopathological work-up of tumor-draining lymph nodes is much more sensitive to identify spread tumor cells compared to a routine histopathological analysis. Moreover, these single tumor cells in the draining lymph nodes were shown to have a strong adverse prognostic impact on the survival of patients with esophageal and lung cancer (Kubuschok et al. 1999; Izbicki et al. 1997). In contrast to immunocytochemistry, molecular markers provide the opportunity to analyze the total volume of a whole lymph node in a one-step biochemical reaction. The time-consuming morphological analysis might thus become dispensable. Preliminary studies on a limited number of patients with colorectal cancer, for example, indicated that using either DNA- (Sanchez-Cespedes et al. 1999b) or RT-PCR-based assays for CEA or CK20 mRNAs can significantly increase the detection rate of lymph node micrometastasis (Weitz et al. 1999) and that this finding is again linked to a worse clinical outcome (Liefers et al. 1998).

Conclusions

Specific and sensitive molecular tools have significantly extended our knowledge of the frequency and type of distribution of disseminated neoplastic cells in patients with solid cancers. The detection of these cells, particularly in early stages of the disease, may have a significant impact on prognosis. This, in turn, suggests that patients with DCC might be ideal candidates for adjuvant therapy modalities, in particular with drugs that eliminate both cycling and dormant cancer cells. In the future, monitoring dynamic changes in the residual tumor cell burden within the context of adjuvant systemic therapies will become an important application of the outlined detection assays.

References

Belinsky, S.A., Nikula, K.J., Palmisano, W.A., Michels, R., Saccomanno, G., Gabrielson, E., Baylin, S.B., and Herman, J.G. (1998). Aberrant methylation of p16(INK4a) is an early event in lung cancer and a potential biomarker for early diagnosis. Proc. Natl. Acad. Sci. U. S. A 95, 11891–11896

Bostick, P.J., Chatterjee, S., Chi, D.D., Huynh, K.T., Giuliano, A.E., Cote, R., and Hoon, D.S. (1998). Limitations of specific reverse-transcriptase polymerase chain reaction markers in the detection of metastases in the lymph nodes and blood of breast cancer patients. J. Clin. Oncol. 16, 2632–2640

Brennan, J.A., Mao, L., Hruban, R.H., Boyle, J.O., Eby, Y.J., Koch, W.M., Goodman, S.N., and Sidransky, D. (1995). Molecular assessment of histopathological staging in squamous-cell carcinoma of the head and neck [see comments]. N. Engl. J. Med. 332, 429–435

Chen, X., Bonnefoi, H., Diebold-Berger, S., Lyautey, J., Lederrey, C., Faltin-Traub, E., Stroun, M., and Anker, P. (1999). Detecting tumor-related alterations in plasma or serum DNA of patients diagnosed with breast cancer [In Process Citation]. Clin. Cancer Res. 5, 2297–2303

Chen, X.Q., Stroun, M., Magnenat, J.L., Nicod, L.P., Kurt, A.M., Lyautey, J., Lederrey, C., and Anker, P. (1996). Microsatellite alterations in plasma DNA of small cell lung cancer patients [see comments]. Nat. Med. 2, 1033–1035

Cheung, I.Y., Cheung, N.K., Ghossein, R.A., Satagopan, J.M., Bhattacharya, S., and Coit, D.G. (1999). Association between molecular detection of GAGE and survival in patients with malignant melanoma: a retrospective cohort study [In Process Citation]. Clin. Cancer Res. 5, 2042–2047

Czegledy, J., Iosif, C., Hansson, B.G., Evander, M., Gergely, L., and Wadell, G. (1995). Can a test for E6/E7 transcripts of human papillomavirus type 16 serve as a diagnostic tool for the detection of micrometastasis in cervical cancer? Int. J. Cancer 64, 211–215

De la, T.A., Olsson, C.A., and Katz, A.E. (1999). Molecular staging of prostate cancer: dream or reality? Oncology (Huntingt) 13, 187–194

Denis, M.G., Lipart, C., Leborgne, J., LeHur, P.A., Galmiche, J.P., Denis, M., Ruud, E., Truchaud, A., and Lustenberger, P. (1997). Detection of disseminated tumor cells in peripheral blood of colorectal cancer patients. Int. J. Cancer 74, 540–544

Fujiwara, Y., Chi, D.D., Wang, H., Keleman, P., Morton, D.L., Turner, R., and Hoon, D.S. (1999). Plasma DNA microsatellites as tumor-specific markers and indicators of tumor progression in melanoma patients. Cancer Res. 59, 1567–1571

Ghossein, R.A., Bhattacharya, S., and Rosai, J. (1999a). Molecular detection of micrometastases and circulating tumor cells in solid tumors [In Process Citation]. Clin. Cancer Res. 5 1950–1960

Ghossein, R.A., Bhattacharya, S., and Rosai, J. (1999b). Molecular detection of micrometastases and circulating tumor cells in solid tumors [In Process Citation]. Clin. Cancer Res. 5 1950–1960

Ghossein, R.A., Coit, D., Brennan, M., Zhang, Z.F., Wang, Y., Bhattacharya, S., Houghton, A., and Rosai, J. (1998). Prognostic significance of peripheral blood and bone marrow tyrosinase messenger RNA in malignant melanoma. Clin. Cancer Res. 4, 419–428

Ghossein, R.A., Rosai, J., Scher, H.I., Seiden, M., Zhang, Z.F., Sun, M., Chang, G., Berlane, K., Krithivas, K., and Kantoff, P.W. (1997). Prognostic significance of detection of prostate-specific antigen transcripts in the peripheral blood of patients with metastatic androgen-independent prostatic carcinoma. Urology 50, 100–105

Goessl, C., Heicappell, R., Munker, R., Anker, P., Stroun, M., Krause, H., Muller, M., and Miller, K. (1998). Microsatellite analysis of plasma DNA from patients with clear cell renal carcinoma. Cancer Res. 58, 4728–4732

Hayashi, N., Arakawa, H., Nagase, H., Yanagisawa, A., Kato, Y., Ohta, H., Takano, S., Ogawa, M., and Nakamura, Y. (1994). Genetic diagnosis identifies occult lymph node metastases undetectable by the histopathological method. Cancer Res. 54, 3853–3856

Hayashi, N., Ito, I., Yanagisawa, A., Kato, Y., Nakamori, S., Imaoka, S., Watanabe, H., Ogawa, M., and Nakamura, Y. (1995). Genetic diagnosis of lymph-node metastasis in colorectal cancer [see comments]. Lancet %20;345, 1257–1259

Hibi, K., Robinson, C.R., Booker, S., Wu, L., Hamilton, S.R., Sidransky, D., and Jen, J. (1998). Molecular detection of genetic alterations in the serum of colorectal cancer patients. Cancer Res. 58, 1405–1407

Izbicki, J.R., Hosch, S.B., Pichlmeier, U., Rehders, A., Busch, C., Niendorf, A., Passlick, B., Broelsch, C.E., and Pantel, K. (1997). Prognostic value of immunohistochemically identifiable tumor cells in lymph nodes of patients with completely resected esophageal cancer [see comments]. N. Engl. J. Med. 337, 1188–1194

Jung, R., Ahmad-Nejad, P., Wimmer, M., Gerhard, M., Wagener, C., and Neumaier, M. (1997). Quality management and influential factors for the detection of single metastatic cancer cells by reverse transcriptase polymerase chain reaction. Eur. J. Clin. Chem. Clin. Biochem. 35, 3–10

Jung, R., Kruger, W., Hosch, S., Holweg, M., Kroger, N., Gutensohn, K., Wagener, C., Neumaier, M., and Zander, A.R. (1998). Specificity of reverse transcriptase polymerase chain reaction assays designed for the detection of circulating cancer cells is influenced by cytokines in vivo and in vitro. Br. J. Cancer 78, 1194–1198

Keilholz, U. (1998). New prognostic factors in melanoma: mRNA tumour markers. Eur. J. Cancer 34 Suppl 3:S37–41, S37-S41

Kobayashi, Y., Yoshinouchi, M., Tianqi, G., Nakamura, K., Hongo, A., Kamimura, S., Mizutani, Y., Kodama, J., Miyagi, Y., and Kudo, T. (1998). Presence of human papilloma virus DNA in pelvic lymph nodes can predict unexpected recurrence of cervical cancer in patients with histologically negative lymph nodes. Clin. Cancer Res. 4, 979–983

Kubuschok, B., Passlick, B., Izbicki, J.R., Thetter, O., and Pantel, K. (1999). Disseminated tumor cells in lymph nodes as a determinant for survival in surgically resected non-small-cell lung cancer. J. Clin. Oncol. 17 19–24

Liefers, G.J., Cleton-Jansen, A.M., van de Velde, C.J., Hermans, J., van Krieken, J.H., Cornelisse, C.J., and Tollenaar, R.A. (1998). Micrometastases and survival in stage II colorectal cancer [see comments]. N. Engl. J. Med. 339, 223–228

Mao, L., Schoenberg, M.P., Scicchitano, M., Erozan, Y.S., Merlo, A., Schwab, D., and Sidransky, D. (1996). Molecular detection of primary bladder cancer by microsatellite analysis. Science 271, 659–662

Mellado, B., Colomer, D., Castel, T., Munoz, M., Carballo, E., Galan, M., Mascaro, J.M., Vives-Corrons, J.L., Grau, J.J., and Estape, J. (1996). Detection of circulating neoplastic cells by reverse-transcriptase polymerase chain reaction in malignant melanoma: association with clinical stage and prognosis. J. Clin. Oncol. 14, 2091–2097

Mellado, B., Gutierrez, L., Castel, T., Colomer, D., Fontanillas, M., Castro, J., and Estape, J. (1999). Prognostic significance of the detection of circulating malignant cells by reverse transcriptase-polymerase chain reaction in long-term clinically disease-free melanoma patients. Clin. Cancer Res. 5, 1843–1848

Millon, R., Jacqmin, D., Muller, D., Guillot, J., Eber, M., and Abecassis, J. (1999). Detection of Prostate-Specific Antigen- or Prostate-Specific Membrane Antigen-Positive Circulating Cells in Prostatic Cancer Patients: Clinical Implications. Eur. Urol. 36, 278–285

Nawroz, H., Koch, W., Anker, P., Stroun, M., and Sidransky, D. (1996). Microsatellite alterations in serum DNA of head and neck cancer patients [see comments]. Nat. Med. 2, 1035–1037

Oefelein, M.G., Ignatoff, J.M., Clemens, J.Q., Watkin, W., and Kaul, K.L. (1999). Clinical and molecular followup after radical retropubic prostatectomy. J. Urol. 162, 307–310

Raj, G.V., Moreno, J.G., and Gomella, L.G. (1998). Utilization of polymerase chain reaction technology in the detection of solid tumors [see comments]. Cancer 82, 1419–1442

Sanchez-Cespedes, M., Esteller, M., Hibi, K., Cope, F.O., Westra, W.H., Piantadosi, S., Herman, J.G., Jen, J., and Sidransky, D. (1999b). Molecular detection of neoplastic cells in lymph nodes of metastatic colorectal cancer patients predicts recurrence [In Process Citation]. Clin. Cancer Res. 5, 2450–2454

Sanchez-Cespedes, M., Esteller, M., Hibi, K., Cope, F.O., Westra, W.H., Piantadosi, S., Herman, J.G., Jen, J., and Sidransky, D. (1999a). Molecular detection of neoplastic cells in lymph nodes of metastatic colorectal cancer patients predicts recurrence [In Process Citation]. Clin. Cancer Res. 5, 2450–2454

Sanchez-Cespedes, M., Monzo, M., Rosell, R., Pifarre, A., Calvo, R., Lopez-Cabrerizo, M.P., and Astudillo, J. (1998). Detection of chromosome 3p alterations in serum DNA of non-small-cell lung cancer patients. Ann. Oncol. 9, 113–116

Sidransky, D. (1997). Nucleic acid-based methods for the detection of cancer. Science 278, 1054–1059

Soeth, E., Vogel, I., Roder, C., Juhl, H., Marxsen, J., Kruger, U., Henne-Bruns, D., Kremer, B., and Kalthoff, H. (1997). Comparative analysis of bone marrow and venous blood isolates from gastrointestinal cancer patients for the detection of disseminated tumor cells using reverse transcription PCR. Cancer Res. 57, 3106–3110

von Knebel, Doeberitz, M. and Lacroix, J. (1999). Nucleic acid based techniques for the detection of rare cancer cells in clinical samples. Cancer Metastasis Rev. 18, 43–64

Weitz, J., Kienle, P., Lacroix, J., Willeke, F., Benner, A., Lehnert, T., Herfarth, C., and von Knebel Doeberitz, M. (1998). Dissemination of tumor cells in patients undergoing surgery for colorectal cancer. Clin. Cancer Res. 4, 343–348

Weitz, J., Kienle, P., Magener, A., Koch, M., Schrodel, A., Willeke, F., Autschbach, F., Lacroix, J., Lehnert, T., Herfarth, C., and von Knebel Doeberitz, M. (1999). Detection of disseminated colorectal cancer cells in lymph nodes, blood and bone marrow. Clin. Cancer Res. 5, 1830–1836

Willeke, F., Mechtersheimer, G., Schwarzbach, M., Weitz, J., Zimmer, D., Lehnert, T., Herfarth, C., von Knebel Doeberitz, M., and Ridder, R. (1998a). Detection of SYT-SSX1/2 fusion transcripts by reverse transcriptase- polymerase chain reaction (RT-PCR) is a valuable diagnostic tool in synovial sarcoma. Eur. J. Cancer 34, 2087–2093

Willeke, F., Ridder, R., Mechtersheimer, G., Schwarzbach, M., Duwe, A., Weitz, J., Lehnert, T., Herfarth, C., and von Knebel Doeberitz, M. (1998b). Analysis of FUS-CHOP fusion transcripts in different types of soft tissue liposarcoma and their diagnostic implications. Clin. Cancer Res. 4, 1779–1784

Zippelius, A., Kufer, P., Honold, G., Kollermann, M.W., Oberneder, R., Schlimok, G., Riethmuller, G., and Pantel, K. (1997). Limitations of reverse-transcriptase polymerase chain reaction analyses for detection of micrometastatic epithelial cancer cells in bone marrow [see comments]. J. Clin. Oncol. 15, 2701–2708

The Clinical Relevance of Molecular Staging for Melanoma

S.C. Shivers, W. Li, J. Lin, A. Stall, M. Stafford, J. Messina, L.F. Glass, and D.S. Reintgen

Cutaneous Oncology Program, H. Lee Moffitt Cancer Center
and Research Institute at the University of South Florida, 12902 Magnolia Drive,
Tampa, FL 33612, USA

Abstract

The presence of metastatic disease in the regional nodal basin is the most important prognostic indicator for patients with malignant melanoma. The metastatic status of the sentinel lymph node (SLN), defined as the first node in the basin to drain a primary tumor, has been shown to represent that of the entire basin. Since routine histologic examination of lymph nodes often underestimates the presence of micrometastatic disease, a more sensitive assay for detecting tumor cells is needed. We have previously shown that a molecular assay based on the reverse transcriptase polymerase chain reaction (RT-PCR) was able to define a population of patients at higher risk for both recurrence and death, compared with routine H&E histology. Recently, we have compared "molecular staging" of patients by RT-PCR with conventional S-100 immunohistochemistry (IHC) staining of the SLNs. In these studies, SLN specimens were bivalved, and half of each specimen was examined by routine histology, including both H&E and S-100 IHC. The other half of each specimen was analyzed by a nested RT-PCR assay. H&E histology alone detected metastatic disease in 36 of 233 (16%) patients tested. Serial sectioning and IHC detected micrometastatic disease in another 16 patients, thus increasing the proportion of patients with nodal disease to 22%. RT-PCR detected micrometastatic disease in 114 of 181 patients who were negative by conventional methods, further increasing the proportion of patients with evidence of nodal disease to 70% overall. The clinical significance of these findings is still uncertain. The value of additional therapy (including elective lymph node dissection and interferon therapy) for patients who are positive only by the molecular method is currently being investigated by the national multi-center Sunbelt Melanoma Trial.

Introduction

For patients with a newly diagnosed melanoma, the metastatic status of the regional nodal basin is the most important prognostic indicator. Once the disease has spread to regional lymph nodes, prognostic factors based on the primary tumor add little to the prediction of recurrence and survival. In fact, the presence of nodal disease (stage III) decreases the overall survival by as much as 40%. In addition to its prognostic significance, patients with nodal disease might benefit from elective lymph node dissection (ELND) [1, 2] and/or adjuvant therapy with interferon (IFN)-α2b [3]. Therefore, accurate nodal staging is critical for determination of the need for further therapy in addition to the prediction of the clinical course of disease.

Unfortunately, standard methods have been shown to commonly underestimate the presence of metastatic disease in lymph nodes [4]. In the past, when the location of the at-risk nodal basin was obvious, ELND followed by histologic examination of all of the regional nodes could be performed as a staging procedure. However, most patients with thin melanomas turn out to be negative for nodal disease [5], which means that ELND is unnecessary for them. The situation is further complicated for many tumors located on the trunk or head and neck, where multiple nodal sites are potentially at risk.

The developments of pre-operative lymphoscintigraphy, intra-operative lymphatic mapping and sentinel lymph node (SLN) biopsy have helped to drastically reduce the number of nodes that need to be examined for full nodal staging information. The SLN is defined as the lymph node(s) that receive the primary lymphatic drainage from the primary tumor. Multiple studies have shown that the metastatic status of the SLN(s) reflects that of the entire lymphatic basin [6–9]. Therefore, in patients without clinical evidence of nodal disease, these new surgical techniques can be used to identify the locations of the nodal basins at risk for metastatic spread, identify the existence of "in-transit" nodes that are found outside of the predictable nodal basins, and allow for the identification and selective biopsy of the nodes that are most likely to contain metastatic cells if they are present [10–12]. Furthermore, since there are fewer nodes to analyze, pathologists can perform more extensive searches for metastatic cells, including serial sectioning, immunohistochemistry (IHC) and molecular assays.

Routine Detection of Micrometastatic Nodal Disease

For routine histologic examination of lymph nodes, the tissue is usually cut into sections, embedded in paraffin, and thin slices from the surface of each section are stained with H&E for microscopic examination. More recently, the use of IHC to detect melanocyte-specific antigens (such as S-100 and HMB-45) has helped to improve the microscopic detection of micrometastatic nodal disease [13, 14].

However, even with IHC, routine histologic examination of lymph nodes is associated with considerable sampling errors. The tissues are normally cut into sections every 1–4 mm, and the tissue sections put onto the slide for staining are only about 3 μm in thickness. Therefore, even with more aggressive serial sectioning protocols (such as 3 slides for every 1 mm section), less than 1% of the tissue is actually examined under the microscope. This sampling error alone probably accounts for the observation that 25–50% of metastatic disease may be missed upon routine examination [4, 10].

Molecular Staging for Melanoma

The use of molecular assays to detect gene expression markers that are specific for metastatic cells in lymph nodes has been termed "molecular staging." Reverse-transcriptase polymerase chain reaction (RT-PCR) can be used to target and amplify mRNA sequences for tissue-specific and/or tumor-specific genes that are not usually expressed in normal lymph nodes or other tissues [15–18]. In general, total cellular RNA is extracted from the lymph node tissue and a cDNA library of the mRNA species is prepared by using reverse transcriptase (RT) in the presence of oligo-d_T primers, which bind to the poly-A tails of mRNAs. PCR is then performed on the resulting cDNA to amplify gene-specific sequences to detectable levels.

Our laboratory primarily uses the tyrosinase gene as the molecular target for detection of micrometastatic numbers of melanoma cells in SLNs. Tyrosinase is a key enzyme involved in melanin pigment production and expression of this gene is mostly unique to melanocytes, including melanoma cells [19]. Tyrosinase appears to be a good tissue-specific marker because all melanocytes and more than 95% of melanoma primary tumors have been shown to express the gene [20]. However, there are two potential sources of false-positive results using this marker: benign nevus cells (observed in approximately 5% of lymph node specimens) and Schwann cells, which produce the myelin sheath of peripheral nerves [21]. Although nerve cells are commonly observed in histologic sections of lymph nodes, it is unclear whether the level of tyrosinase expression by Schwann cells is a problem for the use of RT-PCR assays for this marker.

The use of RT-PCR assays to detect submicroscopic metastases has the potential to increase the sensitivity of detection over routine histology and IHC up to three orders of magnitude. Routine H&E staining of lymph nodes has been shown to detect one metastatic cell per 10^4 normal cells, while IHC using antibodies against tissue- and/or tumor-specific markers can increase the detection to approximately one metastatic cell in 10^5 normal cells. RT-PCR assays have been shown to detect as few as one metastatic cell in 10^6–10^7 normal cells [15, 16, 22].

The biggest advantage to the use of molecular over histologic methods is that the former are not as susceptible to sampling errors, since the entire node has the potential for being assayed. While histologic methods examine

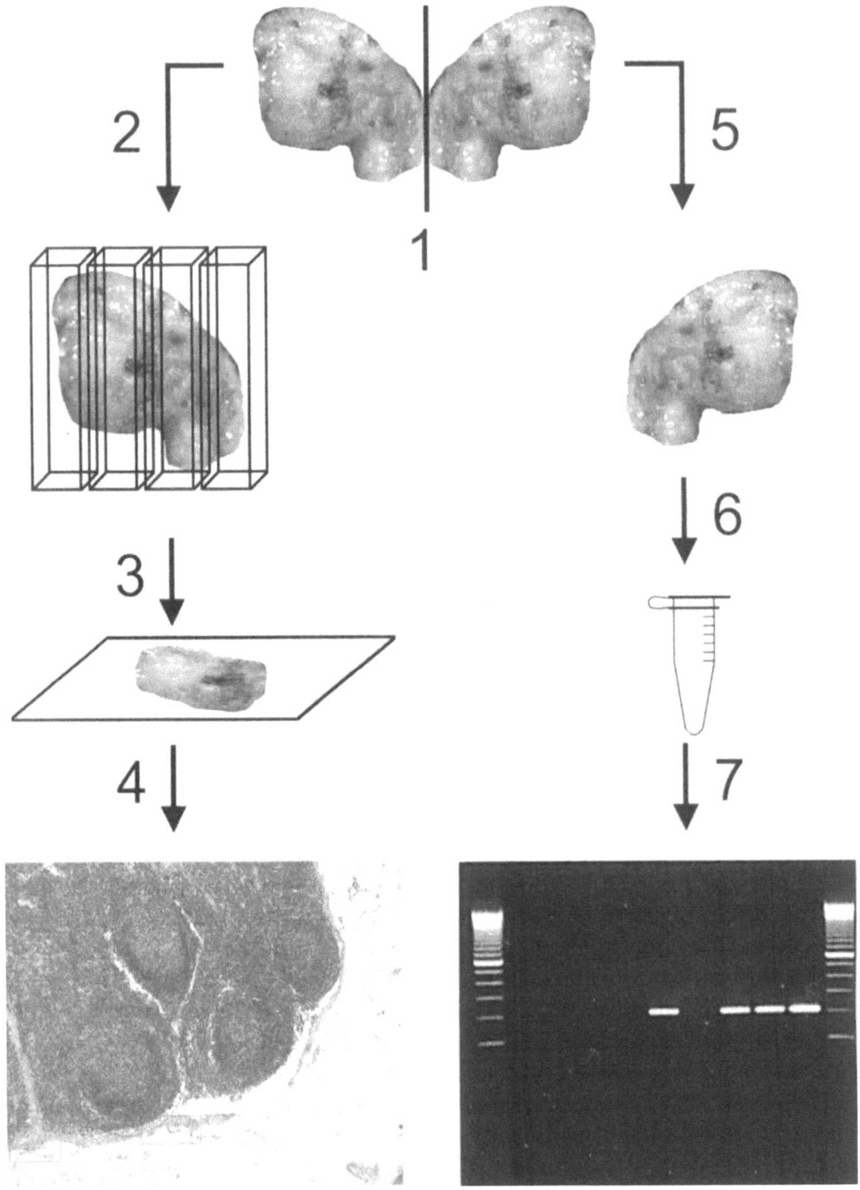

Fig. 1. Tissue sampling for histologic and molecular analysis of the sentinel lymph node (SLN). *1* SLNs were trimmed of excess fat and bivalved by the surgeon in the operating room. Randomly, half of each node was sent to pathology for routine histologic analysis (*2–4*) and the other half was sent to the research lab for RT-PCR analysis (*5–7*). *2* The specimens were cut into sections every 3–4 mm and each section was embedded in paraffin blocks. *3* Thin (3 μm) slices were cut from the surface of each block and mounted on glass slides. *4* Slides were stained with H&E or by S-100 IHC and examined for the presence of metastatic cells under high power by an experienced dermatopathologist. *5* Specimens for RT-PCR analysis were frozen at −70 °C (or lower) within 2 h after harvest in order to slow degradation of the mRNA. *6* Total cellular RNA was extracted from the frozen specimens in the presence of RNAse inhibitors. *7* RT-PCR using tyrosinase- and *β*-actin- (not shown) specific primers was performed and PCR products were visualized by electrophoresis in a 2% agarose gel containing ethidium bromide. A band at 207 bp indicates amplification of cDNA derived from tyrosinase mRNA

only a few micrometers for every 1 mm or so of tissue, molecular methods can detect cells in a much larger proportion of the tissue that is submitted for analysis (Fig. 1). Total cellular RNA is extracted from the entire specimen submitted and a homogeneous solution of the RNA is prepared for assay.

RT-PCR vs Routine H&E Histology

In order to assess the ability of RT-PCR to predict melanoma recurrence and overall survival, we performed the assay on the SLNs from 114 patients with newly diagnosed cutaneous malignant melanoma, but with no evidence of palpable lymph nodes (clinical stage I or stage II disease) [23]. The patients underwent lymphatic mapping and SLN biopsy using both radiocolloid and blue dye techniques. The SLNs were bivalved and, randomly, half of each node was sent to pathology for routine histologic analysis (H&E staining only). The other half of each SLN was frozen at –70 °C to preserve the mRNA for later RT-PCR analysis. Total cellular RNA was extracted from the frozen tissue by a phenolguanidinium thiocyanate method. The presence of amplifiable mRNA in the specimens was confirmed by performing a RT-PCR assay for β-actin, a housekeeping gene [24]. RT-PCR was performed using nested primers for the tyrosinase gene (Fig. 2) [25]. PCR products were detected by electrophoresis in a 2% agarose gel containing ethidium bromide.

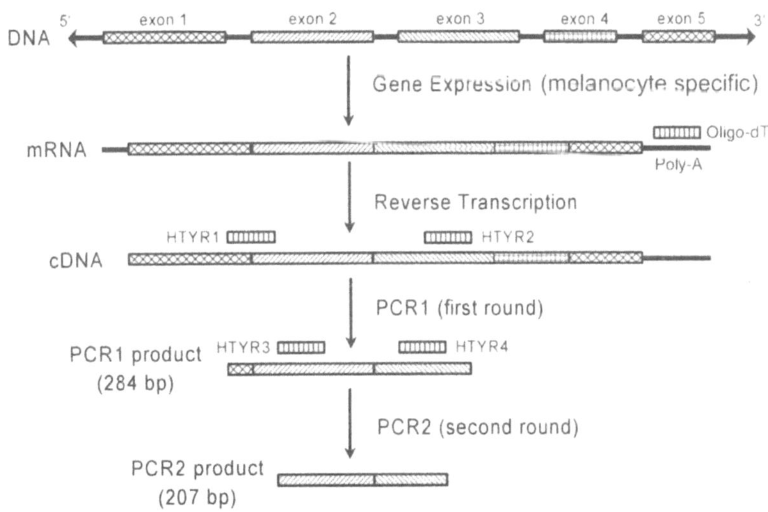

Fig. 2. Tyrosinase RT-PCR. The tyrosinase gene, which consists of five exons, is expressed almost exclusively by melanocytes, including melanoma cells. An oligo-d_T primer is used in the reverse transcriptase step to generate a cDNA library of all of the mRNA present in the sample. The tyrosinase cDNA is amplified by two rounds of PCR using nested primer pairs (HTYR1/HTYR2 and HTYR3/HTYR4), resulting in a final 207-bp product. Note that the HTYR1 primer spans an exon-exon boundary, which favors amplification of sequences derived from mRNA over those from genomic DNA

Table 1. Patient groups defined by SLN status: correlation with clinical outcome

Patient group	SLN status		Patients	Recurrences	Deaths
	Histology	RT-PCR			
Group 1	Neg.	Neg.	44 (39%)	1/44 (2%)	0/44 (0%)
Group 2	Neg.	Pos.	47 (41%)	6/47 (13%)	4/47 (9%)
Group 3	Pos.	Pos.	23 (20%)	14/23 (61%)	9/23 (39%)

Patients were placed into three groups according to the status of their SLNs by both routine H&E histology and tyrosinase RT-PCR (Table 1). Twenty-three patients had histologic evidence of metastatic disease in one or more SLNs and all of these patients were also RT-PCR positive. Therefore, there were no false-negatives for the RT-PCR assay in this patient population. Of the 91 patients who were histology-negative, 47 patients (52%) were positive by the molecular assay.

After an average follow-up of 28 months, the patient groups were analyzed for recurrence-free and overall survival. Some 61% of the histology-positive patients had a recurrence and/or died of malignant melanoma, while only one patient from the histology-negative and PCR-negative group relapsed (with a local recurrence) and none of these patients died. However, the group of patients who would have been upstaged by the molecular assay (histology-negative, PCR-positive) had intermediate rates of recurrence-free and overall survival. Kaplan-Meier analysis (Fig. 3) showed that the differences between the histology-negative patients in group 1 (PCR-negative) and group 2 (PCR-positive) were significant for both recurrence-free ($P=0.02$) and overall ($P=0.02$) survival.

Furthermore, univariate and multivariate regression analyses were performed for disease-free survival (DFS) to determine the prognostic significance of a number of variables (Breslow thickness, Clark level, ulceration of the primary tumor, cutaneous site, sex, age and histologic or RT-PCR status of the SLNs). For both univariate (with each variable acting independently in the model) and multivariate analyses, the histologic status and the RT-PCR status of the SLNs were the only variables that significantly predicted DFS. Therefore, once metastatic disease (detected either by histology or RT-PCR) developed in the SLNs, other factors based on the primary tumor did not significantly contribute to the prognosis.

RT-PCR vs S-100 Immunohistochemistry

One of the problems with the previously referenced study was that the histology did not include IHC for S-100, which has recently been incorporated into the routine analysis of lymph nodes at risk for metastatic melanoma in many pathology labs throughout the country, including our own. Therefore,

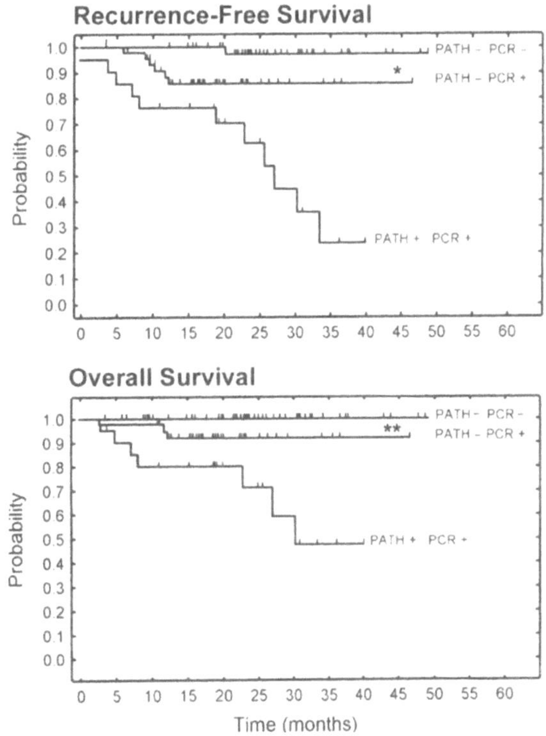

Fig. 3. Clinical relevance of molecular staging: recurrence-free and overall survival. Kaplan-Meier survival analysis showed that the differences between the pathology-negative/PCR-negative and pathology-negative/PCR-positive patient groups were significant for both relapse-free (* $P = 0.0167$) and overall (** $P = 0.0238$) survival

we have been following a more recent population of 233 patients who had their SLNs analyzed by both RT-PCR for tyrosinase and routine histology, including S-100 IHC [26]. As before, these were patients without clinically palpable nodes who underwent lymphatic mapping and SLN biopsy. Again, the half of each SLN sent for histologic analysis was sectioned every 3–4 mm, but this time at least three slides were made from each section. One slide was stained with H&E as before, one was used as a negative control for IHC with an irrelevant antibody and the third was stained by IHC with S-100. If a specimen was negative by H&E staining, but positive by S-100 IHC, the presence of metastatic melanoma cells was confirmed by looking for them on the H&E slide or by doing more sections and staining with H&E. Since the malignant morphology of cells is best determined on H&E sections, finding the cells in retrospection on further H&E-stained slides was a requirement for calling a SLN positive for metastatic disease.

A summary of the results for this study is shown in Table 2. Initial examination of the H&E-stained slides detected metastatic melanoma cells in the SLNs of 36 patients. An additional 16 patients had evidence of disease that

Table 2. Detection of micrometastases: H&E vs S-100 IHC vs RT-PCR

Patient group	*N*	%
H&E+	36	16
H&E–/S-100+	16	7
H&E–/S100–/PCR+	114	49
H&E–/S100–/PCR–	64	27

was detected only by S-100 IHC; however, a closer look with H&E was able to confirm the presence of metastatic cells in all of these patients. Therefore, 31% of the 52 patients with histologically detectable disease would have been missed without the use of S-100 IHC. Out of 178 patients without histologically detectable disease, 114 (64%) were positive by tyrosinase RT-PCR. Note, however, that in this study there were three patients who were positive by routine histology, but negative by RT-PCR. Two of these three patients were initially negative by H&E , but the disease was detected by S-100 IHC. This suggests that the cause of the false-negative RT-PCR assays might be due to sampling errors in which there is a small amount of disease present in one-half of a specimen, but not the other.

Since we do not yet have adequate follow-up to assess the prognostic value of the RT-PCR assay in this patient population, we instead attempted to demonstrate that PCR positivity is at least related to prognostic factors based on the primary tumor that have been previously shown to be important in predicting survival (Fig. 4). When used as a continuous variable, the Breslow thickness of patients who were PCR-positive (mean=2.37 mm) was overall significantly higher than in patients who were PCR-negative (mean = 1.70 mm). Furthermore, when compared to patients with thin tumors (less than 1.5 mm), patients with intermediate-thickness tumors (1.5–4.0 mm) were about twice as likely to be PCR-positive, and patients with thick tumors (greater than 4.0 mm) were almost five times more likely to be PCR-positive. In addition, patients with Clark level IV tumors were two and a half times more likely to be PCR-positive than patients with Clark level III tumors, and patients with ulcerated primary tumors were more than twice as likely to be PCR-positive than patients whose tumors were not ulcerated.

RT-PCR Sensitivity and Specificity

Our data show that the nested RT-PCR assay for tyrosinase is considerably more sensitive for the detection of micrometastatic melanoma in SLN, and at least some of the disease detected by the molecular assay alone has a significant impact on the patient's risk for recurrence and chance for survival. However, even though the follow-up periods are relatively short, a considerably large proportion of patients who would be upstaged by the molecular

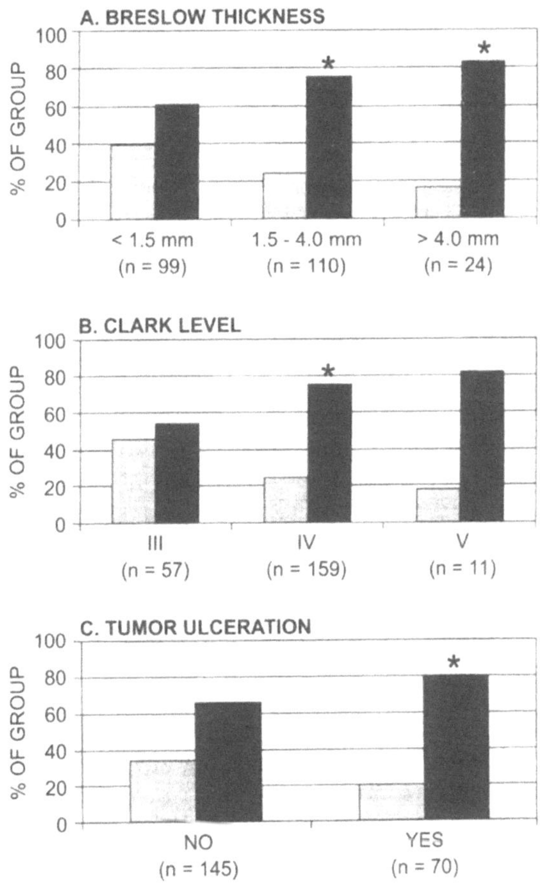

Fig. 4 A–C. Relationship of SLN RT-PCR positivity to prognostic factors based on the primary tumor. **A** When used as a continuous variable, the mean Breslow thickness was 1.70 mm for the PCR-negative patients and 2.37 mm for the PCR-positive patients (*t* test: P=0.010). The proportion of PCR-positive patients was significantly higher among patients with intermediate-thickness (1.5–4.0 mm) tumors (χ^2: odds ratio=1.84, $P=0.050$) and patients with thick (>4.0 mm) tumors (odds ratio=4.77, $P=0.046$) than in patients with thin tumors (<1.5 mm). **B** Patients with a Clark level IV tumor were more likely to be PCR-positive than patients with Clark level III tumors (odds ratio=2.58, $P=0.003$). **C** Patients with an ulcerated primary tumor were also more likely to be PCR-positive than patients whose tumors were not ulcerated (odds ratio=2.11, $P=0.032$)

assay have not yet relapsed. Therefore, we have recently performed further studies to better define the sensitivity and specificity of the assay.

To define the sensitivity of the assay, we have pooled data from the two studies above for all patients with histologically detected disease (Table 3). In the first study, 23 patients were histology-positive and all of these patients were PCR-positive. In the second study, 52 patients were histology-positive, including 16 patients whose disease would have been missed without the use of S-100 IHC, and 49 of these patients were PCR-positive. Therefore, consid-

Table 3. Sensitivity and specificity of the nested RT-PCR assay for tyrosinase

	Fraction	%
Sensitivity (in histology+SLNs)	72/75	96
Specificity (in non-melanoma LNs)	29/36	81

ering all of the histology-positive patients, the sensitivity of the PCR assay was 96% (72/75), and considering only those cases in which S-100 IHC was used, the sensitivity was 94% (49/52).

To define the specificity of the tyrosinase RT-PCR assay, we tested a panel of lymph nodes from 36 patients undergoing lymph node dissection for other non-melanoma cancers (prostate, breast, lung, colon, lymphoma and squamous cell carcinoma.) All of the specimens were histologically negative for the disease being tested. The tyrosinase RT-PCR assay gave an apparent false-positive result in seven patients, which corresponds to a specificity of 81% (29/36). The observed false-positive rate of 19% is higher than what would be expected due to benign nevus cells, which express tyrosinase and are routinely observed in approximately 5% of patients.

Another possible source of the molecular false-positives might be Schwann cells, which have been shown to express low levels of tyrosinase, and are routinely noted in histologic sections of lymph nodes. Colleagues at the John Wayne Cancer Institute (JWCI) have used an in situ RT-PCR method to detect tyrosinase expression in histologic sections [27]. Using this technique, they found that although metastatic melanoma cells were the strongest expressers of tyrosinase, lower but detectable levels of tyrosinase were found in nerve cells. However, when our laboratory sent the JWCI investigators slides from specimens that had been tested by our RT-PCR assay, they found tyrosinase-expressing nerve cells even in three out of five specimens that were PCR-negative by our assay [28]. Therefore, the in situ PCR method detected low levels of tyrosinase expression that were not picked up by the whole-tissue method. It is still possible, however, that higher levels of tyrosinase expression by Schwann cells could result in some false-positive results for the whole-tissue method.

Conclusions

Our results show that use of the RT-PCR assay for tyrosinase expression in SLNs is considerably more sensitive than routine histology (with or without IHC) for the detection of micrometastatic melanoma cells. Overall, tyrosinase RT-PCR detected metastatic disease in the SLNs of up to 64% of patients who were negative by routine histology. Recently, at least two other laboratories have reported similar findings [29, 30]. Furthermore, our data show that the molecular assay has clinical relevance for the prediction of both recurrence-free and overall survival.

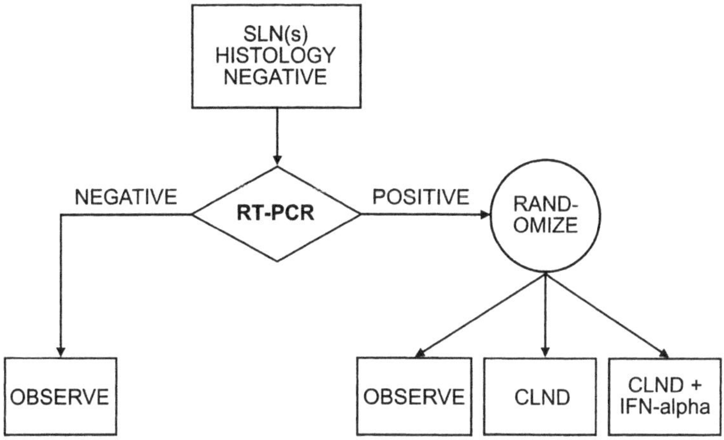

Fig. 5. Protocol B of the Sunbelt Melanoma Trial. Patients with histology-negative, but PCR-positive SLN(s) will be randomized to three arms: observation only, completion lymph node dissection (*CLND*) or CLND with interferon (*IFN*)-α treatment

Although our current follow-up times are relatively short (mean <28 months, overall), only a small proportion of the histology-negative PCR-positive patients have recurred so far. Further follow-up time is needed to determine whether the gap between PCR-positive and PCR-negative survival curves will widen and the PCR-positive patients will fare more like the histology-positive patients. At least some of these patients might be false positive by RT-PCR due to the presence of benign nevus cells, or possibly Schwann cells. In addition, some of these patients might be "biological" false positives, in which a small number of metastatic cells are present, but the patient is cured either by the SLN dissection or by their immune system.

A more important question – whether more aggressive treatment can be used to improve the outcome of the histology-negative, PCR-positive patients – remains to be answered. This question is currently being addressed by the national, multi-center Sunbelt Melanoma Trial (SMT; Fig. 5). Protocol B of the SMT randomizes the histology-negative PCR-positive patients to one of three arms: (1) observation only, which is the standard of care for histology-negative patients, (2) lymph node dissection, which has been shown to benefit certain histology-positive patients and is the standard of care for patients with a histology-positive SLN [1, 2], or (3) lymph node dissection with IFN-α2b therapy, which might benefit some patients with nodal disease [3, 31].

In addition, the SMT is using some improvements and/or modifications to the RT-PCR assay. For instance, the SMT is using a multiple-marker PCR protocol to define PCR-positivity of the SLNs. Specimens must be positive for tyrosinase, as well as at least one other marker (gp100, MART-1/Melan-A, or MAGE-3) to be considered PCR-positive. Benign nevus cells and Schwann cells are usually not positive with any of these last three melanoma-associated markers. Furthermore, the SMT is using a non-nested PCR protocol for the expression of tyrosinase, which might be less sensitive but perhaps more clinically relevant than the nested assay due to better specificity.

Further studies are needed to better define the clinical significance of the tyrosinase and other RT-PCR assays for the detection of metastatic cells in SLNs and other tissues. If it can be shown that completion lymph node dissection and/or adjuvant IFN-α2b can be used to improve the outcome of patients with small amounts of disease detected only by the molecular assays, then molecular staging will undoubtedly become part of the standard pathological analysis of SLNs in the near future.

References

1. Balch C, Soong SJ, Bartolucci AA, et al. (1996) Efficacy of an elective regional lymph node dissection of 1-4 mm thick melanomas for patients 60 years of age and younger. Ann Surg 224:255-66
2. Balch CM. (1999) Randomized surgical trials involving elective node dissection for melanoma. Advances in Surgery 32:255-70.
3. Kirkwood JM, Strawderman MH, Ernstoff MS, et al. (1996) Interferon alfa-2b adjuvant therapy of high-risk resected cutaneous melanoma: The eastern Cooperative Oncology Group Trial EST 1684. J Clin Oncol 14:7-17
4. Cochran AJ, Wen DR, Morton DL. (1988) Occult tumor cells in lymph nodes of patients with pathological stage I melanoma. Am J Surg Path 12:612-8
5. Reintgen DS, Vollmer R, Tso CV, Seigler HF. (1987) Prognosis for Stage I Malignant Melanoma. Arch Surg 122:1338-1342
6. Ross MI, Reintgen DS, Balch C. (1993) Selective lymphadenectomy: emerging role for lymphatic mapping and sentinel node biopsy in the management of early melanoma. Semin Surg Oncol 9:219-223
7. Uren RF, Howman-Giles RB, Shaw HM, Thompson JF, McCarthy WH. (1993) Lymphoscintigraphy in high risk melanoma of the trunk: Predicting draining lymph node groups, defining lymphatic channels and locating the sentinel node. J Nucl Med 34:1435-1440
8. Reintgen DS, Cruse CW, Wells K, et al. (1994) The orderly progression of melanoma nodal metastases. Ann Surg 220:759-767
9. Krag DN, Meijer SJ, Weaver DL, et al. (1995) Minimal-access surgery for staging of malignant melanoma. Arch Surg 130:654-658
10. Wong JH, Cagle LA, Morton DL. (1991) Lymphatic drainage of skin to a sentinel node in a feline model. Ann Surg 214:637-641
11. Morton DL, Wen DR, Wong JH, et al. (1992) Technical details of intra-operative lymphatic mapping for early stage melanoma. Arch Surg 127:392-399
12. Norman J, Cruse CW, Wells K, Berman C, Clark R, Reintgen DS. (1991) A redefinition of skin lymphatic drainage by lymphoscintigraphy for malignant melanoma. Am J Surg 162:432-437
13. Cho KH, Hashimoto K, Taniguchi Y, et al. (1990) Immunohistochemical study of melanocytic nevus and malignant melanoma with monoclonal antibodies against S-100 subunits. Cancer 66:765-771
14. Messina J, Glass F. (1997) Pathologic examination of the sentinel lymph node. J Florida Med Assoc 84:153-156
15. Wang X, Heller R, VanVoorhis N, et al. (1994) Detection of submicroscopic lymph node metastases with polymerase chain reaction in patients with malignant melanoma. Ann Surg 220:768-74
16. Noguchi S, Aihara T, Motomura K, et al. (1996) Detection of breast cancer micrometastases in axillary nodes by means of reverse transcriptase-polymerase chain reaction. Am J Pathol 148:649-656

17. Shivers SC, Stall A, Goscin C, et al. (1999) Molecular staging for melanoma and breast cancer. Surgical Oncology Clinics of North America 8(3):515–526
18. Okegawa T, Yoshioka J, Morita R, et al. (1998) Molecular staging of prostate cancer: comparison of nested reverse transcription polymerase chain reaction assay using prostate specific antigen versus prostate specific membrane antigen as primer. Int J Urol 5(4):349–356
19. Kwon BS, Haq AK, Pomerantz SH, Halaban R. (1987) Isolation and sequence of a cDNA clone for human tyrosinase that maps at the mouse c-albino locus. Proc Natl Acad Sci 84:7473–7477
20. Chen YT, Stockert E, Tsang S, et al. (1995) Immunophenotyping of melanomas for tyrosinase: implications for vaccine development. Proceedings of the National Academy of Sciences of the United States of America 92(18):8125–8129
21. Battyani Z, Xerri L, Hassoun J, et al. (1993) Tyrosinase gene expression in human tissues. Pigment Cell Research 6(6):400–405
22. Fields KK, Elfenbein GJ, Trudeau WL, et al. (1996) Clinical significance of bone marrow metastases detected using the polymerase chain reaction in patients with breast cancer undergoing high dose chemotherapy and autologous bone marrow transplantation. J Clin Oncol 6:1868–1876
23. Shivers S., Wang X., Li W., et al. (1998) Molecular staging of malignant melanoma: correlation with clinical outcome. JAMA 280:1410–1415
24. McLean AG, Hughes D, Welsh KI, et al. (1997) Patterns of graft infiltration and cytokine gene expression during the first 10 days of kidney transplantation. Transplantation 63(3):374–380
25. Smith B, Selby P, Southgate J, et al. (1991) Detection of melanoma cells in peripheral blood by means of reverse-transcriptase and polymerase chain reaction. Lancet 338:1227–1229
26. Li W, Stall A, Shivers S, et al. The clinical relevance of molecular staging for melanoma: comparison of RT-PCR and immunohistochemistry staining in sentinel lymph nodes of melanoma patients. Ann Surg Oncol, in press
27. Guo J, Cheng L, Wen DR, et al. (1998) Detection of tyrosinase mRNA in formalin-fixed, paraffin embedded archival sections of melanoma, using reverse transcriptase in situ polymerase chain reaction. Diagnostic Molecular Pathology 7(1):10–15
28. Guo J, Messina J, Wen DR, Huang RR, Reintgen DS, Cochran A. (1999) Does the PCR detect melanoma in sentinel nodes (SN) that is not detected by immunohistochemistry. US and Canadian Academy of Pathology
29. Blaheta HJ, Schittek B, Breuninger H, et al. (1999) Detection of melanoma micrometastasis in sentinel nodes by reverse transcription-polymerase chain reaction correlates with tumor thickness and is predictive of micrometastatic disease in the lymph node basin. Am J Surg Pathol 23(7):822–828
30. Bieligk SC, Ghossein R, Bhattacharya S, Coit D. (1999) Detection of tyrosinase mRNA by reverse transcription-polymerase chain reaction in melanoma sentinel nodes. Annals of Surgical Oncology 6(3):232–240
31. Agarwala SS, Kirkwood JM. (1998) Adjuvant interferon treatment for melanoma. Hematology – Oncology Clinics of North America 12(4):823–833

Clinical Significance of PCR-Positive mRNA Markers in Peripheral Blood and Regional Nodes of Malignant Melanoma Patients

G. Palmieri[1], M. Pirastu[1], M. Strazzullo[2], P.A. Ascierto[2], S.M.R. Satriano[2], M.L. Motti[2], G. Botti[2], N. Mozzillo[2], G. Castello for the Melanoma Cooperative Group[2], A. Cossu[3], A. Lissia[3], and F. Tanda[3]

[1] Institute of Molecular Genetics, C.N.R., Alghero, Italy
[2] National Tumor Institute "G. Pascale", Naples, Italy
[3] Institute of Pathology, University of Sassari, Italy

Abstract

Reverse-transcriptase polymerase chain reaction (RT-PCR) with multiple markers has been demonstrated to be highly sensitive in detecting metastatic cells in peripheral blood of malignant melanoma (MM) patients, and the circulating MM cells to be significantly correlated with disease stages. We further evaluated the presence of specific PCR-positive mRNA markers in peripheral blood as well as in regional nodes as an expression of tumor progression. Peripheral blood samples from 317 MM patients with either localized ($n=219$) or metastatic ($n=98$) disease were processed to obtain total cellular RNA. RT-PCR was performed using tyrosinase (TYR), p97, and MelanA/MART1 as mRNA markers. PCR products were analyzed by gel electrophoresis and Southern blot hybridization. In addition, paraffin-embedded samples of histologically proven tumor-negative lymph nodes from the subset of patients with localized disease were analyzed by RT-PCR, using radiolabeled primers for TYR and MelanA/MART1. The presence of mRNA markers was significantly correlated with tumor burden with a good correlation between risk of recurrence (evaluated in stage I–III patients) and increasing number of PCR-positive markers ($p=0.0002$). Currently, for each patient, PCR results obtained at different times during follow-up are being analyzed, and any variation in the number of PCR-positive markers is being correlated to the clinical status. Molecular screening of histologically negative nodes for the presence of metastatic MM cells is also under evaluation. Preliminary assessment of a subset of MM patients with higher risk of recurrence will require longer follow-up in order to define the role of RT-PCR in monitoring these patients.

Aims of the Study

Reverse-transcriptase polymerase chain reaction (RT-PCR) using tyrosinase mRNA has been reported to be a useful tool for the detection of circulating

Recent Results in Cancer Research, Vol. 158

tumor cells in the peripheral blood of patients with malignant melanoma (MM) [1, 2]. However, different authors have reported conflicting results on the sensitivity and clinical value of tyrosinase RT-PCR [3–9]. The heterogeneity of tyrosinase expression in melanomas and methodological differences in blood sample preparation, RNA extraction and cDNA synthesis may account for these discrepancies. Therefore, a single mRNA marker assay could be less inclusive than a multi-marker mRNA assay for detecting the heterogeneous population of occult metastatic melanoma cells. RT-PCR with multiple markers has been demonstrated to be highly sensitive in detecting metastatic cells in peripheral blood of MM patients [10, 11], and the MM circulating cells to be significantly correlated with disease stages [12]. We further evaluated the presence of specific PCR-positive mRNA markers in peripheral blood as well as in regional nodes as an expression of tumor progression.

Patients and Methods

Peripheral blood samples from 317 MM patients with either localized ($n=219$) or metastatic ($n=98$) disease were processed to obtain total cellular RNA, following the indications of the European Organization for Research and Treatment of Cancer's Melanoma Cooperative Group (EORTC-MCG) [13]. No clinical decisions were made based on the result of the RT-PCR assay. All stage I–III patients were visited every 4 months after the diagnosis. RT-PCR was performed using tyrosinase (TYR), p97, and MelanA/MART1 as mRNA markers. Primer sequences were as previously described [12]. In each RT-PCR assay, respective controls included a melanoma cell line RNA as reaction-positive control, PCR reagents and primers without RNA as reaction-negative control (to reveal abnormal PCR-mixture contamination), and amplification control for the housekeeping gene GAPDH (to facilitate quantitative and qualitative assessment of both RNA extraction and cDNA synthesis). PCR products were analyzed by gel electrophoresis and Southern blot hybridization. In addition, paraffin-embedded samples of histologically proven tumor-negative lymph nodes from the subset of patients with localized disease were analyzed by RT-PCR, using radiolabeled primers for TYR and MelanA/MART1.

Results

A high sensitivity of the RT-PCR assay with multiple markers was demonstrated, detecting one melanoma cell in 10^7 peripheral blood nucleated cells. Among the gene markers used, we did not observe any TYR mRNA transcript in non-melanoma controls, confirming the highspecificity of this marker (Table 1). Nonetheless, p97 and MelanA/MART1 showed a good specificity, with only 5–7% false-positive results in non-melanoma controls (Table 1). Significant correlation with disease stage for each mRNA marker (P of linearity ranged from 0.004 of TYR to <0.00001 of p97), and for patients positive

Table 1. RT-PCR analysis of non-melanoma controls

	TYR (%)	p97 (%)	MelanA (%)
Healthy donors ($n=20$)	0	0	0
Cancer patients ($n=21$)	0	3 (14)	2 (12)
All patients ($n=41$)	0	3 (7)	2 (5)

Table 2. RT-PCR results for each individual mRNA marker and total number of PCR-positive markers: correlation to the disease stage

AJCC stage (patients)	PCR-positive markers (%)			No. of PCR-positives (%)			
	TYR	p97	MelanA	0	1	2	3
I (114)	29 (25)	57 (50)	21 (18)	40 (35)	43 (38)	27 (24)	4 (3)
II (105)	35 (33)	67 (64)	26 (25)	27 (26)	46 (44)	22 (21)	10 (9)
III (66)	28 (42)	54 (82)	25 (38)	9 (14)	20 (30)	21 (32)	16 (24)
IV (32)	24 (75)	31 (97)	20 (63)	0	4 (12)	13 (41)	15 (47)
Total (317)	116 (37)	209 (66)	92 (29)	76 (24)	113 (36)	83 (26)	45 (14)

Table 3. Preliminary data on histologically negative regional lymph nodes

AJCC stage (number of patients)	No. of PCR-positive markers (%)	
	0	≥1
I (8)	6 (75)	2 (25)
IIA (24)	8 (33)	16 (67)
IIB (9)	2 (22)	7 (78)
Total (41)	16 (39)	25 (61)

to all markers ($P<0.0001$) was demonstrated (Table 2). A significant preliminary observation in our series was the association between increasing number of PCR-positive markers and risk of relapse in stage I–III patients with no evidence of clinical disease ($P=0.0002$; median follow-up 23 months). Currently, for each patient, PCR results obtained at different times during follow-up are being analyzed and any variation in the number of PCR-positive markers is being correlated to the clinical status. Preliminary data regarding the molecular screening of histologically negative nodes for the presence of metastatic MM cells are reported in Table 3.

Conclusion

Our results establish the existence of statistically significant associations between clinical stage of malignant melanoma and detection by RT-PCR of tumor-associated antigens in peripheral blood as an expression of circulating neoplastic cells. Assessment of a subset of patients with higher risk of recurrence requires further evaluation in order to define the role of RT-PCR in monitoring MM patients.

ACKNOWLEDGEMENTS. The authors would like to thank Dr. Assunta Criscuolo for data management and Dr. Egidio Celentano for statistical analysis. The work was supported by the Italian Ministry of Health.

Melanoma Cooperative Group: Aprea P., Ascierto P.A., Botti G., Caraco' C., Castello G., Celentano E., Comella C., Daponte A., Graziano F., Mozzillo N., Parasole R., Picone A., National Tumor Institute, Naples, Italy; Bosco L., Satriano R., 2nd University of Naples, Italy; Palmieri G., Muresu R., Institute of Molecular Genetics, C.N.R., Alghero, Italy; Cossu A., Lissia A., Massarelli G., Tanda F., University of Sassari, Italy.

References

1. Smith B, Selby P, Southgate J, et al. (1991) Detection of melanoma cells in peripheral blood by means of reverse transcriptase and polymerase chain reaction. Lancet 338:1227–1229
2. Brossart P, Schmier J, Kruger S, et al. (1995) A PCR-based semiquantitative assessment of malignant melanoma cells in peripheral blood. Cancer Res 55:4065–4068
3. Battayani Z, Grob J, Xerri R, et al. (1995) PCR detection of circulating melanocytes as a prognostic marker in patients with melanoma. Arch Dermatol 131:443–447
4. Kunter U, Buer J, Probst M, et al. (1996) Peripheral blood tyrosinase messenger RNA detection and survival in malignant melanoma. J Natl Cancer Inst 88:590–594
5. Pittman K, Burchill S, Smith B, et al. (1996) Reverse transcriptase-polymerase chain reaction for expression of tyrosinase to identify malignant melanoma cells in peripheral blood. Ann Oncol 7: 97–301
6. Reinhold U, Ludtke Handjery HC, Schnautz S, et al. (1997) The analysis of tyrosinase specific mRNA in blood samples of melanoma patients by RT-PCR is not a useful test for metastatic tumor progression. J Invest Dermatol 108:166–169
7. Mellado B, Colomer D, Castel T, et al. (1996) Detection of circulating neoplastic cells by reverse-transcriptase polymerase chain reaction in malignant melanoma: association with clinical stage and prognosis. J Clin Oncol 14:2091–2097
8. Glaser R, Rass K, Seiter S, et al. (1997) Detection of circulating melanoma cells by specific amplification of tyrosinase complementary DNA is not a reliable tumor marker in melanoma patients: a clinical two-center study. J Clin Oncol 15:2818–2825
9. Jung FA, Buzaid AC, Ross MI, et al. (1997) Evaluation of tyrosinase mRNA as a tumor marker in the blood of melanoma patients. J Clin Oncol 15:2826–2831
10. Hoon DSB, Wang Y, Dale PS, et al. (1995) Detection of occult melanoma cells in blood with a multiple-marker polymerase chain reaction assay. J Clin Oncol 13:2109–2116
11. Sarantou T, Chi DDJ, Garrison DA, et al. (1997) Melanoma-associated antigens as messenger RNA detection markers for melanoma. Cancer Res 57:1371–1376
12. Palmieri G, Strazzullo M, Ascierto PA, et al. (1999) PCR-Based Detection of Circulating Melanoma Cells as an Effective Marker of Tumor Progression. J Clin Oncol 17:304–311
13. Keilholz U (1996) Diagnostic PCR in melanoma: methods and quality assurance. Eur J Cancer 32 A:1661–1663

Decrease in Circulating Tumor Cells as an Early Marker of Therapy Effectiveness

J.-C. Bystryn[1], J. Albrecht[2], S.R. Reynolds[1], M.C. Rivas[1], R. Oratz[1], R.L. Shapiro[1], D.F. Roses[1], M.N. Harris[1], and A. Conrad[2]

[1] The Kaplan Comprehensive Cancer Center, NYU School of Medicine, New York, NY, USA
[2] The National Genetics Institute, Santa Monica, CA, USA

Abstract

As melanoma cells are present in the circulation of many patients with this cancer, decreases in their number could provide an early indication of therapy effectiveness. To evaluate this possibility, we examined the effect of treatment with a melanoma vaccine on the number of melanoma cells present in the circulation. PCR was used to detect melanoma cells that expressed the melanoma-associated antigens MART-1, MAGE-3, tyrosinase and/or gp100 in 91 patients with melanoma. Melanoma cells that expressed one or more of these markers were present more often in advanced disease, i.e. in 80% of patients with advanced stage IV compared to in less than one-third of patients with less advanced disease. We then measured circulating melanoma cells in a subset of 43 of these patients who were treated with a polyvalent, shed antigen, melanoma vaccine. The vaccine contains multiple melanoma-associated antigens including MART-1, MAGE-3, tyrosinase and gp100. Immunizations were given intradermally q2–3 weeks ×4 and then monthly ×3. Prior to vaccine treatment, circulating melanoma cells were detected in 14 (32%) patients. Following 4 and 7 months of vaccine treatment, melanoma cells that expressed any of these markers were present in only nine (21%) and three (7%) of patients, respectively. Thus, vaccine therapy was associated with clearance of melanoma cells from the circulation in 78% of initially positive patients. As the number of these cells declined steadily with increasing length of therapy, it is unlikely that this was due to a random change in their number. Rather it suggests that the decline was a result of the therapy.

These observations suggest that the presence of melanoma cells in the circulation is related to the extent of the melanoma, and that their disappearance may provide an early marker of the efficacy of therapy. However, the practical utility of assaying circulating tumor cells as a guide to the effectiveness of therapy or of prognosis will need to be confirmed by correlations with clinical outcome.

Recent Results in Cancer Research, Vol. 158

There is a need for improved procedures to evaluate the clinical effectiveness of new cancer treatments, particularly of those administered in the adjuvant setting. The current procedures use as end-points disease recurrence and overall survival. Unfortunately, reaching these end-points is lengthy, which markedly increases the time and expense required to evaluate new therapies.

The rationale for measuring circulating tumor cells as an early marker of treatment effectiveness is based on two considerations: tumor cells are present in the circulation of some patients with cancer, and their incidence increases with increasing tumor load. A reasonable hypothesis is that the converse is true: a decrease in circulating tumor cells indicates a decreased tumor load, and hence provides an indirect marker of therapy effectiveness. In addition, it can be assumed that therapies that kill tumor cells in the circulation should also be able to kill these cells in metastatic deposits outside the circulation.

To test this hypothesis, we examined the impact of immunotherapy with a melanoma vaccine on the presence of circulating melanoma cells and the relation between the clearance of these cells and clinical outcome. The study was conducted in 91 patients with malignant melanoma: 45 had AJCC stage IIB (primary melanoma, ≥4 mm thick) or early stage III disease (regional nodes clinically negative, and only one histologically positive nodes), 28 had advanced stage III disease (clinically positive nodes and/or two or more histologically positive), 15 had low tumor volume stage IV disease, and five had more advanced stage IV disease as evidenced by recurrence of stage IV disease after initial resection. All patients had resected disease, apart for those with recurrent stage IV disease.

All patients were treated with a polyvalent, shed antigen, melanoma vaccine prepared from antigens released into culture medium by a pool of four melanoma cell lines. The procedure used to prepare the vaccine has been published [1]. Immunizations were given every 2–3 weeks for four cycles, monthly for three cycles, every 3 months for two cycles, and then every 6 months for 5 years or until disease recurrence. The presence of melanoma cells in the peripheral blood of all patients was measured by PCR, at baseline and at intervals following vaccine treatment, looking at four markers: MART-1, MAGE-3, gp100 and tyrosinase.

Prior studies have shown that the vaccine contains multiple melanoma-associated antigens, including the marker antigens measured in this study, i.e. MART-1, MAGE-3, gp100 and tyrosinase. The vaccine is immunologically active and stimulates antibody and CD8+ T cell responses to antigens expressed by human melanoma cells in vivo [2–4]. The vaccine appears to be clinically effective, as the recurrence-free and overall survival of vaccine-treated patients with resected AJCC stage III disease are both prolonged by approximately 50% compared to historical controls [5]. More compellingly, in a double-blind, placebo-controlled, randomized clinical trial in advanced stage III disease, the median recurrence-free survival of patients treated with the melanoma vaccine was two and a half times longer than that of similar control patients treated with a placebo (human albumin) vaccine [6]. This difference in

Table 1. Effect of vaccine RX on circulating melanoma cells

Interval from onset of vaccine treatment	No. (%) patients with circulating melanoma cells ($n=43$)	Decrease (%)
Baseline	14 (32.5)	
3–4 months	9 (21)	35
5–7 months	3 (6.9)	78

outcome was statistically significant ($p=0.03$) after adjusting for differences in risk factors between the two groups by Cox multivariate analysis.

We found that there was a great deal of heterogeneity in the pattern of marker antigens expressed by circulating melanoma cells. None of the circulating cells we detected expressed more than one of the four marker antigens studied. Consequently, the frequency with which circulating melanoma cells were detected depended on the marker studied. The most sensitive marker for detecting circulating melanoma cells was MART-1, which was positive at baseline in 18% of the 91 patients. The least sensitive markers were MAGE-3 and gp100, each of which was positive in only 2% of the patients at baseline. The incidence of circulating melanoma cells depended in part on the extent of the tumor, although such cells were present in a surprisingly high proportion (28%) of patients with thick primary melanomas even though the tumor had been completely resected. The incidence of circulating melanoma cells remained in the same range in patients with more advanced stage III disease and in patients with limited stage IV disease; but increased to 80% of patients with more advanced recurrent stage IV melanoma.

Following vaccine treatment, there was a steady decline in the proportion of patients with circulating melanoma cells (Table 1). This analysis was conducted in a subset of 43 patients in whom sequential analysis of circulating melanoma cells was available at baseline immediately prior to vaccine treatment and at least two time points thereafter, i.e. following 3–4 months and 5–7 months of therapy. At baseline, circulating melanoma cells were present in 14 (32%) of the patients. Some 3–4 months later, such cells were detected in only nine (21%) of the patients; 5–7 months following initiation of therapy, such cells were present in only three (7%) of the patients, i.e. a 78% reduction in the proportion of patients with circulating melanoma cells.

Overall, there was a correlation between the presence of circulating melanoma cells and clinical outcome. The median recurrence-free survival of patients with circulating melanoma cells at baseline was 12.6 months compared to over 20 months for patients without circulating melanoma cells. There was also a correlation between the clearance of circulating melanoma cells following vaccine treatment and prognosis. The median recurrence-free survival of patients who were initially negative for circulating melanoma cells, and remained negative, was over 20 months. The recurrence-free survival of patients who were initially positive for melanoma cells, but who became negative following vaccine treatment, was 11 months. By contrast, the median recurrence-free survival of patients who were initially negative for circulating melanoma cells, but who became positive after treatment, was only 7 months.

In summary, there is a marked heterogeneity in the expression of marker antigens by circulating melanoma cells in different patients, and there is a steady decline in the number of melanoma cells in the circulation following treatment with a shed, polyvalent, melanoma vaccine. Because the percentage of positive patients declined steadily with time of treatment, it is unlikely that this represents random changes in the number of these cells. Rather, it suggests that the decline is a result of vaccine therapy. In addition, we have found that there is a relation between vaccine-associated decline in circulating melanoma cells and improved clinical outcome.

The implications of these findings are that the detection of circulating tumor cells is optimized by using multiple markers to identify these cells, and that the sequential assay of tumor cells in the circulation may provide an early marker of the effectiveness of cancer therapy, particularly in patients with no measurable disease. The fact that treatment with a polyvalent, shed melanoma antigen vaccine correlates with clearance of melanoma cells from the circulation suggests that this vaccine is clinically effective.

ACKNOWLEDGEMENTS. Supported in part by The Rita and Stanley Kaplan Foundation, The Gaisman Foundation, The Skin Cancer Foundation, The Blair O. Rogers Medical Research Fund, and NIH grants nos. 1 R21 CA78659 and 5 R21 CA75317.

References

1. Bystryn J-C, Jacobsen S, Harris M, Roses D, Speyer J, Levin M. Preparation and characterization of a polyvalent human melanoma antigen vaccine. J Biol Resp Modif 5:211-224, 1986
2. Gershman N, Johnston D, Bystryn J-C. Potentiation of B16 melanoma vaccine immunogenicity by IL-2 liposomes. Vaccine Res 3(2):83-92, 1994
3. Reynolds Sr, Oratz R, Shapiro RL, Fotino M, Hao P, Vukmanovic S, Bystryn J-C. Stimulation of CD8+ T cell responses to MAGE-3 and MELAN A/MART-1 by immunization to a polyvalent melanoma vaccine. Int J Cancer 72:972-976, 1997.
4. Reynolds Sr, Celis E, Sette A, Oratz R, Shapiro RL, Johnston D, Fotino M, Bystryn J-C. HLA-independent heterogeneity of CD8+ T cell responses to MAGE-3, Melan A/MART-1, gp100, tyrosinase, MC1R and TRP-2 in vaccine-treated melanoma patients. J Immunol 161:6970-6976, 1998.
5. Bystryn J-C, Shapiro RL, Oratz R. Cancer vaccines: Clinical applications: Partially purified tumor antigen vaccines. In: Biologic Therapy of Cancer, 2nd Edition, ed by V DeVita, S Hellman and SA Rosenberg; JB Lippincott:Philadelphia, pp 668-679, 1995
6. Bystryn J-C, Oratz R, Shapiro RL, Harris MN, Roses DF, Zeleniuch-Jacquotte A, Chen Dl, Rivas MC. Double-blind, placebo-controlled, trial of a shed, polyvalent, melanoma vaccine in stage III melanoma. Proc Am Soc Clin Oncol 434(1673), 1999

VI. Therapeutic Strategies Against Residual Melanoma Cells

Utility of Tests for Circulating Melanoma Cells in Identifying Patients Who Develop Recurrent Melanoma

B.J. Curry, K. Myers, and P. Hersey

Oncology and Immunology Unit, Mater Misericordiae Hospital,
Newcastle and Sydney Melanoma Unit, Sydney, New South Wales, Australia

Abstract

Prospective studies were carried out on 186 patients with AJCC stage I (13), II (76) and III (97 patients) melanoma before and after surgical removal of their tumour. The goal was to determine if PCR tests on blood samples for MART-1 and tyrosinase were predictive of recurrence of melanoma in a 2-year follow-up period. (PCR assays for MUC-18, p97 and gp100 were positive in blood samples from normal subjects and excluded from the study.) PCR tests for MART-1 and tyrosinase were most commonly positive in the first 3 months following surgical removal of melanoma, and three tests over this period gave maximum sensitivity in the identification of patients who subsequently developed recurrences. Positive tests for the first time in the second year of follow-up had similar predictive power. The tests identified 68.5% of patients who developed recurrences in the 2-year follow-up period. Assays for MART-1 were mainly positive in patients with locoregional recurrences, whereas tyrosinase was detected in blood samples from patients with both locoregional and disseminated recurrences. (Positivity rate for tyrosinase in 48 patients with disseminated melanoma was 60.4% compared to 14.6% for MART-1.) Tests for MART-1 and tyrosinase were strongly predictive of disease-free survival (DFS) and were more powerful predictors of DFS than lymph node status or thickness of the primary melanoma. (Hazard ratios by Cox analysis were 2.97 in patients with disseminated recurrences and 2.93 in those with locoregional recurrences.) These results indicate that PCR tests for MART-1 and tyrosinase are powerful prognostic indicators, but their practical utility for selecting patients for adjuvant therapy is limited by the high false-negative rate of approximately 30%. Intermittent shedding of melanoma cells into the circulation would appear to be the most likely explanation for the latter.

Recent Results in Cancer Research, Vol. 158

Introduction

Melanoma differs from other skin cancers because of the greater potential for metastasis to distant organs. The risk of the latter is related to the thickness of the primary tumour and whether it has metastasised to regional lymph nodes (LNs) [1]. The route of metastasis to distant organs in most instances is through the bloodstream [2]; therefore, detection of melanoma cells in the circulation after removal of primary melanoma or melanoma metastatic to regional LNs might be a useful indicator of patients who will subsequently develop overt metastases.

The detection of circulating melanoma cells (CMCs) was facilitated by the introduction of polymerase chain reaction (PCR) tests to detect products specifically associated with the melanin biosynthesis pathway. Smith et al. [3] described the identification of CMCs by PCR detection of tyrosinase, and we and others have reported a general correlation between CMCs and clinical stage of melanoma [4–9]. We have shown that other potential markers for detection of CMCs (i.e. gp100, MUC-18 and p97) lacked sufficient specificity to be of use [9], but the addition of RT-PCR tests for MART-1 was found to increase the sensitivity of detection of melanoma cells in the circulation [9].

Assays to detect CMCs would, on theoretical grounds, appear superior in the prediction of metastatic potential compared to assays that detect tumour cell products, because the latter are related to the mass of the tumour [10–13] and not necessarily to the metastatic potential of the melanoma cells. Such assays might have a practical use, e.g., to select patients who might benefit from adjuvant therapy or to monitor response to treatment. CMC assays might also provide an early indication of patients who are about to develop recurrent disease or assist in identifying subgroups of patients with disseminated melanoma who have a particularly bad prognosis.

We have focused in our studies on evaluating the reliability of assays aimed at identifying patients who will develop recurrent melanoma after apparent complete surgical removal of their disease. If the assays were found to be reliable predictors of recurrence, they would allow more selective use of adjuvant therapies and have a significant impact on the management of melanoma.

Materials and Methods

Patients

Patients eligible for the study were those who presented with a localised primary tumour (AJCC stage I or II), or regional LN metastases (AJCC stage III). No previous distant metastases were permitted. Patients were recruited through the Sydney and Newcastle Melanoma Units (New South Wales, Australia), and consent was obtained after a full written and verbal explanation of the study. The protocol for the study was approved by the Central Sydney and Hunter Regional Institutional Review Committees. When possible, blood samples were drawn the day before surgery, and 1–2 weeks, 4–6 weeks and 8–12 weeks post-surgery, and then routinely at 3-month intervals.

Control blood samples were drawn from 50 outpatients who attended the Royal Newcastle and Newcastle Mater Hospitals. There were five, four, and one patients with colon, breast and bladder carcinoma, respectively; 18 patients had a history of dysplastic naevi, 12 patients had a past history of limb fractures, and 10 patients had various inflammatory dermatologic disorders. Blood samples were taken from nine patients within 2 months of surgery that involved a general anaesthetic (two patients with colon carcinoma, three patients with breast carcinoma and four patients with limb fractures).

Blood Collection and RNA Extraction

Approximately 10 ml of blood was taken from each patient into heparinised or plain tubes and centrifuged at 2000 rpm. Total RNA was extracted from 2 ml of packed blood using RNAzol, as described previously [9].

RT-PCR for Melanoma Markers

Synthesis of cDNA from mRNA was carried out using the Advantage-for-PCR cDNA synthesis kit from Clontech Laboratories (Palo Alto, CA), as described previously [9]. The sequences of the oligonucleotide primers used for PCR and the conditions for PCR of the melanoma markers were also as described previously [9]. PCR products were analysed by electrophoresis on a 2% agarose/ethidium bromide gel (1.5% NuSieve, 0.5% Seakem, FMC, Rockland, ME). PCR products for tyrosinase, gp100, p97, MART-1 and MUC18 were sequenced by the dideoxy termination method on an Applied Biosystems 377 prism DNA sequencer (Applied Biosystems, Foster City, CA).

The integrity of each cDNA sample was checked by PCR amplification using primers specific for the housekeeping gene human β-actin. For PCR of this gene, 1 µl of patient cDNA was added to a 20-µl reaction volume containing the β-actin primers, overlaid with mineral oil and heated at 94 °C for 5 min. Forty cycles of PCR were then carried out (95 °C for 65 s; 60 °C for 65 s; 72 °C for 2 min), with a final extension of 72 °C for 10 min. Products were run on a 1% agarose/ethidium bromide gel as described above.

Blood samples that contained melanoma cells were also used as a positive control. Five hundred MM200 cells were added to 100 ml of blood from a healthy donor, and 2-ml aliquots were stored under the same conditions used for patient samples. One of these control samples was processed at the same time as the batches of patient samples to control for variations in RNA processing, cDNA synthesis and PCR quality. A negative blood sample was also included with each batch of patient blood samples. This was to control for any cross-contamination of samples throughout the RNA extraction and RT-PCR procedure.

Results

When Were the Tests Most Frequently Positive?

To answer this question, we examined the results obtained from serial samples of blood taken before and at regular intervals after surgical removal of AJCC stage II–III melanoma. The results shown in Fig. 1 indicated that the tests were most frequently positive in the first 3 months following surgery,

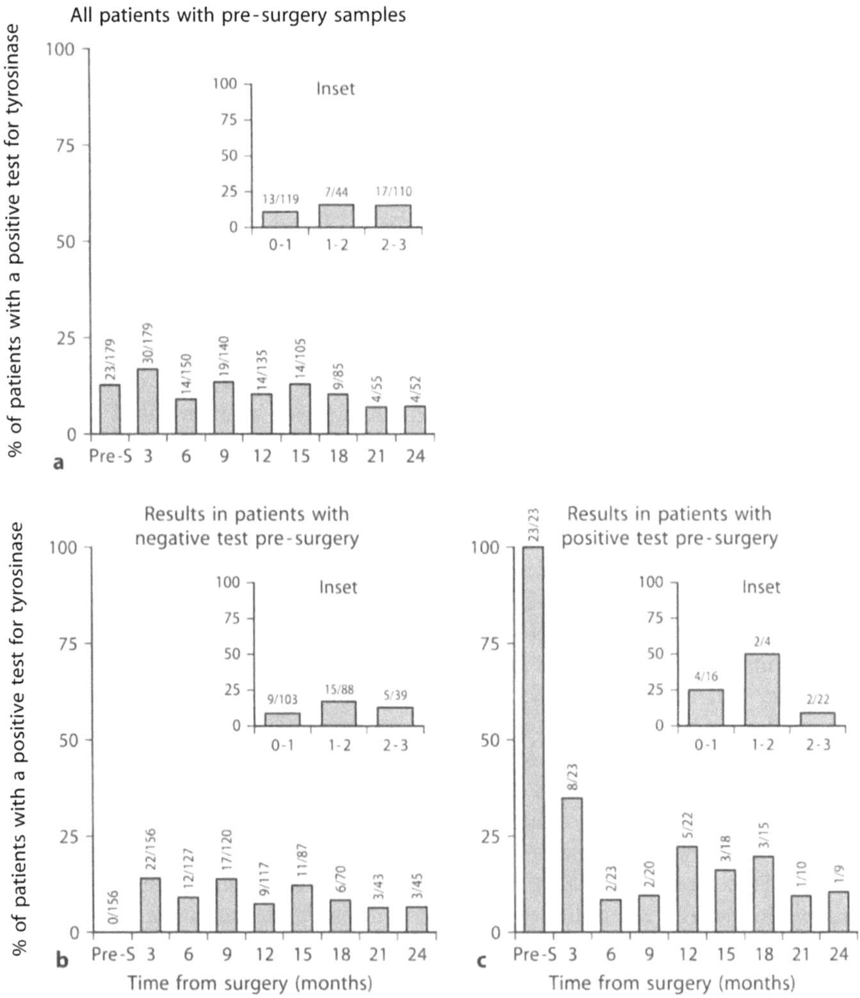

Fig. 1 a–c. Percentage of positive tests for tyrosinase in relation to time before and after surgery for AJCC stage I–III patients. **a–c** 179 patients with pre-surgery samples, including patients; **b** negative or **c** positive pre-surgery. *Insets* show a breakdown of data within 3 months of surgery, indicating the percentage of positive tests for tyrosinase at 0–1, 1–2, and 2–3 months post-surgery but it is notable that low levels of positivity continued during the 2-year period. Figure 1b shows that 14% of patients with a negative test prior to surgery became positive after surgery. This may be evidence that surgery precipitated the entry of melanoma cells into the circulation. Figure 1c shows that 15 of the 23 (65%) patients with a positive test before surgery became negative in the tests performed within 3 months after surgery. These results suggest that the tumour removed by the surgeon was the source of the CMCs.

What Are the Best Markers to Use for Detection of Melanoma Cells in the Circulation?

To be useful in a clinical setting, a marker must be both sensitive, i.e., detected in a high proportion of patients with CMCs, and specific, i.e., not detected in normal subjects or patients with other diseases. In view of reports by others [14], we examined MART-1, gp100, p97 and MUC-18 to see how well they satisfied the criteria. The latter three markers failed the specificity test in that all were detected in blood samples from normal subjects.

Sequencing of the cDNA products from the PCR amplification of tyrosinase, MART-1 and p97 showed the expected sequence, whereas with MUC-18 the product in normal blood was a splice variant that included intron 3. It was unlikely that this was due to genomic DNA contamination, because intron 4 splits the antisense-nested primer binding site. gp100 was also larger than expected because of a splice variant that included intron 8, similar to what has been described elsewhere [15]. Primer pairs with different sequences were investigated for gp100 and were found to give the expected size; however, gp100 was still found in normal blood (Fig. 2b). Tests for p97 were negative in RNA extracts from whole blood, and RNA from mononuclear cells was only detected after separation of these cells from blood and subsequent RNA extraction. The PCR assays for MUC-18, p97 and gp100 were repeated over a wide range of conditions but remained positive in samples from healthy subjects.

In contrast, MART-1 was not detected in normal blood samples and, as shown in Fig. 2c, had a sensitivity for the detection of CMCs that was similar to that for PCR detection of tyrosinase (Fig. 2d). In view of this, MART-1 was selected for further studies, together with tyrosinase.

As shown elsewhere, the sensitivity of PCR tests for MART-1 to detect CMCs in patient samples was similar but slightly lower than that for tyrosinase. These studies also found that there was no apparent correlation between the two assays, which suggested they were detecting CMCs in different patients [9].

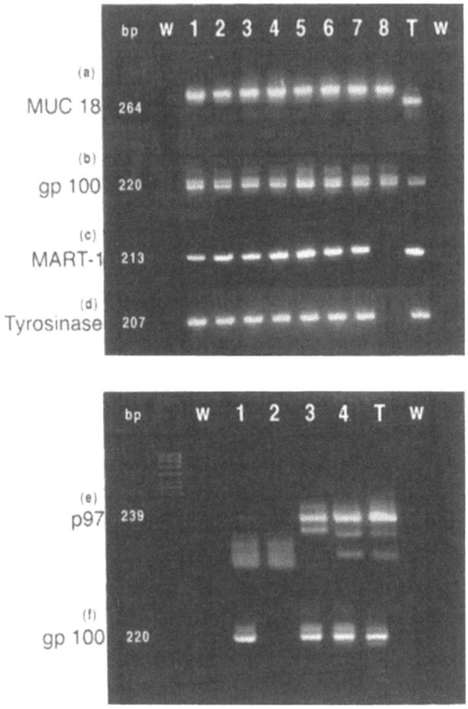

Fig. 2 a–f. Sensitivity and specificity of detection of markers by PCR. **a–d** *Lanes 1–7, 8*, 1–10^6 and 0 tumour cells. **e** *Lanes 1, 3*, RNA from whole blood or mononuclear cells, respectively. *Lanes 2, 4*, as above plus 10^6 tumour cells. **f** *Lanes 1–4*, healthy subjects. *W*, water controls; *T*, tumour cell controls. (Reproduced with permission from JCO 16:1760–1769, 1998)

What Is the Optimal Number of Tests Needed To Identify Patients Who Subsequently Develop Recurrences?

This question was examined in a cohort of patients who had developed a positive test at some time over the 2-year post-operative period. As shown in Fig. 3, when the results of the assays in the first 3 months were examined, it was found that three tests appeared to give the maximum sensitivity. This was also apparent in tests on patients with known recurrence of disease (Fig. 3 b), in that one test would have identified only 49.1% of patients who subsequently developed recurrence, whereas two and three tests identified 65.6% and 67.2%, respectively. There was a small increase (approximately 10%) in the number of positive results in those without recurrence at 2 years, but some of the latter patients may still develop recurrences.

Do Tests at Different Time Periods Have More Predictive Power?

It might be asked whether tests that are positive at certain time periods are more significant in terms of identifying patients who will subsequently develop recurrences. As shown in Fig. 4, when the assay results for MART-1 and tyrosinase were combined, the tests at 3 months identified the highest pro-

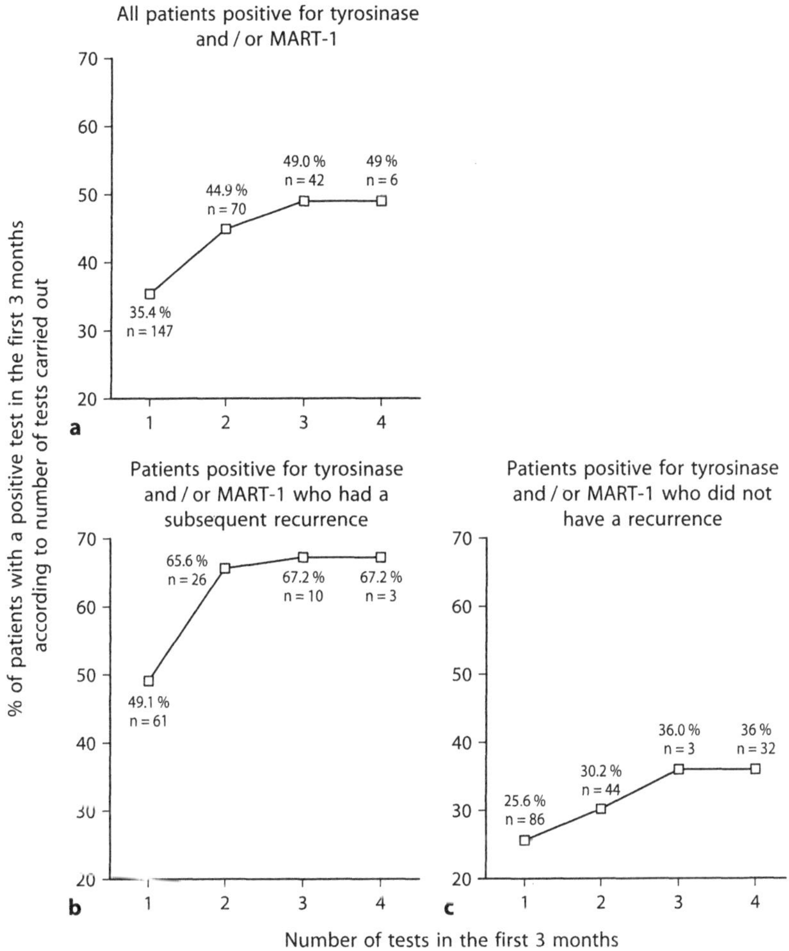

Fig. 3 a–c. The percentage of positive tests for each test in the first 3-month time period in 147 patients with AJCC stage I–III melanoma who were followed for a minimum of 2 years post-surgery. **a** All 147 patients; **b** 61 patients who had a recurrence; **c** 86 patients without a recurrence after at least 2 years post-surgery

portion of patients with a subsequent recurrence. Another estimate of optimum timing of tests was calculated by multiplying the percentage of positive tests at a certain time by the proportion of patients with a positive test who subsequently developed a recurrence. For example, from Fig. 4 it can be seen that 56/147 patients, or 38%, had a positive test, and 35/56 of these, or 62.5%, subsequently developed a recurrence. The tests at this time, therefore, identified 23.8 patients from 100 original patients who subsequently developed a recurrence. Values at other time periods are shown in Table 1.

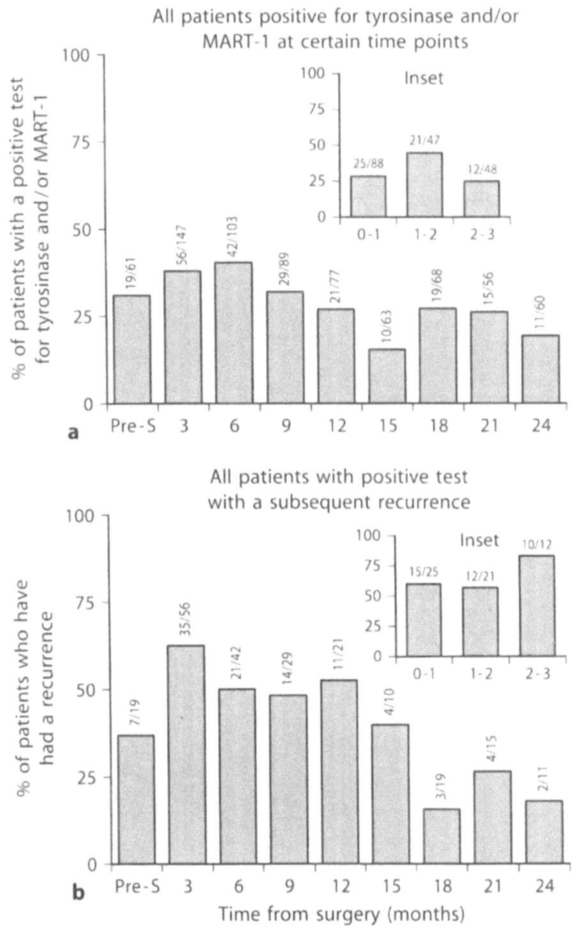

Fig. 4 a,b. The recurrence rate of patients for each time period post-surgery, in relation to the positivity rate post-surgery, for patients followed for at least 2 years post-surgery. **a** The percentage of positive tests for tyrosinase and/or MART-1 at each time period post-surgery; *inset*, the percentage of positive tests at 0–1, 1–2 and 2–3 months post-surgery. **b** The percentage of patients with positive tests who had a recurrence at each time point post-surgery; *inset*, the percentage of patients with positive tests who had a recurrence at 0–1, 1–2, and 2–3 months post-surgery

Does the Time at Which a Test First Became Positive Have Predictive Power for Identifying Patients with Subsequent Recurrences?

The results of an analysis of this question are shown in Fig. 5. For both tests combined, the first 3 months remained the most predictive, although tests that became positive for the first time at 12 months after surgery appeared to have similar predictive power.

Table 1. The predictive recurrence value for tyrosinase, MART-1 and tyrosinase and/or MART-1, for patients followed for at least 2 years after surgery

Time from surgery	Tyrosinase	Marker	
		MART-1	Tyrosinase+MART-1
Pre-surgery	8.20	3.28	11.44
3 months	19.43	7.58	23.81
0–1 months	12.36	6.90	17.05
1–2 months	16.67	10.88	25.52
2–3 months	20.83	0.0	20.83
6 months	15.74	8.08	20.40
9 months	10.53	6.09	15.75
12 months	9.87	9.74	14.31
15 months	4.84	1.59	6.36
18 months	4.0	1.56	4.41
21 months	3.51	3.70	7.16
24 months	2.96	0.0	1.82

Do patients with Ulcerated Primary Melanoma Have a Higher Incidence of CMCs?

Data relating to this question are shown in Table 2. There was a trend for a higher percentage of CMCs in patients with ulcerated melanoma, but this was not statistically significant ($p > 0.05$ for CMCs detected by tyrosinase, MART-1, or tyrosinase and MART-1 combined; McNemar test). Analysis of this question was limited by the lack of information regarding the ulceration status of most of the melanomas.

Reliability of Tests for MART-1 and Tyrosinase in the Identification of Patients Who Subsequently Develop Recurrent Melanoma

The sensitivity of the assays on samples taken within 3 months of surgery from 186 patients to identify those who subsequently developed recurrences is shown in Fig. 6. RT-PCR with tyrosinase and MART-1 identified 49.3% and 23.3%, respectively, of patients whose disease recurred. Combining the results of each test on one sample increased the sensitivity to 68.5%. Presurgery samples were available in the case of 23 of the 75 patients with disease recurrence. In these presurgery samples, tyrosinase was expressed in 30.3% of cases, MART-1 in 13.0% of cases, and both markers combined in 43.5%.

The clinical data relating to the 186 patients are described elsewhere [16]. Melanoma recurred in 33% of patients with stage II disease and 49% of patients with stage III disease. Of the 24 patients with stage II disease whose melanoma recurred, 14 had locoregional recurrence, and ten had disseminated recurrence. Samples from only one patient (10%) of the ten who had disseminated (stage IV) metastases were positive for MART-1, whereas

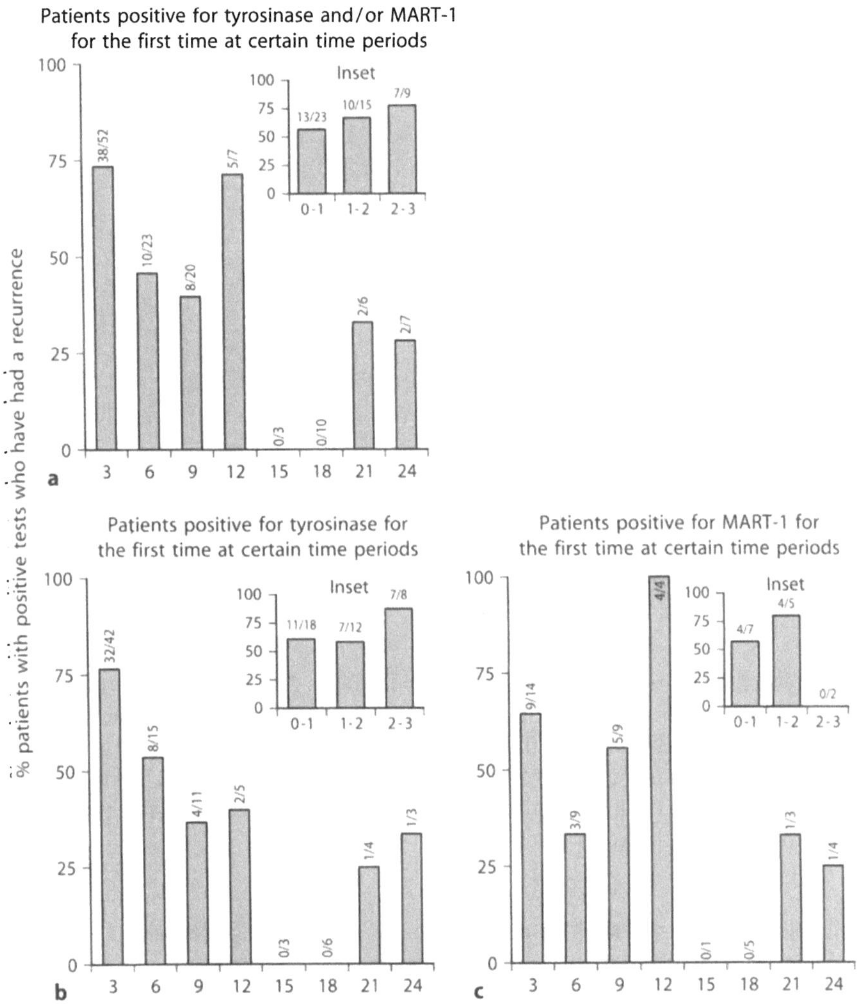

Fig. 5 a–c. The recurrence rate of patients for each time period post-surgery, in relation to the first positive test post-surgery, for patients followed for at least 2 years post-surgery. **a** The percentage of patients with a first positive test for tyrosinase and/or MART-1 who had a recurrence at each time period post-surgery; inset, the percentage of first positive tests at 0–1, 1–2 and 2–3 months post-surgery. **b, c** The percentage of patients with a first positive test for **b** tyrosinase, **c** MART-1 who had a recurrence at each time point post-surgery; insets, the percentage of patients with a first positive test for **b** tyrosinase, **c** MART-1 who had a recurrence at 0–1, 1–2, and 2–3 months post-surgery

among those patients with locoregional recurrence, samples from three were positive for tyrosinase and samples from seven were positive for MART-1. Of the 48 patients with stage III disease and recurrent metastases, ten had a locoregional recurrence and 38 had disseminated stage IV metastases. Among patients with locoregional recurrence, samples from three were positive for

Table 2. Detection of melanoma cells in the circulation in terms of ulceration of primary melanoma

	n	Tyrosinase	MART-1	Combined[a]
Ulcerated	36	56	31	78
Nonulcerated	49	43	39	71
Unknown	101	44	36	60

[a] Percentage of patients positive for tyrosinase, MART-1 or tyrosinase and/or MART-1 (combined) in the first 12 months post-surgery.

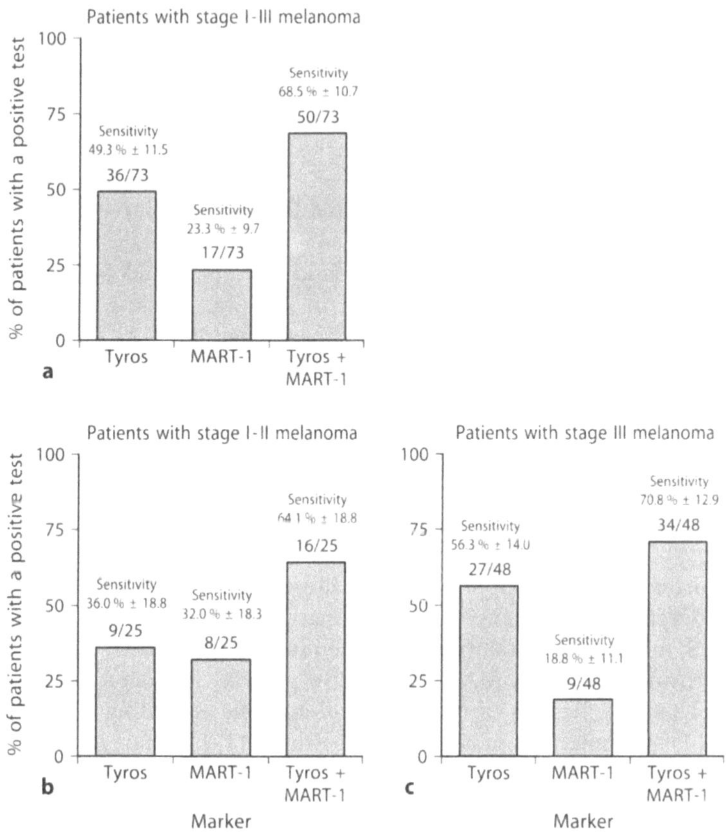

Fig. 6. Percentage of positive tests in samples taken in the first 3 months after surgery from 73 patients with stage I–III melanoma and a known recurrence. Sensitivity given as a percentage ± the 95% confidence interval. *Tyros*, tyrosinase. (Reproduced with permission from JCO 17:2562–2572, 1999)

tyrosinase, and samples from three were positive for MART-1, whereas among patients with disseminated recurrences, samples from 63% were positive for tyrosinase and from 16% were positive for MART-1.

Overall, samples from 71% of patients with disseminated recurrence were positive for CMCs compared with samples from 64% of patients with locoregional disease. Samples from 29 (60.4%) of 48 patients with disseminated recurrence were positive for tyrosinase, but samples from only seven (14.6%) were positive for MART-1. The difference in tyrosinase and MART-1 expression in samples from patients with disseminated recurrence compared to locoregional disease was statistically significant ($p<0.0001$, McNemar test). There was no obvious difference in the combined results of the tests according to the site of metastases. However only seven (16%), of 43 patients with first metastases to skin, lung, liver, brain, or intestine tested positive for MART-1; 25 (58%) of 43 tested positive for tyrosinase ($p<0.01$, McNemar test).

Relation Between the RT-PCR Tests and Disease-Free Survival

Disease-free survival, using the method of Kaplan and Meier [16], for all patients with recurrence is shown in Fig. 7a. Among tyrosinase-negative, MART-1-positive patients and tyrosinase-positive, MART-1-negative patients, DFS was significantly shorter ($p=0.0003$ and $p<0.0001$, respectively; log-rank test) than among those patients who tested negative for both markers. The 75% DFS of patients who tested negative for both tyrosinase and MART-1 was 38 months compared to 10 months for tyrosinase-positive, MART-1 negative patients.

The DFS for the 25 patients with locoregional recurrence is shown in Fig. 7b. Only tyrosinase-negative, MART-1-positive patients had significantly shorter DFS ($p=0.0007$). However, there was no significant difference in DFS between these patients and tyrosinase-positive, MART-1-negative patients. DFS for the 48 patients with disseminated recurrence is shown in Fig. 7c. Tyrosinase-positive, MART-1-negative patients had significantly shorter DFS ($p<0.0001$). Results of the statistical analysis according to disease stage and RT-PCR results are summarised elsewhere [17]. When markers were considered in isolation for patients with locoregional recurrence, only MART-1-positive patients with stage II disease had significantly shorter DFS ($p=0.012$). The same analysis for patients with disseminated recurrence showed that only tyrosinase-positive patients with stage III disease had significantly shorter DFS ($p<0.0001$).

To determine whether a positive test within 3 months of surgery was an independent prognostic determinant of recurrence, univariate hazard ratios were calculated using the Cox proportional hazards model [18]. The presence of positive tests was controlled for by the variables thickness of the primary melanoma, number of lymph nodes, age and sex. When these determinants of prognosis were taken into account, positive tests for tyrosinase and/or MART-1 remained significant determinants of recurrence (data not shown).

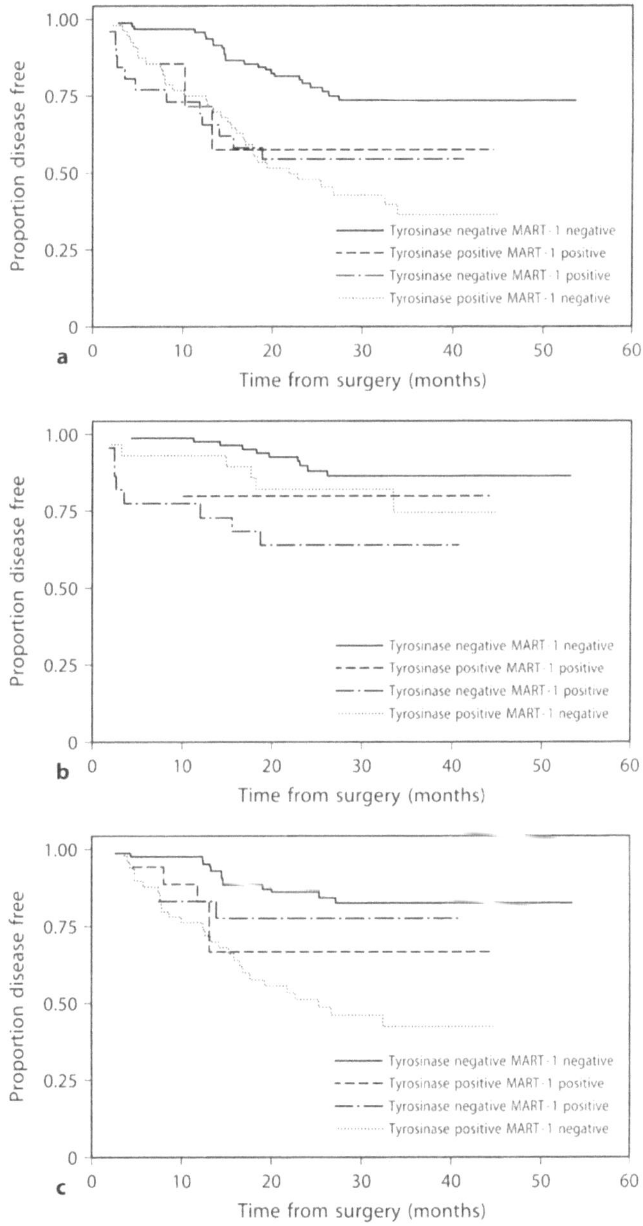

Fig. 7 a–c. Relationship between disease-free survival and results of tests performed within 3 months of surgery in 186 patients with stage I, II or III melanoma. **a** All 73 patients with recurrence; **b** 25 patients with locoregional recurrence; **c** 48 patients with disseminated recurrence. Survival curves start from 1 at time 0. (Reproduced with permission from JCO 17:2562–2572, 1999)

Table 3. Cox proportional hazards model analysis of the prognostic significance of results of PCR with tyrosinase and MART-1 for all patients with recurrence

	Hazards ratio	95% confidence interval	*P*
Thickness of primary melanoma	0.92	0.82–1.03	0.136
No. of lymph nodes involved	1.07	1.00–1.14	0.056
Sex	0.56	0.28–1.15	0.113
Age	1.01	0.99–1.04	0.356
Tyrosinase expression[a]	2.97	1.49–5.93	0.002
MART-1 expression[a]	1.22	0.50–2.99	0.657

[a] In the first 3 months after surgery. (Reproduced with permission from JCO 17:2562–2572, 1999).

Analysis of overall DFS using the Cox proportional hazards model was performed to determine the effect of interaction of the known prognostic factors with the results of PCR. As shown in Table 3, positive tests for tyrosinase alone and MART-1 alone were associated with a 2.97- and 1.22-fold increase in the relative hazard, respectively. Only tests for tyrosinase alone indicated that the ability of the test to identify patients whose disease would recur was independent of other known prognostic factors ($p=0.002$). Tests for tyrosinase and/or MART-1 were associated with a 3.9-fold increase in the relative hazard. Results of Cox model analysis of the tests in patients with locoregional and distant recurrence showed that tyrosinase expression was an independent prognostic factor in patients with disseminated disease ($p=0.001$), but not in those with locoregional disease ($p=0.226$), whereas MART-1 expression was an independent prognostic factor in patients with locoregional disease ($p=0.017$), but not in those with disseminated disease ($p=0.570$).

Do Tests Between 3 and 12 Months Add to the Sensitivity of Identifying Patients Who Subsequently Relapse?

There were 37 patients who developed recurrences after 12 months. Tests between 3 and 12 months were found to detect an extra 12 patients who developed recurrence 12 months post-surgery (20/37 for tests in the first 3 months after surgery, compared to 32/37 for tests in the first 12 months after surgery). Tests between 3 and 12 months did not identify any additional patients who had recurrences in the first 12 months post-surgery. As shown in Fig. 8 the sensitivity of detection in the second year resulting from summation of all tests up to 12 months post-surgery was 32/37 or 86%. Tyrosinase alone had a sensitivity of 76%.

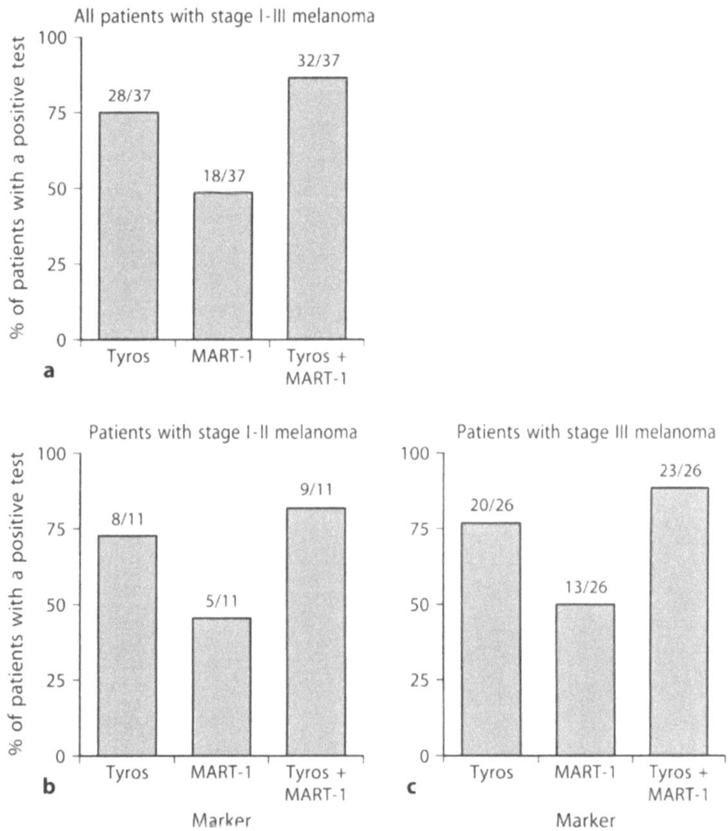

Fig. 8 a–c. Percentage of positive tests in the first 12 months in 37 patients with a known recurrence, and who had a recurrence at least 12 months after surgery. Sensitivity given as a percentage ± the 95% confidence interval

Preliminary Assessment of False-Positive Rate

Positive tests in patients who had not developed recurrence after 2 years occurred in 40 (35.4%) of 113 patients (Fig. 9). With regard to tyrosinase and MART-1 alone, the percentages of positive tests were 21.2% and 15.9% respectively. The corresponding specificities for the detection of CMCs by tyrosinase and MART-1 in samples taken within 3 months of surgery were 78.8% and 84.1% respectively. Performing each test on one sample decreased the specificity to 64.6%.

On the basis of hazard rates calculated by Kirkwood et al. [19], 2 years after surgery, 20% of disease-free patients who had stage I, II or III melanoma could be expected to have recurrence at some later time. On this basis, 23 of 113 patients who were recurrence-free could expect to have recurrence, which means the false-positive rate may be as low as 15%. This corresponds to a specificity of 85%.

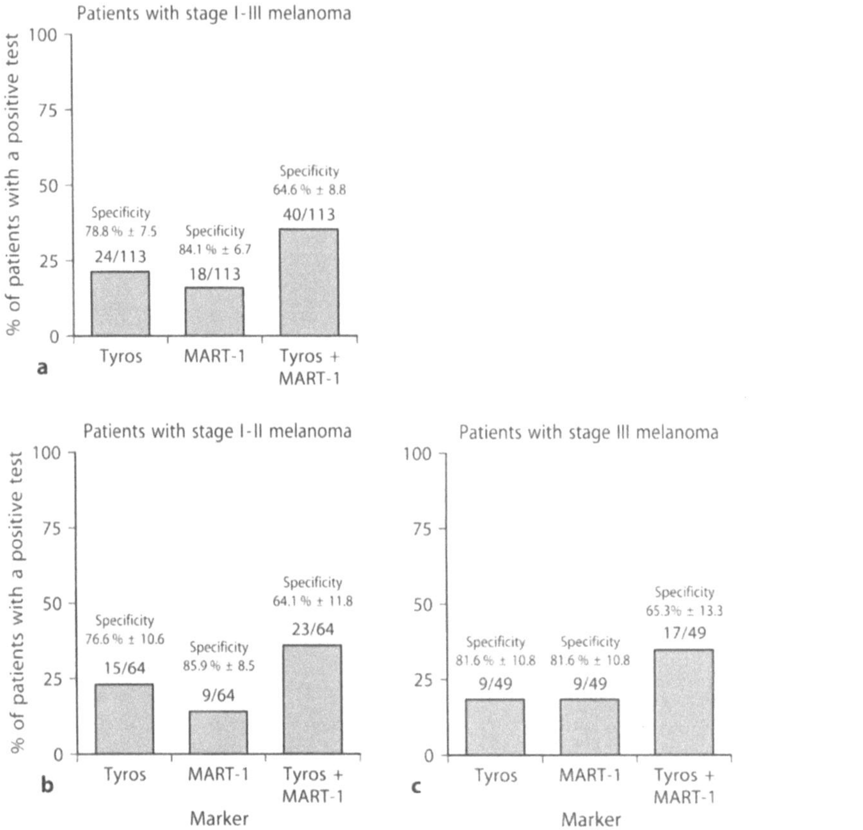

Fig. 9. Percentage of positive tests in samples taken in the first 3 months after surgery from 113 patients without a known recurrence. Sensitivity given as a percentage ± the 95% confidence interval. (Reproduced with permission from JCO 17:2562–2572, 1999)

Discussion

The introduction of RT-PCR with tyrosinase and MART-1 has made it possible to detect low numbers of melanoma cells in the circulation. In spiking experiments, as few as one cell per 10^7 leukocytes, or one cell in 2 ml of blood, could be detected [3, 9, 20–22]. A number of investigators have reported that detection of CMCs by RT-PCR relates to the clinical stage of disease [4–9]. We have confirmed this in previous studies and have shown that combined results of PCR with tyrosinase and MART-1 showed a good correlation with disease stage [9, 17]. We have also shown that assays on whole blood, as described by Smith et al. [3], are reproducible from day to day and feasible for routine monitoring [9, 17].

The main purposes of the present study were to assess whether RT-PCR with these markers identifies patients in the preoperative or early postoperative period who will subsequently develop recurrence of melanoma, and to investigate differences in patterns of expression of tyrosinase and MART-1 between patients with locoregional and those with distant recurrence. Seventy-three of the 186 patients followed for more than 2 years developed recurrent melanoma. Among 50 patients with recurring disease (68.5%), blood samples drawn in the first 3 months after surgery tested positive for markers. Assays for tyrosinase alone predicted recurrence in 49.3 of patients, and assays for MART-1 alone predicted recurrence in 23.3%. Given the false-negative results of this study and of our previous study involving a similar cohort [9], it is questionable whether the assays are a reliable means of determining which patients are suitable for immunotherapy. It is still too early to assess the false-positive rate of the tests, but extrapolating from estimates, one might suggest that 10–15% of patients with positive tests will not develop recurrent disease.

We found that the optimal number of tests in the first 3 months needed to achieve maximum sensitivity was three. We also found that tests at other time periods in the first 12 months would not have increased the sensitivity of detection of recurrence during this time, but if results of all tests in the first 12 months were summed, their sensitivity for identifying patients developing recurrence in the second year after surgery was 86%. Again however, it would be difficult to incorporate these findings into management decisions.

As in our previous study [9], and in studies by others [5, 6, 23], the presence of CMCs in disease-free patients was found to be an independent prognostic predictor of recurrence. In univariate analysis, controlling separately for tumour thickness, number of positive lymph nodes, sex and age, the relative hazard of the presence of CMCs was statistically significant, and it remained significant when multivariate analysis was performed with these variables. There was a 3.9-fold increase in the risk of recurrence when CMCs were present in patients with stage I, II or III disease in the first 3 months after surgery, and the presence of CMCs was by far the strongest prognostic indicator in patients with stage II and III disease.

The results suggested that RT-PCR with tyrosinase was more sensitive than RT-PCR with MART-1 in terms of detection of distant metastases. Of 48 patients with a distant recurrence, 29 (60.4%), were positive for tyrosinase within 3 months of surgery, yet only seven patients (14.6%) were positive for MART-1. The difference in the pattern of expression of the two markers was statistically significant and suggests that MART-1 expression was low or absent in CMCs of patients who developed distant metastases. In contrast, of the patients who had locoregional recurrence, seven (28%) were positive for tyrosinase and ten (40%) were positive for MART-1. Most recurrences in the latter group were in lymph nodes, the first capillary bed encountered on the melanoma cells' journey in the circulation.

The association of the tests with the different patterns of recurrence was also reflected in patient DFS. The presence of CMCs by either test was associated with a significantly shorter overall DFS. However, among patients with locoregional recurrence, the shorter DFS was associated only with MART-1-positive, tyrosinase-negative patients. The pattern was reversed in patients with distant recurrence, in that short DFS was seen predominantly in tyrosinase-positive, MART-1-negative patients. These findings were derived from results of assays on samples from 50 of 73 patients with disease recurrence, 16 with locoregional and 34 with distant metastases. The statistical tests suggest that it is unlikely that the results were due to chance, but a longer follow-up, particularly in patients with stage I or II disease, is needed if these findings are to be confirmed.

The lack of MART-1 expression on the CMCs of patients with recurrence at distant sites may be explained by the higher immunogenicity of MART-1 than of tyrosinase. MART-1 was recognised by the majority of HLA-A2-restricted, melanoma-specific, cytotoxic T lymphocytes that were generated from tumour-infiltrating lymphocytes [24]. The same laboratory showed that among ten HLA-A2-restricted, melanoma-specific, tumour-infiltrating lymphocyte lines, nine reacted with MART-1, four with gp100, and none with tyrosinase [24]. Evidence for selection of MART-1-negative melanoma cells comes from studies by Maeurer et al. [25], who found that MART-1 was expressed on an autologous melanoma lesion resected in 1987, but not on a recurrent metastatic melanoma resected in 1993. Development of MART-1-negative melanoma has also been reported during immunotherapy with melanoma peptides [26]. It is also possible that MART-1 may be associated with a more differentiated melanoma phenotype that has less propensity to metastasise through the bloodstream. In subsequent studies, CMCs from patients with locoregional and those with distant metastases will need to be analysed to determine whether the cells differ in expression of adhesion molecules and other factors associated with the metastatic process.

Acknowledgement. Supported in part by the New South Wales State Cancer Council, the J.P. Morgan Fund, the Sydney Melanoma Foundation, and the Melanoma and Skin Research Institute, Sydney, Australia.

References

1. Balch CM, Soong S-J, Shaw HM, Urist MM, and McCarthy WH. (1992) An analysis of prognostic factors in 8500 patients with cutaneous melanoma. In Balch CM, Houghton AN, Milton GW, Sober AJ, and Soong S-J. (eds). Cutaneous melanoma. J. B. Lippincott Co. Philadelphia, USA. pp 165–187
2. Hart IA, and Saini A. (1992) Biology of tumour metastasis. Lancet. 339: 1453–1457
3. Smith B, Selby P, Southgate J, Pittman K, Bradley C, and Blair GE. (1991) Detection of melanoma cells in peripheral blood by means of reverse transcriptase and polymerase chain reaction. Lancet. 338: 1227–1229
4. Brossart P, Keilholz U, Willhauck M, Scheibenbogen C, Mohler T, and Hunstein W. (1993) Hematogenous spread of malignant melanoma cells in different stages of disease. J. Invest. Dermatol. 101: 887–889
5. Battayani Z, Grob JJ, Xerri L, Noe C, Zarour H, Houvaeneghel G, Delpero JR, Birmbaum D, Hassoun J, and Bonerandi JJ. (1995) Polymerase chain reaction detection of circulating melanocytes as a prognostic marker in patients with melanoma. Arch. Dermatol. 131: 443–447

6. Mellado B, Colomer D, Castel T, Munoz M, Carballo E, Galan M, Mascaro JM, Vives-Corrons JL, Grau JJ, and Estape J. (1996) Detection of circulating neoplastic cells by reverse-transcriptase polymerase chain reaction in malignant melanoma: association with clinical stage and prognosis. J. Clin. Oncol. 14: 2091–2097
7. Reinhold U, Ludtke-Handjery H-C, Schnautz S, Kreysel H-W, and Abken H. (1997) The analysis of tyrosinase-specific mRNA in blood samples of melanoma patients by RT-PCR is not a useful test for metastatic tumour progression. J. Invest. Dermatol. 108: 166–169
8. Farthmann B, Eberle J, Krasagakis K, Gstottner M, Wang N, Bisson S, and Orfanos CE. (1998) RT-PCR for tyrosinase-mRNA-positive cell in peripheral blood: evaluation strategy and correlation with known prognostic markers in 123 melanoma patients. J. Invest. Dermatol. 110: 263–267
9. Curry BJ, Myers K, and Hersey P. (1998) Polymerase chain reaction detection of melanoma cells in the circulation: Relation to clinical stage, surgical treatment, and recurrence from melanoma. J. Clin. Oncol. 16: 1760–1769
10. Reintgen D, Cruse C, Wells K, Saba HI, and Fabri PJ. (1992) The evaluation of putative tumour markers for malignant melanoma. Ann. Plast. Surg. 28: 55–59
11. Buzaid A, Sandler A, Hayden C, Scinto J, Poo WJ, Clark MB, and Hotchkiss S. (1994a) Neuron-specific enolase as a tumour marker in metastatic melanoma. Am. J. Clin. Oncol. 17: 430–431
12. Buzaid A, Sandler A, Hayden C, Scinto J, Poo WJ, Clark MB, and Hotchkiss S. (1994b) Correlation of lipid-associated sialic acid and tumour burden in melanoma. Int. J. Biol. Markers. 9: 247–250
13. von Schoultz E, Hansson LO, Djureen E, Hansson J, Karnell R, Nilsson B, Stigbrand T, and Ringborg U. (1996) Prognostic value of serum analyses of S-100β protein in malignant melanoma. Melanoma Res. 6: 133–137
14. Hoon DSB, Wang Y, Dale PS, Conrad AJ, Schmid P, Garrison D, Kuo C, Foshag LJ, Nizze AJ, and Morton DL. (1995) Detection of occult melanoma cells in blood with a multiple-marker polymerase chain reaction assay. J. Clin. Oncol. 13: 2109–2116
15. Adema GJ, de Boer AJ, Vogel AM, Loenen WAM, and Figdor CG. (1994) Molecular characterisation of the melanocyte lineage-specific antigen gp100. J. Biol. Chem. 269: 20126–20133
16. Kaplan FL, and Meier P. (1958) Nonparametric estimation from incomplete observations. J. Am. Stat. Assoc. 52: 457–481
17. Curry BJ, Myers K, and Hersey P. (1999) MART-1 is expressed less frequently on circulating melanoma cells in patients who develop distant compared with locoregional metastases. J. Clin. Oncol. 17: 2562–2571
18. Cox DR. (1972) Regression models and life tables. J. R. Stat. Soc. Ser. B 34: 187–220
19. Kirkwood JM, Strawderman MH, Ernstoff MS, Smith TJ, Borden EC, and Blum RH. (1996) Interferon alfa-2b adjuvant therapy of high-risk resected cutaneous melanoma: the Eastern Cooperative Oncology Group trial EST 1684. J. Clin. Oncol. 14: 7–17
20. Curry BJ. The detection of melanoma cells and the melanoma cell product S-100b in the circulation: Relation to clinical stage, surgical treatment and recurrence from melanoma. Newcastle, New South Wales, Australia, University of Newcastle 1998 (doctoral thesis)
21. Burchill SA, Bradbury MF, Pittman K, SouthgateJ, Smith B, and Selby P. (1995) Detection of epithelial cancer cells in peripheral blood by reverse transcriptase-polymerase chain reaction. Br. J. Cancer 71: 278–281
22. Keilholz U, Willhauck M, Scheibenbogen C, de Vries TJ, Burchill S. (1997) Polymerase chain reaction detection of circulating tumour cells. Melanoma Res. 7: S133-S141
23. Ghossein RA, Coit D, Brennan M, Zhang ZF, Wang Y, Bhattacharya S, Houghton A, and Rosai J. (1998) Prognostic significance of peripheral blood and bone marrow tyrosinase messenger RNA in malignant melanoma. Clin. Cancer Res. 4: 419–428
24. Kawakami Y, Eliyahu S, Sakaguchi K, Robbins PF, Rivoltini L, Yannelli JR, Appella E, and Rosenberg SA. (1994) Identification of the immunodominant peptides of the MART-1 human melanoma antigen recognised by the majority of HLA-A2-restricted tumour infiltrating lymphocytes. J. Exp. Med. 180: 347–352

25. Maeurer MJ, Gollin SM, Martin D, Swaney W, Bryant J, Castelli C, Robbins P, Parmiani G, Storkus WJ, and Lotze MT. (1996) Tumour escape from immune recognition. Lethal recurrent melanoma in a patient associated with downregulation of the peptide transporter protein TAP-1 and loss of expression of the immunodominant MART-1/Melan-A antigen. J. Clin. Invest. 98: 1633–1641
26. Jager E, Ringhoffer M, Altmannsberger M, Arand M, Karbach J, Jager D, Oesch F, and Knuth A. (1997) Immunoselection in vivo: independent loss of MHC class I and melanocyte differentiation antigen expression in metastatic melanoma. Int. J. Cancer 71: 142–147

Active Specific Immunotherapy of Malignant Melanoma and Peptide Mimics of the Human High-Molecular-Weight Melanoma-Associated Antigen

S. Ferrone and X. Wang

Department of Immunology, Roswell Park Cancer Institute,
Elm and Carlton Streets, Buffalo, NY 14263, USA

Abstract

The realization that tumor cells utilize multiple mechanisms to escape from immune recognition and destruction has stimulated interest in developing and applying immunotherapeutic strategies which target both humoral and cellular immunity to malignant cells. As a result, the tumor-associated antigens (TAA) used as targets have to be expressed on the cell surface membrane of malignant cells. Furthermore, since most of the TAA used for active specific immunotherapy are self-antigens, a challenge facing tumor immunologists is to develop strategies which are effective in breaking tolerance to self-antigens. This chapter describes one strategy which relies on the use of peptide mimics of the human high-molecular-weight melanoma-associated antigen (HMW-MAA) as immunogens to implement active specific immunotherapy in patients with malignant melanoma. These mimics, which are isolated from phage display peptide libraries by panning with anti-HMW-MAA monoclonal antibodies, are expected to induce both humoral and cellular anti-HMW-MAA immunity.

The identification and molecular characterization of human tumor-associated antigens (TAA) during the last few years [1–4] have provided well defined moieties to implement active specific immunotherapy in patients with malignant diseases [5, 6]. For several years the emphasis has been on T cell-defined TAA because of the general belief that T cells are the major, if not the only, players in the control of tumor growth and because of the disappointing results of the early clinical trials relying on anti-TAA antibodies [7]. The realization that the multiple mechanisms utilized by malignant cells to escape from T cell recognition represent a major limitation in the successful application of T cell-based immunotherapy of malignant diseases [8] has rekindled interest in the utilization of anti-TAA antibodies, by themselves or in combination with $CD4^+$ and/or $CD8^+$ T cells, to control tumor growth. This trend has been strengthened by the association between induction of anti-

Recent Results in Cancer Research, Vol. 158

TAA antibodies in patients with malignant diseases and improved prognosis [9–11] and by the recent favorable results of passive immunotherapy of malignant diseases with anti-TAA antibodies, by themselves or in combination with chemotherapy [12–14].

The large majority of TAA identified in malignant cells with T cells or with antibodies have been found to be self-antigens [15, 16] which are expressed in larger amounts in malignant cells than in their normal counterparts, most likely because of abnormalities in gene regulation associated with the transformation process. Therefore a challenge facing tumor immunologists in applying active specific immunotherapy of malignant diseases is to develop and utilize approaches which are effective in breaking tolerance to self-antigens.

Among the many approaches which are being tested, we have selected one relying on the utilization of mimics of TAA as immunogens. The rationale for our choice derives from the results of our previous clinical trials in malignant melanoma utilizing mouse anti-idiotypic monoclonal antibodies which mimic the HMW-MAA [9, 17]. In those investigations we found that anti-idiotypic monoclonal antibodies were more effective than the original TAA in breaking tolerance to a self-antigen. Anti-idiotypic antibodies elicited anti-HMW-MAA antibodies in more than 50% of the immunized patients, while the HMW-MAA was not immunogenic. This finding is likely to reflect the deletion, during the establishment of self-identity, of B cell clones that recognize the HMW-MAA with high affinity. In contrast the immunogenicity of the corresponding anti-idiotypic antibodies is likely to reflect their ability to stimulate clones which have not been deleted during the establishment of self-identity, since they secrete antibodies reacting with the corresponding antigen with an affinity below the threshold required for their deletion. We have selected the HMW-MAA as a target of immunotherapy because of its high frequency of expression in patients with melanoma [18, 19], its high expression by melanoma cells with limited intra- and inter-lesional heterogeneity [19, 20], its restricted distribution in normal tissues [18, 19] and its suggested role in the metastatic potential of melanoma cells [21, 22]. Furthermore the expression of HMW-MAA by pericytes [23] suggests that the effect of anti-HMW-MAA immunity on melanoma lesions may be mediated not only by a direct interaction with melanoma cells, but also by disturbing the blood supply.

The mimics of HMW-MAA we plan to use as immunogens are represented by peptides we have isolated by panning phage display peptide libraries with mouse anti-HMW-MAA monoclonal antibodies and with human anti-HMW-MAA single chain Fv fragments. Analysis of the isolated peptides has shown that most of them do not display a significant homology in their sequence with the published amino acid sequence of the HMW-MAA [24]. Furthermore the isolated peptides have distinct sequences. Most of the peptides react only with the antibody used for their isolation and do not cross-react even with antibodies which display a high degree of homology in the amino acid sequence of the variable regions of their heavy and light chains with

Table 1. Homology with the human HMW-MAA and with the rat NG2 antigen of peptides isolated from the phage display peptide library X15 by panning with the anti-HMW-MAA monoclonal antibodies 149.53 and 225.28

Monoclonal antibody	Homology with HMW-MAA and NG2 antigen of peptides isolated with monoclonal antibodies	
149.53	Peptide	EELHPP**GSRAPS** **IRK**
	HMW-MAA	PLRLTR**GSRAP**ISR**A**
	NG2	P LRITR**GSRAP**VSR**A**
225.28	Peptide	TQYTRTDPWGL**EPPK**
	HMW-MAA	PT CLGLSLQ V**LEPPQ**
	NG2	GTCPGLVLQ V**LEPPQ**

Amino acids which are identical in the isolated peptides and in the antigen analyzed are in bold.

those of the antibodies used for their isolation. Only the peptides isolated from the phage display peptide library X15 [25] with the mouse monoclonal antibodies 149.53 and 225.28 display homology with the amino acid sequence of HMW-MAA. As shown in Table 1, the sequences of the peptides isolated with the monoclonal antibodies 149.53 and 225.28 are identical to that of the HMW-MAA at positions 1846–1850 and 1852 and at positions 1457–1460, respectively. It is noteworthy that the monoclonal antibodies 149.53 and 225.28 cross-react with the rat antigen NG2, a chondroitin sulfate proteoglycan isolated from a chemically induced rat neuronal tumor [26]. The human HMW-MAA displays an approximately 80% homology with the rat NG2 antigen in its amino acid sequence [24, 27]. The amino acids shared by the peptides isolated with the monoclonal antibodies 149.53 and 225.28 with the HMW-MAA are also present in the NG2 antigen [27], therefore strengthening the possibility that these amino acids play an important role in the expression of the determinants recognized by the two monoclonal antibodies. Interestingly both monoclonal antibodies are less reactive with the rat NG2 antigen than with the human HMW-MAA. Whether this finding reflects the differences in the amino acid sequences of the flanking regions of the identical amino acid sequence stretches remains to be determined.

The large number of peptide mimics of the HMW-MAA we have isolated with the panel of human and mouse anti-HMW-MAA antibodies from phage display peptide libraries represents a useful source of immunogens to implement active specific immunotherapy in patients with melanoma. One of the major challenges we are facing is to develop an effective strategy to select the peptides which are most likely to be immunogenic in patients with melanoma. Hopefully this information may be derived from the analysis of the immunogenicity of the peptides mimics of HMW-MAA in mice transgenic for human HMW-MAA (we plan to construct) and in rabbits which express a molecule with the tissue distribution and with the antigenic profile similar to those of the HMW-MAA in humans [23].

One might ask which advantages we expect by replacing mouse anti-idiotypic monoclonal antibodies with peptide mimics of HMW-MAA as immunogens in our trials of active specific immunotherapy in malignant melanoma. We expect that these peptides will improve our immunization strategy in patients with malignant melanoma, since: (1) they may induce HLA class I antigen-restricted, HMW-MAA-specific cytotoxic T lymphocytes in addition to anti-HMW-MAA antibodies; (2) they eliminate the induction of antibodies to constant and variable regions of mouse anti-idiotypic monoclonal antibodies; and (3) they facilitate the development of immunogens resulting from the fusion of peptide(s) with cytokines which are likely to display an increased immunogenicity. Lastly, from a practical view point, it is easier and less expensive to prepare synthetic peptides to be used as immunogens in clinical trials than mouse anti-idiotypic monoclonal antibodies.

ACKNOWLEDGEMENTS. The authors wish to acknowledge the excellent secretarial assistance of Mrs. Charlene DeMont, Mrs. Marilyn Balon and Mrs. Barbara Nanna.

This work was supported by PHS Grants CA37959, CA51814 and CA85184 awarded by the National Cancer Institute, DHHS.

References

1. Reisfeld RA, Cheresh DA (1987) Human tumor antigens. Adv Immunol:40;323–377
2. Boon T, Cerottini JC, Van den Eynde B, Van der Bruggen P, Van Pel A (1994) Tumor antigens recognized by T lymphocytes. Annu Rev Immunol 12:337–365
3. Tureci O, Sahin U, Pfreundschuh M (1997) Serological analysis of human tumor antigens: molecular definition and implications. Mol Med Today 3:342–349
4. Rosenberg SA (1999) A new era for cancer immunotherapy based on the genes that encode cancer antigens. Immunity10:281–287
5. Bystryn J-C, Ferrone S, Livingston P (1993) (editors) Specific immunotherapy of cancer with vaccines. Ann NY Acad Sci 690:1–401
6. Greten TF, Jaffee EM (1999) Cancer vaccines. J Clin Oncol 17:1047–1060
7. Milstein C, Waldmann H (1999) Curr Opin Immunol 11:589–591
8. Marincola FM, Jaffee EM, Hicklin DJ, Ferrone S (1999) Escape of human solid tumors from T cell recognition: molecular mechanisms and functional significance. Adv Immunol In press
9. Mittelman A, Chen ZJ, Yang H, Wong GY, Ferrone S (1992) Human high molecular weight melanoma-associated antigen (HMW-MAA) mimicry by mouse anti-idiotypic monoclonal antibody MK2-23: Induction of humoral anti-HMW-MAA immunity and prolongation of survival in patients with stage IV melanoma. Proc Natl Acad Sci USA 89:466–470
10. Livingston PO, Wong GY, Adluri S, Taó Y, Padavan M, Parente R, Hanlon C, Calves MJ, Helling F, Ritter G, Oettgen HF, Old LJ (1994) Improved survival in AJCC stage III melanoma patients with GM2 antibodies: A randomized trial of adjuvant vaccination with GM2 ganglioside. J Clin Oncol 12:1036–1044
11. Maclean GD, Reddish MA, Koganty RR, Longenecker BM (1996) Antibodies against Mucin-associated sialyl-Tn epitopes correlate with survival of metastatic adenocarcinoma patients undergoing active specific immunotherapy with synthetic STn vaccine. J Immunother 19:59–68
12. Riethmuller G, Schneider-Gadicke E, Schlimok G, Schmiegel W, Raab R, Hoffken K, Gruber R, Pichlmaier H, Hirche H, Pichlmayr R, Buggisch P, Witte J and the German Cancer Aid 17-1A study group (1994) Randomised trial of monocloncal antibody for adjuvant therapy of resected Dukes' C colorectal carcinoma. Lancet 343:1177–1183

13. Pegram MD, Lipton A, Hayes DF, Weber BL, Baselga JM, Tripathy D, Baly D, Baughman SA, Twadddell T, Glaspy JA, Slamon DJ (1998) Phase II study of receptor-enhanced chemosensitivity using recombinant humanized anti-p185HER2/neu monoclonal antibody plus cisplatin in patients with HER/2neu-overexpressing metastatic breast cancer refractory to chemotherapy treatment. J Clin Oncol 16:2659–2671
14. Mendelsohn J, Shin DM, Donato N, Khuri F, Radinsky R, Glisson BS, Shin HJ, Metz E, Pfister D, Perez-Soler R, Lawhorn K, Matsumoto T, Gunnett K, Falcey J, Waksal H, Hong WK (1999) A phase I study of chimerized anti-epidermal growth factor receptor (EGFr) monoclonal antibody, C225, in combination with cisplatin (CDDP) in patients (PTS) with recurrent head and neck squamous cell carcinoma (SCC). Proc Am Soc Clin Oncol 18:389a
15. Houghton AN (1994) Cancer antigens: immune recognition of self and altered self. J Exp Med 180:1–4
16. Old LJ, Chen YT (1998) New paths in human cancer serology. J Exp Med187:1163–1167
17. Mittelman A, Chen GZJ, Wong GY, Liu C, Hirai S, Ferrone S (1995) Human high molecular weight-melanoma associated antigen mimicry by mouse anti-idiotypic monoclonal antibody MK2-23: Modulation of the immunogenicity in patients with malignant melanoma. Clin Cancer Res 1:705–713
18. Natali PG, Imai K, Wilson BS, Bigotti A, Cavaliere R, Pellegrino MA, Ferrone S (1981) Structural properties and tissue distribution of the antigen recognized by the monoclonal antibody 653.40 S to human melanoma cells. J Natl Cancer Inst 67:591–601
19. Ferrone S, Temponi M, Gargiulo D, Scassellati GA, Cavaliere R, Natali PG (1988) Selection and utilization of monoclonal antibody defined melanoma associated antigens for immunoscintigraphy in patients with melanoma. In: Radiolabeled monoclonal antibodies for imaging and therapy, NATO ASI Series, (Srivastava, SC, ed) Plenum Press New York and London 152:55–78
20. Giacomini P, Natali PG, Ferrone S (1985) Analysis of the interaction between a human high molecular weight melanoma-associated antigen and the monoclonal antibodies to three distinct antigenic determinants. J Immunol 135:696–702
21. Chattopadhyay P, Kaveri S-V, Byars N, Starkey J, Ferrone S, Raychaudhuri S (1991) Human high molecular weight-melanoma associated antigen mimicry by an anti-idiotypic antibody: Characterization of the immunogenicity and the immune response to the mouse monoclonal antibody IMEL-1. Cancer Res 51:6045–6051
22. Kageshita T, Kuriya N, Ono T, Horikoshi T, Takahashi M, Wong GY, Ferrone S (1993) Association of high molecular weight melanoma-associated antigen expression in primary acral lentiginous melanoma lesions with poor prognosis. Cancer Res 53:2830–2833
23. Schlingemann RO, Rietveld FJR, de Waal RMW, Ferrone S, Ruiter DJ (1990) Expression of the high molecular weight melanoma-associated antigen by pericytes during angiogenesis in tumors and in healing wounds. Am J Pathol 136:1393–1405
24. Pluschke G, Vanek M, Evans A, Dittmar T, Schmid P, Itin P, Filardo EJ, Reisfeld RA (1996) Molecular cloning of a human melanoma-associated chondroitin sulfate proteoglycan. Proc Natl Acad Sci USA 93:9710–9715
25. Bonnycastle LL, Mehroke JS, Rashed M, Gong X, Scott JK (1996) Probing the basis of antibody reactivity with a panel of constrained peptide libraries displayed by filamentous phage. J Mol Biol 258:747–762
26. Schubert D, Heinemann S, Carlisle W, Tarikas H, Kimes B, Patrick, J, Steinbach JH, Culp W, Brandt BL (1974) Clonal cell lines from the rat central nervous system. Nature 249:224–227
27. Nishiyama A, Dahlin KJ, Prince JT, Johstone SR, Stallcup WB (1991) The primary structure of NG2, a novel membrance-spanning proteoglycan. J Cell Biol 114:359–371

Autologous Dendritic Cells for Treatment of Advanced Cancer – An Update

D. Schadendorf[1] and F.O. Nestle[2]

[1] Clinical Cooperation Unit for Dermatooncology (DKFZ), Department of Dermatology, Mannheim Clinics, Mannheim, Germany
[2] Department of Dermatology, University Hospital Zurich, Zurich, Switzerland

Abstract

Dendritic cells (DC) are commonly viewed as the professional antigen-presenting cell. They capture antigens, migrate to appropriate lymphoid organs and initiate an antigen-specific CD4 and CD8 T cell response. Much is known about DC physiology, and it is now possible to culture, maintain and expand DC from different human sources, including hematopoietic progenitors in bone marrow and peripheral blood. Combined with the detection of an increasing number of tumor-associated antigens and T cell-recognized peptide epitopes, this has led to a new enthusiasm in the field of tumor immunotherapy and to various clinical applications in phase I/II studies on the treatment of different malignancies. This chapter will review the latest developments and give a brief update of the results obtained in studies of advanced melanoma, as well as provide a short overview of published results for other tumors.

Melanoma and Tumor Immunology

Melanoma is a malignant tumor of neuroectodermal origin with an increasing incidence and mortality. It needs to be detected and eliminated early, since melanoma is characterized by its high resistance to conventional therapies including surgery and chemotherapy (Ahmann et al. 1989; Johnson et al. 1995; Garbe, 1993). Nonetheless,, melanoma is considered to be one of the most immunogenic tumors, as demonstrated by tumor-infiltrating lymphocytes (TIL), which destroy melanoma cells (Oettgen and Old 1991; Parkinson et al. 1992; Dagleish 1996). This response may also explain the occurrence of spontaneous partial or complete melanoma regression and for concomitant destruction of melanocytes in benign lesions, leading to clinical phenomena such as halo nevi, uveitis and vitiligo in melanoma patients.

Nevertheless it became clear that immune responses to tumor antigens are frequently not observed because of tolerance and immunological non-respon-

Recent Results in Cancer Research, Vol. 158

siveness to cancer. In order to overcome this hurdle, cancer vaccines must break tolerance and activate "cryptic" T cell populations that escaped tolerance induction by low-affinity binding, which is critically dependent on the proper activation of the encountering antigen-presenting cell (APC). Danger signals will lead to appropriate co-stimulation and T cell activation (reviewed in Bell et al. 1999). The critical role of CD4 cells and CD40/CD40L interaction in delivering help to CD8 and providing an adequate cytokine milieu has been recognized to be of great importance in recent years (Bennett et al. 1997; Mackey et al. 1998).

In order to fight cancer, the idea of using the destructive power of immune responses can be easily visualized in autoimmune diseases and by the rejection of allografts. A number of clinical observations in human malignant melanoma suggest a particularly vigorous immune response (Oettgen and Old 1991; Parkinson et al. 1992; Mackensen et al. 1994; Dagleish, 1996). CD8+ T lymphocytes derived from melanoma lesions or the peripheral blood and tumor tissue were shown to be capable of mediating impressive tumor regressions in vivo (Kawakami et al. 1994; Robbins et al. 1994). The availability and further characterization of such tumor-specific T cell clones in recent years has led to the identification of several melanoma-associated antigens (reviewed in Sun et al.; Table 1), providing tools which allow the rationale design of vaccination strategies.

Dendritic Cells and the Control of Immunity

Basic immunology demonstrates the pivotal role of dendritic cells in generating an immune response. Dendritic cells (DC) are APC specialized for the induction of a primary T cell response (Banchereau and Steinman 1998; Bell et al. 1999). DC derived from various sources such as bone marrow or peripheral blood are responsible for initiating T cell responses in vivo, including CD4 and CD8 responses, by their unique capability to present antigens to naive T cells (reviewed in Banchereau and Steinman 1998; Bell et al. 1999). Differentiation of monocytes into DC was shown to be accelerated by contact with the endothelium and phagocytosis (Randolph et al. 1998).

Since DC can now easily be generated from different sources including peripheral blood (Romani et al. 1994; Sallusto and Lanciavecchia 1994), these cells can either be used after pulsing with peptides or after transfection with a tumor antigen for vaccination of cancer patients (Alijagic et al. 1995; Mayordomo et al. 1995, 1996; Celuzzi et al. 1996, Paglia et al. 1996; Porgador et al. 1996). The implication for vaccine design is that DC would be more potent than tumor cells as immunogens. Alternative approaches to stimulate the immune system such as immunization with naked DNA are dependent on DC (Beckerleg and Pardoll, 1995; Casares et al. 1997).

Both cytotoxic T lymphocytes and natural killer cells are essential effectors of anti-tumor immunity. DC were shown not only to prime antigen-specific T cells but also to trigger innate, NK cell-mediated anti-tumor immunity

Table 1. Melanoma-associated antigens recognized by cytotoxic T lymphocytes

Target antigen	Restricting HLA molecule	Peptides recognized	Amino acid position	Reference
MAGE-1	HLA-A1	EADPTGHSY	161–169	van der Bruggen et al. (1991)
	HLA-A3	SLFRAVITK	96–104	Chaux et al. (1999)
	HLA-A24	NYKHCFPEI	135–143	Fujie et al. (1999)
	HLA-A28	EVYDGREHSA	222–231	Chaux et al. (1999)
	HLA-B53	DPARYEFLW	258–266	Chaux et al. (1999)
	HLA-Cw2	SAFPTTINF	62–70	Chaux et al. (1999)
	HLA-Cw3/-Cw16	SAYGEPRKL	230–238	van der Bruggen et al. (1994)
	HLA-DR13	LLKYRAREPVTKAE	121–134	Chaux et al. (1999)
MAGE-2	HLA-A2	KMVELVHFL	112–120	Visseren et al. (1997)
		YLQLVFGIEV	157–106	Visseren et al. (1997)
	HLA-24	EYLQLVFGI	156–164	Tahara et al. (1999)
	HLA-DR13	LLKYRAREPVTKKE	212–134	Chaux et al. (1999)
MAGE-3	HLA-A1	EVDPIGHLY	168–176	Gaugler et al. (1994)
	HLA-A2	FLWGPRALV	271–279	van der Bruggen et al. (1994)
	HLA-A24	IMPKAGLLI	195–203	Tanaka et al. (1997)
	HLA-B44	MEVDPIGHLY	163–176	Herman et al. (1996)
	HLA-DR13	(RKV)AELVHFLLLKYR (AR)	(111) 114–125 (-127)	Chaux et al. (1999)
	HLA-DR13	(FL)LLKYRAREPVTKAE	(119) 212–134	Chaux et al. (1999)
	HLA-DR11	TSYVKVLHHMV KISG	281–295	Manici et al. (1999)
MAGE-4	HLA-A2	GVYDGREHTV	230–239	Duffour et al. (1999)
MAGE-6	HLA-A3402(A10)	MVKISGGPR		Zorn and Hercend (1999)
	HLA-DR13	LLKYRAREPVTKKE	212–134	Chaux et al. (1999)
BAGE	HLA-Cw16	AARAVFLAL	2–10	Boël et al. (1995)
RAGE	HLA-B7	SPSSNRIRNT		Gaugler et al. (1996)
GAGE-1	HLA-Cw6	YRPRPRRY	9–16	van den Eynde et al. (1995)
	HLA-A29	YYWPRPRRY		
	HLA-A24	LYVDSLFFL	301–309	Ikeda et al. (1997)
NY-ESO-1/ CAG-3/	HLA-A2 (ORF-1)	(QL)SLLMWITQC(FL)	157–165 (-167)	Jäger et al. (1998)
	HLA-A31 (ORF-1)	ASGPGGGAPR	53–62	Wang et al. (1998)
	HLA-A31 (ORF-2)	LAAQERRYPR	Alternative ORF	Wang et al. (1998)
LAGE/CAMEL	HLA-A2 (ORF-2)	MLMAQEALAPL	Alternative ORF	Lethé et al. (1998
pMel-34/ tyrosinase	HLA-A2	YM*D*GTMSQV	368–376	Skipper et al. (1996)
		YM*N*GTMSQV	368–376	Wölfel et al. (1994)
		MLLAVLYCL	1–9	Wölfel et al. (1994)
	HLA-A24	AFLPWHRLF	206–214	Kang et al. (1995)
	HLA-B44	SEIWRDIDF	192–200	Brichard et al. (1996)
	HLA-A1	KCDICTDEY	243–251	Kittlesen et al. (1998)
	HLA-A1	SSDYVIPIGTY	146–156	Kawakami et al. (1998)

Table 1 (continued)

Target antigen	Restricting HLA molecule	Peptides recognized	Amino acid position	Reference
	HLA-DR4	QNILLSNAPLGPQFP	56–70	Topalian et al. (1996)
	HLA-DR4	SYLQDSVPDSFQD	448–462	Topalian et al. (1996)
	HLA-DR15	FLLHHAFVDSI-FEQWLQRHRP	386–406	Kobayashi et al. (1998)
TRP-1/gp75	HLA-A31*(ORF-3)	MSLQRQFLR (ORF-3)	1–9	Wang et al. (1996)
TRP-2	HLA-A0201	SVYDFFVWL	180–188	Parkhurst et al. (1998)
	HLA-A0201	SLHNLYHSFL	367–376	Reynolds et al. (1998)
	HLA-A31,A33	LLPGGTPYR	197–205	Wang et al. J (1996, 1998)
	HLA-CW8	ANDPIFVVL	387–395	Castelli et al. (1999)
TRP-2 (int2)	HLA-A68011/-3301	EVISCKLIKR	222–231	Lupetti et al. (1998)
pMel-17/ gp100	HLA-A2	VLYRYGSFSV	476–485	Kawakami et al. (1994)
		KTWGQYWQV	154–162	Kawakami et al. (1994)
		YLEPGPVTA	280–288	Kawakami et al. (1994)
		LLDGTATLRL	457–466	Kawakami et al. (1994)
		SLADTNSLAV		
		ITDQVPFSV	209–217	Kawakami et al. (1994)
		RLMKQDPSV		Kawakami et al. (1998)
		RLPRIFCSC		Kawakami et al. (1998)
		(A)MLGTHTMEV		Tsai et al. (1997)
	HLA-A3	SLIYRRRLMK		Kawakami et al. (1998)
	HLA-A3	ALLAVGATK	17–25	Castelli et al. (1998); Skipper et al. (1996)
	HLA-A3, -A11	(I)ALNFPGSQK	(86-)87–95	Kawashima et al. (1998)
	HLA-Cw8	SNDGPTLI	71–78	Castelli et al. (1999)
	HLA-(DR1), DR4,(DR3)	WNRQLYPEWTEAQRLD	44–59	Li et al. (1998)
gp100 (int-4)	HLA-A24	VYFFLPDHL	170–178	Robbins et al. (1994)
gp43	HLA-A2	DLTMKYQIF		Takahashi et al. (1997)
Melan-A/ MART-1	HLA-A2	ILTVILGVL	32–40	Castelli et al. (1995)
		(E)AAGIGILTV	(26)27–35	Kawakami et al. (1994); Romero et al. (1997)
		GIGILTVL	29–36	
		GILTVILGV	31–38	
	HLA-B45.1	ALMDKSLHV		
		AEEAAGIGIL(T)	24–33(34)	Schneider et al. (1998)
707-AP	HLA-A2	RVAALARDAP		Takahashi et al. (1997)
N-acetyl-Gn-transferase V	HLA-A2	VLPDVFIRC(V)	(Intron sequence)	Guilloux et al. (1996)
p15	HLA-A24	AYGLDFYIL		Robbins et al. (1995)
β-catenin	HLA-A24	SYLDSGIHF	29–37	Robbins et al. (1996)

Table 1 (continued)

Target antigen	Restricting HLA molecule	Peptides recognized	Amino acid position	Reference
SR-2	HLA-A3	KIFSEVTLK		
MUM-1	HLA-B44	EEKLIVVLF	782–808	Coulie et al. (1995)
Myosin class I	HLA-A3	KINKNPKYK		Zorn and Hercend (1999)
CDK4	HLA-A2.1	ACDPHSGHFV		Wölfel et al. (1995)
TPI (triose phosphate isomerase)	HLA-DR1	GELIGILNAAKVPAD	23–37	Pieper et al. (1999)
Fusion protein LDLR/FUT	HLA-DR1	(PVI)WRRAPA(PGA)	315–323	Wang et al. (1999)
CDC27	HLA-DR4	FSWAMDLDPKGA	760–771	Wang et al. (1999)

via cell-to-cell contact by DC and resting NK cells (Fernandez et al. 1999). Furthermore, the functional state of DC is critical for the outcome of the immune response. It was not known whether subsets of DC provide different cytokine microenviroments that determine the differentiation of either T_{H1}- or T_{H2} cells. Recently, Rissoan et al. (1999) demonstrated that monocyte-derived DC induce T_{H1} differentiation. In addition, the critical role of CD40/CD40L interaction for DC maturation and interleukin (IL)-12 production was pointed out and shown to be critical for the generation of protective anti-tumor immunity (Mackey et al. 1998).

DC as Therapeutic Vehicle

Mouse studies have demonstrated the potent capacity of DC to induce anti-tumor immunity (Flamand et al. 1994, Mayordomo et al. 1995, 1996; Celuzzi et al. 1996, Paglia et al. 1996; Porgador et al. 1996). In a mouse tumor model, systemic administration of IL-2 enhanced the therapeutic efficacy of DC-based tumor vaccines' inducing of tumor regressions in s.c. tumors and pulmonary micro- and macrometastases (Shimizu et al. 1999). The potency of the DC-based immunization approach was further documented by the fact that it was capable of breaking immunodominance against minor histocompatibility and synthetic peptide antigens (Grufman et al. 1999). However, it was pointed out that, depending on the nature of the material (peptides, RNA, DNA), the optimal sequence of antigen-loading differs and is critical (Morse et al. 1998).

In the human system, autologous DC were used in vitro to generate cytotoxic T lymphocytes (CTL) against various targets including p53 and CEA by peptide loading (Chikamatsu et al. 1999; Alters et al. 1998;). Besides pulsing DC with known peptides or with unfractionated peptides eluted by mild acid treatment (Storkus et al. 1993) from 10^9 or more tumor cells, tumor lysates prepared from autologous tumor samples were used for DC loading especially in clinical situations where no tumor-associated antigens are known. Pulsing of DC with tumor lysate led to an augmented T cell-restricted, HLA-dependent tumor lysis in various tumor systems in vitro (Mulders et al. 1999; Abdel-Wahab et al. 1998). Recently it was shown that the physical interaction between DC and tumor cells results in an antigen transfer that is sufficient to induce a protective and therapeutic tumor rejection in mice (Celuzzi and Falo 1998). A report by Nair and co-workers (1999) suggests that CTL activity generated after peptide pulsing of DC is comparable to activity after RNA-loading of DC, opening a new avenue of treatment options.

Of great clinical importance were recent scintigraphic investigation demonstrating that intradermally administered, immature monocyte-derived DCs had an excellent in vivo migratory capacity. Technetium-labeled, peptide-loaded DC traveled within 10 min to the draining lymph node (Thomas et al. 1999). Similar results were obtained by Morse et al. (1999b), who used ^{111}indium-labeled DC to compare i.v., s.c. and intradermal administration. Whereas after i.v. injection of DC, the cells localized in lungs and then redistributed to the liver, spleen and bone marrow, no DC were found in lymph nodes or tumors. These results are in agreement with data published by Sozzani et al. (1998), demonstrating that the lack of receptors such as CCR7 might be necessary for extravasation from blood vessels into the tissue and lymph nodes.

Clinical Application of DC

Results of Vaccination with Dendritic Cells for Melanoma Treatment

In a clinical pilot study, DC were generated in the presence of granulocyte/macrophage colony-stimulating factor (GM-CSF) and IL-4 and were pulsed with tumor lysate or a cocktail of peptides known to be recognized by CTLs depending on the patient's HLA haplotype (Nestle et al. 1998). Almost 50 patients with advanced melanoma have been immunized on an outpatient basis so far. Multiple peptides (MAGE-1 and MAGE-3 for HLA-A1, gp100-, tyrosinase- and MelanA-derived peptides for HLA-A2, MAGE-3 and tyrosinase for HLA-B44) were used. Due to a lack of defined tumor helper antigens, we added keyhole limpet hemocyanin (KLH) to all vaccine preparations as helper antigen to induce a potent KLH-specific memory T cell response. KLH has also the advantage of being a neo-antigen and can therefore serve as an immunological tracer molecule. In 11 patients, tumor lysate was used instead of peptide as source of tumor antigen. Thirty-two patients were eligible for evaluation. Vaccination was well tolerated in all patients. Occasionally, mild fever or swelling of the injected lymph node occurred, lasting for 1–2 days. No physical signs of autoimmune disease were observed in any of the patients. In six patients, anti-thyroid-stimulating hormone (TSH) receptor antibodies became detectable after initiation of DC vaccination, however, without clinical effect on thyroid function. In five patients, anti-nuclear antibodies were observed after treatment, also without clinical relevance. In two patients, a vitiligo was induced, and in another patient an individual melanocytic nevus regressed and lost pigmentation under vaccination. Therefore, we conclude that DC pulsed with antigen can be repeatedly injected into patients without significant toxicity.

We used DTH reactions as a convenient method to detect antigen-specific immunity. Vaccination of patients with DC pulsed with: (1) a globular protein antigen (KLH), (2) peptides binding to the HLA- molecules, or (3) autologous tumor lysate was capable of inducing significant delayed-type hypersensitivity (DTH) skin reactions. Significant DTH reactivity (>10 mm in diameter) against DC pulsed with KLH was observed in 90% of patients. Furthermore, a positive DTH reaction to peptide-pulsed DC was elicited in two out of three patients. DTH reactivity to peptides alone was seen in only six of 21 patients.

A stabilization of disease over 3 months was considered beneficial and was reached in nearly half of the patients. Regression of any metastasis was achieved in a total of one out of three patients, with eight patients experiencing a major clinical response (3CR, 5PR). Partial responders had a mean response duration of 7.3 months; however, the complete responders have been disease-free for up to 38 months until now. Tumor regressions were noted primarily in skin, lung and soft tissue, and remission in one case each in lymph node and pancreas. Responders were treated in six of 21 cases with peptides and in five of 11 cases with lysates, suggesting that both techniques are effective. However, patients expressing HLA-A2 had a much better chance of response than patients carrying HLA-A1. The number of patients treated with a HLA-B44 phenotype was too small, but two patients responded clinically to vaccination.

In conclusion, these data indicate that vaccination of advanced melanoma patients with peptide-pulsed as well as tumor lysate-pulsed DC is well tolerated and is able to induce anti-tumor immunity in vivo which is associated with measurable DTH-reactivity and clinical responses. Major clinical responses were seen in about a quarter of patients. Analysis of non-responding patients revealed several immune escape mechanisms, including loss of individual HLA alleles, and loss of tumor antigens and molecules involved in protein transport. Further studies are necessary to demonstrate the clinical effectiveness and impact on the survival of melanoma patients. A prospective, randomized clinical trial to compare a standard chemotherapy to vaccination with peptide-pulsed DC is currently underway.

Further Clinical Studies

In an early study, four patients with follicular lymphoma were treated with immature DC pulsed with idiotypic proteins (Hsu et al. 1994). However, no further data were reported so far. In a similar approach idiotypic protein from multiple myeloma was pulsed onto monocyte-derived, autologous DC in one patient. The induction of Id-specific immune response was documented by the generation of tumor-specific T cells associated with a transient fall of serum Id levels (Wen et al. 1999). Murphy and co-workers (1996) treated patients with advanced prostate cancer using autologous DC pulsed with HLA-A2-specific peptides derived from prostate-specific antigen (PSA) with some success. DC pulsed with autologous tumour lysate derived from metastatic renal cell cancer were shown to increase growth expansion of TIL and to augment T cell-restricted tumor lysis (Mulders et al. 1999). A first clinical pilot study reported one responding patient out of four (Hötl et al. 1998).

Immunization with tumor cell lysate loaded onto immature autologous APC-based vaccine was performed in 17 patients with advanced melanoma. No major clinical responses were observed; however, a stabilization was seen in 13 patients for more than 30 months. In five out of nine patients, vaccine-infiltrating lymphocytes were shown to be predominantly CD8+ (Chakraborty et al. 1998). In a pilot study, nine healthy donors were injected s.c. with mature, autologous monocyte-derived DC loaded with KLH, influenza matrix peptide or tetanus toxoid, demonstrating priming of CD4+ T cells to KLH (9/9), boosting of tetanus toxoid immunity (5/6) and a several-fold increase of influenza matrix peptide T cell reactivity after a single injection of mature DC (Dhodapkar et al. 1999). More recently, mature antigen-pulsed DC (cell lysate) were shown to elict strong cellular and humoral immune responses in patients with metastatic renal cell cancers in a phase I study involving 12 patients (Höltl et al. 1999).

Interestingly, in the only trial published so far, in which DC were infused i.v., no clinical benefit was detected. In that phase I protocol, patients with advanced CEA-positive malignancies were treated with CEA CAP-1-loaded onto DC by escalating cell infusions i.v. (up to 1×10^8 cells/dose) without major response (Morse et al. 1999a).

Whether the route of administration is critical is currently not clear, however, s.c. injections were shown in several studies to induce antigen-specific T cell responses.

Conclusion and Perspectives

Tumor immunology has made great progress in recent years. Recent animal studies have indicated that a potent protective immune response can be generated in vivo using DC loaded with peptides or tumor lysate. This response was shown to mediate tumor rejection and long-lived anti-tumor immunity (Flamand et al. 1994, Mayordomo et al. 1995, 1996; Celuzzi et al. 1996, Paglia et al. 1996; Porgador et al. 1996). Based on these successful animal studies, various clinical protocols for the treatment of human cancer have recently been initiated.

It is clear that the definition of tumor-associated antigens – starting a decade ago – has elicited a plethora of novel therapeutic options, including peptide vaccination, the use of APC or the utilization of recombinant viruses or bacteria to expose the patient's immune system to tumor antigens. At present, it seems safe to conclude that vaccination with DC can influence the immunological tumor-host relationship. The role of CD4 cells and additional ways to fully activate the anti-tumour immune response including CD40 activation needs more careful attention and is of particular interest. Clinical phase I/II studies are still in the early stages but have shown some interesting clinical results, and the first phase III trials are being planned. There is still enormous room for improvement including our understanding of how to induce a reliable and sufficiently strong immune response and how to maintain it. This is connected to choosing the correct adjuvant, the best dosing schedule and route as well as the boosting scheme. Although there is a lot of enthusiasm, one should keep in mind that standard therapy modalities such as chemotherapy needed decades before at least a few cancer entities could be cured.

ACKNOWLEDGEMENTS. The work would not have been possible without the contributions of Y. Sun, M. Gilliet, A Tunkyi, A. Musial, and the excellent assistance of A. Sucker, W. Eickelbaum, M. Vazansky, S. Manolio. Supported by grants from the Swiss Cancer League, the Zürich Cancer League and "Stiftung für wissenschaftliche Forschung der Universität Zürich" and DFG.

References

Abdel-Wahab Z et al. (1998) Human dendritic cells, pulsed with either melanoma tumor cell lysates or the gp100 peptide (280–288), induce pairs of T-cell cultures with similar phenotype and lyric activity. Cell Immunol 186: 63–74

Ahmann DL et al. (1989) Complete responses and long-term survivals after systemic chemotherapy for patients with advanced malignant melanoma. Cancer 63: 224–227

Alijagic S et al. (1995) Dendritic cells generated from peripheral blood transfected with human tyrosinase induce specific T cell activation. Eur J Immunol 25, 3100–3107

Banchereau J and Steinman RM (1998) Dendritic cells and the control of immunity. Nature 392: 245–252

Bell D et al. (1999) Dendritic cells. Adv Immunol 72: 255–324

Bennett SRM et al. (1997) Induction of a CD8+ cytotoxic T lymphocyte response by cross-priming requires cognate CD4+ help, J Exp Med 186, 65–70

Boel P., et al. (1995) BAGE: A new gene encoding an antigen recognized on human melanomas by cytolytic T lymphocytes. Immunity 2: 167–175

Brichard VG., et al. (1996) A tyrosinase nonapeptide presented by HLA-B44 is recognized on a human melanoma by autologous cytolytic T lymphocytes. Eur J Immunol 26: 224–230

Castelli C., et al. (1995) Mass spectrometric identification of a naturally processed melanoma peptide recognized by CD8 (+) cytotoxic T lymphocytes. J Exp Med 183: 363–368

Castelli C., et al. (1998) Immogenicity of the ALLAVGATK ($gp100^{17-25}$) peptide in HLA-A3.1 melanoma patients. Eur J Immunol 28: 1143–1154

Castelli C., et al. (1999) Novel HLA-Cw8-restricted T cell epitopes derived from tyrosinase-related protein-2 and gp100 melanoma antigens. J Immunol 162: 1739–1748

Cella M et al (1997) Inflammatory stimuli induce accumulation of MHC class II complexes dendritic cells. Nature 388: 782–783

Celluzzi C et al. (1996) Peptide-pulsed dendritic cells induce antigen-specific, CTL-mediated protective tumor immunity. J Exp Med 183, 283–287
Celluzzi CM and Falo LD (1998) Physical interaction between dendritic cells and tumor cells results in an immunogen that induces protective and therapeutic tumor rejection. J Immunol 160: 3081–3085
Chaux P., et al. (1999) Identification of five MAGE-A1 epitopes recognized by cytolytic T lymphocytes obtained by in vitro stimulation with dendritic cells transduced with MAGE-A1. J Immunol 163: 2928–2936
Chaux P., et al. (1999) Identification of MAGE-3 epitopes presented by HLA-DR molecules to CD(+) T lymphocytes. J Exp Med 189: 767–778
Chikamatsu K et al. (1999) Generation of anti-p53 cytotoxic T lymphocytes from human peripheral blood using autologous dendritic cells. Clin Cancer Res 5: 1281–1288
Coulie P.G, et al. (1995) A mutated intron sequence codes for an antigenic peptide recognized by cytolytic T lymphocytes on a human melanoma. Proc Natl Acad Sci USA 92: 7976–7980
Dagleish A (1996) The case for therapeutic vaccines. Melanoma Res 6: 5–10
Dhodapkar MV et al. (1999) Rapid generation of broad T cell immunity in humans after a single injection of mature dendritic cells. J Clin Invest 104: 173–180
Fernandez NC et al (1999) Dendritic cells directly trigger NK cell function: cross talk relevant in innate anti-tumor immune responses in vivo. Nature Med 5: 405–411
Flamand V et al. (1994) Murine dendritic cells pulsed in vitro with tumor antigen induce tumor resistance in vivo. Eur J Immunol 24, 605–610
Fujie T., et al. (1999) A MAGE-1-encoded HLA-A24-binding synthetic peptide induces specific anti-tumor cytotoxic T lymphocytes. Int J Cancer 80: 169–172
Garbe C. (1993) Chemotherapy and chemoimmunotherapy in disseminated malignant melanoma. Melanoma Res. 3: 291–299
Gaugler B., et al. (1994) Human gene Mage-3 codes for an antigen recognized on a melanoma by autologous cytolytic T lymphocytes. J Exp Med 179: 921–930
Gaugler B., et al. (1996) A new gene coding for an antigen recognized by autologous cytolytic T lymphocytes on a human renal carcinoma. Immunogenetics 44: 323–330
Grabbe S et al. (1995) Dendritic cells as initiators of tumor immune responses – a possible strategy for tumor immunotherapy ? Immunol Today 16, 117–121
Guilloux Y., et al. (1996) A peptide recognized by human cytolytic T lymphocytes on HLA-A2 melanomas is encoded by an intron sequence of the N-acetylglucosaminyltransferase V gene. J Exp Med 183: 1173–1183
Herman J., et al. (1996) A peptide encoded by the human MAGE3 gene and presented by HLA-B44 induces cytolytic T lymphocytes that recognize tumor cells expressing MAGE3. Immunogenetics 43: 377–383
Höltl L et al (1997) Cellular and humoral immune responses in patients with metastatic renal cell carcinoma after vaccination with antigen pulsed dendritic cells. J Urol 16: 777–782
Höltl L, et al. (1998) CD83+ blood dendritic cells as a vaccine for immunotherapy of metastatic renal-cell cancer. Lancet 352: 1358
Hsu et al. (1994) Vaccination of patients with B-cell lymphoma using autologous dendritic cells. Nat Med 2: 52–58
Ikeda H., et al. (1997) Characterization of an antigen that is recognized on a melanoma showing partial HLA loss by CTL expressing an NK inhibitory receptor. Immunity 6: 199–208
Jäger E., et al. (1998) Simultaneous humoral and cellular immune response against cancer-testis antigen NY-ESO-1: definition of human histocompatibility leukocyte antigen (HLA)-A2-binding peptide epitopes. J Exp Med 187: 265–270
Johnson TM et al. (1995) Current therapy for cutaneous melanoma. J Am Acad Dermatol 32: 689–707
Kang XQ, et al. (1995) Identification of a tyrosinase epitope recognized by HLA-A24-restricted tumor-infiltrating lymphocytes. J Immunol 155: 1343–1348

Kawakami Y., et al. (1994) Identification of a human melanoma antigen recognized by tumor-infiltrating lymphocytes associated with in vivo tumor rejection. Proc Natl Acad Sci USA 91: 6458–6462
Kawakami Y., et al. (1994) Identification of the immunodominant peptides of the MART-1 human melanoma antigen recognized by the majority of HLA-A2-restricted tumor infiltrating lymphocytes. J Exp Med 180: 347–352
Kawakami Y., et al. (1998) Identification of new melanoma epitopes on melanosomal proteins recognized by tumor infiltrating T lymphocytes restricted by HLA-A1, -A2 and -A3 alleles. J Immunol 161: 6985–6992
Kawakami, YS et al. (1994). Identification of a human melanoma antigen recognized by tumor-infiltrating lymphocytes associated with in vivo tumor rejection. Proc Natl Acad Sci USA 91: 6458–6462
Kawashima I., et al. (1998) Identification of gp100-derived, melanoma-specific cytotoxic T-lymphocyte epitopes restricted by HLA-A3 supertype molecules by primary in vitro immunization with peptide-pulsed dendritic cells. Int J Cancer 78: 518–524
Kittlesen DJ, et al. (1998) Human melanoma patients recognize an HLA-A1-restricted CTL epitope from tyrosinase containing two cysteine residues: implications for tumor vaccine development. J Immunol 160: 2099
Kobayashi H., et al. (1998) CD4+ T cells from peripheral blood of a melanoma patient recognize peptides derived from nonmutated tyrosinase. Cancer Res 58: 296–301
Lethe B., et al. (1998) LAGE-1, a new gene with tumor specificity. Int J Cancer 76: 903–908
Li K., et al. (1998) Tumour-specific MHC-class-II-restricted responses after in vitro sensitization to synthetic peptides corresponding to gp 100 and Annexin II eluted from melanoma cells. Cancer Immunol Immunother 47: 32–38
Lupetti R., et al. (1998) Translation of a retained intron in tyrosinase-related protein (TRP) 2 mRNA generates a new cytotoxic T lymphocyte (CTL)-defined and shared human melanoma antigen not expressed in normal cells of the melanocytic lineage. J Exp Med 188: 1005–1016
Mackensen A et al. (1994) Direct evidence to support the immunosurveillance concept in a human regressive melanoma. J Clin Invest 93: 1391–1402
Mackey MF et al. (1998) Dendritic cells require maturation via CD40 to generate protective antitumor immunity. J Immunol 161: 2094–2098
Manici S., et al. (1999) Melanoma cells present a MAGE-3 epitope to CD4(+) cytotoxic T cells in association with histocompatibility leukocyte antigen DR11. J Exp Med 189: 871–876
Mayordomo JI et al. (1995) Bone marrow-derived dendritic cells pulsed with synthetic tumor peptides elicit protective and therapeutic antitumor immunity. Nature Med 1, 1297–1302
Mayordomo JI et al. (1996) Therapy of murine tumors with p53 wild-type and mutant sequence peptide-based vaccines. J Exp Med 183, 1357–1365
Morse MA et al (1999a) A phase I study of active immunotherapy with carcinoembryonic antigen peptide (CAP-1)-pulsed, autologous human cultured dendritic cells in patients with metastatic malignancies expressing carcinoembryonic antigen. Clin Cancer Res 5: 1331–1338
Morse MA et al. (1999b) Migration of human dendritic cells after injection in patients with metastatic malignancies. Cancer Res 59: 56–58
Mulders P et al. (1999) Presentation of renal tumor antigens by human dendritic cells activates tumor-infiltrating lymphocytes against autologous tumor: implications for live kidney cancer vaccines. Clin Cancer Res 5: 445–454
Nestle FO et al. (1998) Vaccination of melanoma patients with peptide or tumor lysate pulsed dendritic cells. Nat. Med. 4: 328–332
Oettgen H. F., and Old L. J. (1991) The history of cancer immunotherapy. In deVita V. T., Hellman S., and Rosenberg S. A. eds. Biologic Therapy of Cancer, Principles and Practice. J. B. Lippincott pp 87 ff.
Paglia P et al. Murine dendritic cells loaded in vitro with soluble protein prime cytotoxic T lymphocytes against tumor antigen in vivo. J Exp Med 183; 317–3 22 (1996)

Parkhurst MR., et al. (1998) Identification of a shared HLA-A*0201-restricted T cell epitope from the melanoma antigen tyrosinase-related protein 2 (TRP2). Cancer Res 58: 4895–4901
Parkinson, DR, Houghton AN, Hersey P, and Borden EC. 1992. Biologic therapy for melanoma. In Cutaneous Melanoma Balch C.M., A.N. Houghton, G.W. Milton, A.J. Sober, and S.J. Soong. eds. JB Lippincott Co; Philadelphia, p. 522
Peters JH et al. (1996) Dendritic cells: from ontogenetic orphans to myelomonocytic descendants. Immunol Today 17, 273–278
Pieper R., et al. (1999) Biochemical identification of a mutated human melanoma antigen recognized by CD4(+) T cells. J Exp Med 189: 757–766
Porgador A et al. (1996) Induction of antitumor immunity using bone marrow-generated dendritic cells. J Immunol 156, 2918–2926
Randolph GJ et al. (1998) Differentiation of monocytes into dendritic cells in a model of transendothelial trafficking. Science 282: 480–483
Rissoan M-C et al. (1999) Reciprocal control of T helper cell and dendritic cell differentiation. Science 283: 1183–1186
Robbins PF et al. (1994) Recognition of tyrosinase by tumor-infiltrating lymphocytes from a patient responding to immunotherapy. Cancer Res 54: 3124–3126
Robbins PF, et al. (1994) Recognition of tyrosinase by tumor-infiltrating lymphocytes from a patient responding to immunotherapy. Cancer Res 54: 3124–3126
Robbins PF., et al. (1996) A mutated β-catenin gene encodes a melanoma-specific antigen recognized by tumor infiltrating lymphocytes. J Exp Med 183: 1185–1192
Robbins PF., et al. (1995) Cloning of a new gene encoding an antigen recognized by melanoma-specific HLA-A2-restricted tumor-infiltrating lymphocytes. J Immunol 154: 5944–5950
Romani N et al. Proliferating dendritic cell progenitors in human blood. J Exp Med 180, 83–93 (1994)
Romero P., et al. (1997) Cytolytic T lymphocyte recognition of the immunodominant HLA-A*0201-restricted Melan-A/MART-1 antigenic peptide in melanoma. J Immunol 159: 2366–2374
Salgaller ML et al. (1998) Dendritic cell-based immunotherapy of prostate cancer. Crit Rev Immunol 18: 109–119
Sallusto F. and Lanzavecchia A. (1994) Efficient presentation of soluble antigen by cultured human dendritic cells is maintained by granulocyte/macrophage colony-stimulating factor plus interleukin-4 and downregulated by tumor necrosis factor-alpha. J Exp Med 179, 1109–111
Schneider J., et al. (1998) Overlapping peptides of melanocytc differentiation antigen melan-A/MART-1 recognized by autologous cytolytic T lymphocytes in association with HLA-B45.1 and HLA-A2.1. Int J Cancer 75: 451–458
Schoell WM et al. (1999) Generation of tumor-specific cytotoxic T-lymphocytes by stimulation with HPV type 16 E7 peptide-pulsed dendritic cells. An approach to immunotherapy of cervical cancer. Gynecol Oncol 74: 448–455
Shimizu et al. (1999) Systemic administration of interleukin 2 enhances the therapeutic efficacy of dendritic cell-based tumor vaccines. Proc Natl Acad Sci USA 96: 2268–2273
Skipper JCA., et al. (1996) An HLA-A2-restricted tyrosinase antigen on melanoma cells results from posttranslational modification and suggests a novel pathway for processing of membrane proteins. J Exp Med 183: 527–534
Skipper JCA., et al. (1996) Shared epitopes for HLA-A3-restricted melanoma-reactive human CTL include a naturally processed epitope from Pmel-17/gp100. J Immunol 157: 5027–5033
Sozzani et al. (1998) Differential regulation of chemokine receptors during dendritic maturation: a model for their trafficking properties. J Immunol 161: 1083–1086
Storkus WP et al. (1993) Identification of T cell epitopes: rapid isolation of class I-presented peptides from viable cells by mild acid elution. J Immunother 14: 94–103
Sun Y. et al. (1999) Cell-based vaccination against melanoma – background, preliminary results, and perspective J Mol Med 77: 593–608
Tahara K., et al. (1999) Identification of a MAGE-2-encoded human leukocyte antigen-A24-binding synthetic peptide that induces specific antitumor cytotoxic T lymphocytes. Clin Cancer Res 5: 2236–2241

Takahashi T., et al. (1997) 707-AP peptide recognized by human antibody induces human leukocyte antigen A2-restricted cytotoxic T lymphocyte killing of melanoma. Clin Cancer Res 3: 1363–1370
Takahashi T., et al. (1997) Recognition of gp43 tumor-associated antigen peptide by both HLA-A2 restricted CTL lines and antibodies from melanoma patients. Cell Immunol 97: 162–171
Tanaka F., et al. (1997) Induction of antitumor cytotoxic T lymphocytes with a MAGE-3 encoded synthetic peptide presented by human leukocytes antigen-A24. Cancer Res 57: 4465
Thomas R et al. (1999) Immature human monocyte-derived dendritic cells migrate rapidly to draining lymph nodes after intradermal injection for melanoma immunotherapy. Melanoma Res 9: 474–481
Topalian S. L., et al. (1996) Melanoma-specific CD4+ T cells recognize nonmutated HLA-DR-restricted tyrosinase epitopes. J Immunol 183: 1965–1971
Tsai V., et al. (1997) Identification of subdominant CTL epitopes of the gp100 melanoma-associated tumor antigen by primary in vitro immunization with peptide-pulsed dendritic cells. Cell Immunol 158: 1796–1802
van den Bruggen P., et al. (1991) A gene encoding an antigen recognized by cytolytic T on a human melanoma. Science 254: 1643–1647
van den Bruggen P., et al. (1994) A peptide encoded by human gene MAGE-3 and presented by HLA-A2 induces cytolytic T lymphocytes that recognize tumor cells expressing MAGE-3. Eur J Immunol 24: 3038–3043
van den Bruggen P., et al. (1994) Autologous cytolytic T lymphocytes recognize a MAGE-1 nonapeptide on melanomas expressing HLA Cw*1601. Eur J Immunol 24: 2134–2140
Van den Eynden B., et al. (1995) A new family of genes coding for an antigen recognized by autologous cytolytic T lymphocytes on a human melanoma. J Epx Med 182: 689–698
Visseren M. J. W., et al. (1997) Identification of HLA-A*0201-restricted CTL epitopes encoded by the tumor-specific MAGE-2 Gene product. Int J Cancer 73: 125–130
Wang R.- F., et al. (1996) Identification of TRP-2 as a human tumor antigen recognized by cytotoxic T lymphocytes. J Exp Med 184: 2207–2216
Wang R.- F., et al. (1996) Utilization of an alternative open reading frame of a normal gene in generating a novel human cancer antigen. J Exp Med 183: 1131–1140
Wang R.- F., et al. (1998) A breast and melanoma-shared tumor antigen: T cell responses to antigenic peptides translated from different open reading frames. J Immunol 162: 3596–3605
Wang R.- F., et al.. (1998) Recognition of an antigenic peptide derived from tyrosinase-related protein-2 by CTL in the context of HLA-A31 and -A33. J Immunol 160: 890–897
Wang R.-F., et al. (1999a) Cloning genes encoding MHC class II-restricted antigens: mutated CDC27 as a tumor antigen. Science 284: 1351–1354
Wang R.-F., et al. (1999b) Identification of a novel MHC class II-restricted tumor antigen resulting from a chromosomal rearrangement recognized by CD4+ T cells. J Exp Med 189: 1659–1667
Wen Y-J et al (1998) Idiotypic protein-pulsed adherent peripheral blood monouclear cell-derived dendritic cells prime immune immune system in multiple myeloma. Clin Cancer Res 4: 957–962
Wölfel T et al. (1994) Two tyrosinase nonapeptides recognized on HLA-A2 melanomas by autologous cytolytic T lymphocytes. Eur J Immunol 24: 759–764
Wölfel T., et al. (1995) A $p16^{INK4a}$-insensitive CDK4 mutant targeted by cytolytic T lymphocytes in a human melanoma. Science 269: 1281–1284
Zitvogel L et al. (1996) Therapy of murine tumors with tumor peptide-pulsed dendritic cells: Dependence on T cells, B7 costimulation, and T helper cell 1-associated cytokines. J Exp Med 183, 87–97
Zorn E., Hercend T. (1999) A MAGE-6-encoded peptide is recognized by expanded lymphocytes infiltrating a spontaneously regressing human primary melanoma lesion. Eur J Immunol 29: 602–607
Zorn E., Hercend T. (1999) A natural anti-tumor cytotoxic T cell response in a spontaneously regressing human melanoma targets a neoantigen resulting from a somatic point mutation. Eur J Immunol 29: 592–601

A Novel Strategy in the Elimination of Disseminated Melanoma Cells: Chimeric Receptors Endow T Cells with Tumor Specificity

H. Abken[1], A. Hombach[1], C. Heuser[1], and U. Reinhold[2]

[1] Labor für Tumorgenetik, Klinik I für Innere Medizin, Universität zu Köln, 50924 Cologne, Germany
[2] Universitätshautklinik, Universitätskliniken des Saarlandes, 66421 Homburg/Saar, Germany

Abstract

The application of immunotherapy to the treatment of micrometastases of melanoma has attracted growing interest in recent years. This trend reflects, at least in part, the disappointing results of conventional chemotherapy, the identification of melanoma-associated antigens suitable to be used as targets for immunotherapy, and the significant progress in our understanding of molecular processes involved in the development of an immune response. Because of the general belief that T cell immunity plays a major part in the control of tumor growth, we have recently applied a novel strategy to target cytolytic T cells to melanoma cells. The strategy bypasses the requirement of presentation of melanoma-associated-antigen-derived peptides by the major histocompatibility complex to the T cell receptor complex by permanent grafting of T cells with a recombinant, chimeric T cell receptor. The extracellular moiety of the grafted receptor contains the antigen-binding domain, consisting of a single-chain antibody fragment (scFv) derived from a monoclonal antibody specific for the high-molecular-weight melanoma-associated antigen (HMW-MAA). The intracellular receptor moiety contains the cellular activation domain, consisting of the γ-signaling chain derived from the FcεRI receptor. Cytotoxic T cells grafted with the chimeric anti-HMW-MAA scFv-γ signaling receptor specifically lyse HMW-MAA-positive melanoma cells in a human leukocyte antigen class I-independent fashion. The chimeric T cell receptor strategy is designed to eliminate disseminated tumor cells by the power of cytolytic T cells that physiologically penetrate tissues and that are specifically activated by the grafted receptor after binding to antigen-positive melanoma cells.

Recent Results in Cancer Research, Vol. 158

Micrometastasis: The Need To Eliminate Disseminated Melanoma Cells Beyond the Blood Stream

The clinical course of patients with melanoma indirectly indicates that systemic metastases of melanoma cells may occur even in early stages of the disease. A panel of different physical methods have been applied to monitor metastasis of melanoma. The modalities, although informative, do not detect micrometastases that pose a major risk for relapse of the disease. Based on the assumption that a growing tumor sheds viable cells into the blood circulation, it has been suggested that circulating melanoma cells in the peripheral blood may function as a sensitive and prognostic tumor marker (Smith et al. 1991). The analysis of tyrosinase-specific mRNA in blood samples of melanoma patients by RT-PCR, although capable of detecting a single melanoma cell in a blood sample, turned out to be of limited impact for the early diagnosis of metastatic tumor progression (Reinhold et al. 1997). In this analysis, we did not detect tyrosinase mRNA in blood samples of patients with primary melanoma, not even in patients with regional lymph node metastases. In 5/13 patients with visceral metastases, we found at least one blood sample positive for tyrosinase mRNA during a 2- to 4-month interval. Analyses of different blood samples of patients with visceral metastases taken in 2-h intervals indicate that tumor cells are only transiently present in the peripheral blood. Viable melanoma cells indeed circulate in the peripheral blood with retained proliferative capacity in vitro, as demonstrated by successful outgrowth of melanoma cells from blood samples derived from different patients with visceral melanoma metastases (Reinhold et al. 1997) and from bone marrow (Joshi et al. 1987). From the view of therapeutic strategies of metastatic melanoma, this scenario indicates the requirement of elimination of micrometastases during early stages of the disease irrespective of melanoma cells that are detected in the peripheral blood.

Prophylactive lymph node dissections have revealed occult and clinically undetectable metastases (micrometastases) in patients with various types of solid tumors, including cutaneous melanoma (Crowley and Seigler 1992). Micrometastases probably account for disease-free intervals of variable length and may account for the failure of the wide surgical resection margins and elective lymph node dissection to influence prognosis of metastatic melanoma (Piepkorn and Barnhill 1996; Piepkorn et al. 1997). Micrometastases that have not acquired properties required for progressive tumor growth are suggested to be the cellular pool of melanoma cells giving rise to a clinical relapse of the disease. The concept of "dormant" cells in micrometastases was hypothesized to explain why solid tumors may develop metastases after disease-free intervals as long as 10–40 years after resection of the primary tumor. The immunological and/or cellular mechanisms that keep metastatic melanoma cells in a dormant state or facilitate escape therefrom are still unknown. It has been observed that the subsequent survival of patients with melanoma is largely unrelated to disease-free intervals; i.e., once melanoma recurs, the subsequent prognosis is fairly predictable, irrespective of the antecedent disease-free interval. The failure of wide surgical margins and elective lymph node dissection to clearly influence prognosis also supports the idea of occult metastases in other anatomic locations.

Micrometastases of melanoma were recently found to lack significant tumor vascularity and to have low cellular proliferative and programmed cell death rates (Barnhill et al. 1998). These characteristics may explain the dormant state of the malignant cell population and account for their being viable for long periods of time without progressive growth. The observations, on the other hand, suggest that micrometastases may not have acquired properties needed for progressive tumor growth, e.g., vascularization, as have macrometastases with significantly greater rates of proliferation than cell death, consistent with progressive tumor growth.

Taken together, the following biological characteristics account for the need of therapeutic strategies to eliminate micrometastases of melanoma:

1. Micrometastases of melanoma cells are strongly implied to be the source of a clinical relapse even after long periods of time.
2. Micrometastases are poorly or not vascularized.
3. Micrometastases have a low but balanced rate of cellular proliferation and programmed death.

Melanoma is considered to be a chemotherapy-refractory tumor with a high degree of resistance against a variety of cytostatic agents (Schadendorf et al. 1994) potentially due to intrinsic cellular resistance mechanisms in the apoptosis pathways (Serrone and Hersey 1999). Accordingly, commonly used anticancer drugs do not seem to influence favorably the prognosis of metastatic melanoma (Guerry and Schuchter 1992). The particular biology of melanoma, on the other hand, leads to the general belief that T cell immunity plays a major part in the control of the melanoma lesion. The understanding of processes of immune surveillance and the escape of melanoma cells therefrom will open novel strategies in the treatment of melanoma micrometastases, as discussed below.

The Immune Surveillance at Work to Force Back Melanoma

Melanoma cells elicit a potent immunological response that, although rarely, succeeds in "spontaneous" tumor regression and elimination of melanoma cells. Cytolytic T lymphocyte (CTL) clones with specificity for autologous tumor cells can successfully be isolated from peripheral blood samples or melanoma lesions, i.e., tumor-infiltrating lymphocytes (TIL), and maintained in culture (Boon et al. 1994). Melanoma-specific CTLs recognize tumor-associated antigens (TAA), and the increasing number of melanoma TAA identified so far can be grouped according to their expression pattern.

Melanoma are Associated Antigens

1. Encoded by genes that are silent in most normal tissues but activated in different types of tumors ("activation antigens"), e.g., MAGE proteins
2. Encoded by genes that are expressed only in melanocytes and melanomas ("differentiation antigens"), e.g., tyrosinase, Melan A/MART-1, gp100/ Pmel17, gp75/TRP-1
3. Encoded by mutated genes, some of them suggested to be involved in oncogenesis ("mutated antigens"), e.g., MUM-1, cdk4
4. Encoded by nonmutated genes expressed in normal tissues but overexpressed in many tumors ("overexpressed antigens"), e.g., HER2/neu
5. Encoded by viral genes ("viral antigens"), e.g., HPV.

While it is becoming increasingly clear that most, if not all, human tumors carry TAA, questions remain as to why the immune system is obviously not capable of eliminating the antigenic melanoma cells. Explanations proposed pertain either to an absence of stimulation of the immune system, e.g., tolerance, ignorance, no access of lymphocytes to the tumor cells, presence of suppressive soluble factors, or to tumor cells escaping immune attack, e.g., by loss of antigen expression or Fas-mediated killing of T cells. Although the relationships between tumor cells and the immune system display great diversity, it becomes more and more apparent that melanoma cells escape immune surveillance by down-regulation of their target epitopes for CTLs, particularly by shutting down the MHC I presentation pathway (Maeurer et al. 1996; Seliger et al. 1997). Longitudinal analyses of anti-tumor immune responses in a very few patients who enjoy a favorable clinical course despite recurrent metastases revealed strong CTL responses against melanoma cell antigens presented by various HLA class I molecules, whereas subsequent metastases resisted CTL-mediated lysis by loss of expression of most HLA class I molecules (Coulie et al. 1999). Circulating T cells with specificity for MART-1 or tyrosinase, recently identified in patients with metastatic melanoma, were found to be of two phenotypically distinct types, one typical for memory/effector T cells, the other expressing both naive and effector cell markers (Lee et al. 1999). The paradox of TAA-specific T cells in melanoma patients raises the question what part these T cells play in vivo, as they exist in patients with metastatic disease, and thus have not successfully induced tumor regression. This question has been partially resolved, as the naive effector T cell population was found to be functionally unresponsive, unable to directly lyse melanoma cells or to produce cytokines in response to mitogens. This implies that the clonally expanded, TAA-specific T cell population seems to have been selectively rendered anergic in vivo. Although TAA-specific T cell responses can develop de novo in cancer patients, antigen-specific unresponsiveness may explain why such cells are unable to control tumor growth (Lee et al. 1999).

These findings have profound implications for melanoma immunotherapy. The heterogeneity of T cell responses in different patients, i.e., some have T cells specific for TAA and some do not, may be important in stratifying patients into different treatment groups. Studies have shown increases in precursor frequencies of TAA-specific CTLs after vaccination, without evidence of clinical regression in some patients (Yee et al. 1997; Maio and Parmiani, 1996; Maeurer et al. 1996). One possible explanation for this discordance is that TAA-specific T cells may be selectively rendered anergic in vivo (Lee et al. 1999). This indicates the requirement for strategies to prevent such cells from becoming anergized in vivo.

Immunotherapeutic Strategies for the Treatment of Melanoma

Most immunotherapeutic strategies are based on the concept of targeting TAA with monoclonal antibodies to elicit an anti-tumor effect:

1. Anti-tumor antibodies as vehicles to deliver cytotoxic substances, such as radionuclides, chemotherapeutic drugs, or toxins, to the tumor cell
2. Anti-tumor antibodies used as activators of complement-dependent cellular cytotoxicity and as attractants of phagocytic cells for antibody-dependent cellular cytotoxicity directed against the tumor cell
3. Anti-idiotypic antibodies mimicking the antigenic determinant of the tumor cell antigen and resulting in production of tumor-specific antibodies.

While intralesional injection with an human monoclonal antibody to ganglioside GD2 induced regression of cutaneous metastatic melanoma (Irie and Morton 1986), interest was focused on combinations of antibody- and cell-based immunotherapeutic strategies to amplify the efficacy of anti-tumor responses observed with monoclonal antibodies alone. The benefit of additional use of immunomodulatory agents, particularly cytokines, became obvious in clinical trials based on the rationale of increasing cellular and anti-idiotypic immune responses by locally accumulated pro-inflammatory cytokines (Bajorin et al. 1990). Interleukin-2 (IL-2), alone and in combination with TIL, demonstrated anti-tumor activity in patients with melanoma (Rosenberg et al. 1988, 1994). Systemic administration of IL-2 in pharmacological doses, however, was frequently accompanied by suboptimal levels in the tumor microenvironment and high concentrations at sites distant from the tumor, resulting in potentially life-threatening side effects.

This problem was partially overcome by the antibody-directed delivery of immunomodulators, i.e., by antibody-cytokine fusion proteins that achieve both high cytokine concentrations in the tumor microenvironment and effective stimulation of the cellular immune response. The effectiveness of an antibody-IL-2 immunocytokine on disseminated pulmonary and skin metastases of melanoma was demonstrated in a classical mouse melanoma model (Becker et al. 1996a, b). The effects of T cell growth factors on T cell responses to melanoma cells in vitro, however, remain contradictory (Nguyen et al. 1997).

The identification of antigens recognized by cytolytic T cells that mediate rejection responses (Boon, 1992) has attracted interest in immunotherapeutic strategies for elimination of tumor cells, particularly as CTL clones with specificity for autologous melanoma cells can be derived from the peripheral blood or TIL of melanoma patients (Boon et al. 1994). The adoptive immunotherapy for melanoma makes use of TIL that physiologically penetrate tissues and migrate to the tumor site, where they are specifically activated to express their cytolytic activities. The success of this approach, however, was limited, mostly due to the difficulty in obtaining sufficient amounts of specific CTLs. Therefore, considerable attention has been given to combining the generation of large amounts of tumor-specific CTLs with the generation of CTLs with specificity for the particular tumor. The latter strategy, tumor-specific T cell targeting, is limited by the variety of TAA defined by monoclonal antibodies that can be effectively used to target tumor cells. Bispecific antibodies with dual specificity for the tumor cell and the effector cell combine the effector function of CTLs with the antigen specificity of antibodies. The inefficient penetration of antibodies into solid tumors and the rapid dissociation from the cell surface, however, limit their therapeutic use. This situation, particularly in view of the requirement to eliminate disseminated micrometastases of melanoma, has attracted interests in a T-cell-based, antibody-mediated immunotherapy.

Strategies were recently developed that combine the cellular activation potential of the T cell receptor (TCR) complex and the effector function of CTLs with the antigen specificity and MHC independence of monoclonal antibodies in order to target and activate T cells by binding to antigen in a MHC-independent fashion. This is achieved by modifying the TCR itself or by grafting T cells with a recombinant, chimeric receptor (review: Abken et al. 1997, 1998). The approaches are based on endowing autologous T cells with a TCR that is composed of both an extracellular binding domain with specificity for a TAA and an intracellular signaling domain for cellular activation. The strategy makes use of the autologous cellular defense system, the antibody-like and MHC-independent interaction of the effector cell with the target cell, and the self-limitation of the immune response in the absence of antigen. The concept is currently being evaluated in the framework of combined immuno- and gene therapy of melanoma with respect to its potential in eliminating residual, disseminated melanoma cells in micrometastases.

The Chimeric T Cell Receptor Design

The chimeric TCR strategy combines the effector function of CTLs with the antigen-binding specificity of antibodies (Fig. 1). The strategy is based on permanent grafting of immunological effector cells with a chimeric receptor molecule that mediates specific binding to a TAA. Upon antigen-mediated cross-linking, the intracellular signaling domain of the receptor initiates cellular activation, resulting in specific cytolysis of the antigen-positive tumor cell. Cellular activation, moreover, results in limited cell division and expansion of receptor-grafted cells that amplify the immune defense towards the

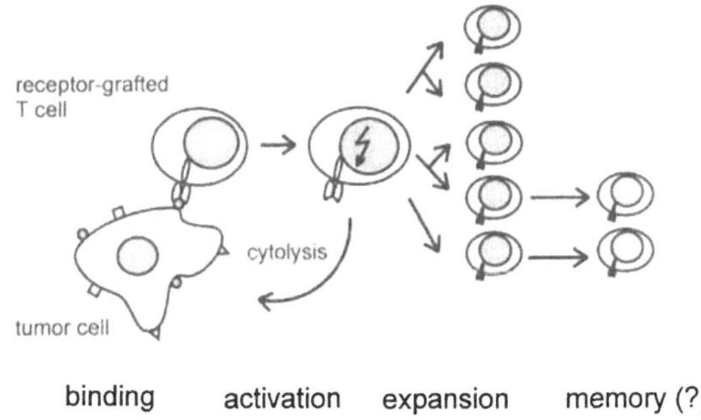

Fig. 1. The chimeric T cell receptor strategy. T cells are grafted with a recombinant T cell receptor that consists of an extracellular binding domain with specificity for a melanoma-associated antigen and an intracellular activation domain. After binding to melanoma-associated antigen and after antigen-mediated cross-linking of the receptor, the T cell is activated to both specific lysis of the melanoma cell and limited cell expansion. It still remains a matter of speculation whether receptor-grafted T cells convert to long-living memory cells that can be re-activated after binding to antigen

tumor cells until no cell-bound antigen remains available for sustaining cellular activation. In this situation, the cell enters apoptosis, thereby limiting the immune reaction. It is a matter of speculation whether memory cells with antigen specificity are generated during expansion of responsive cells.

The molecular design of the chimeric TCR is based on the similarity of the primary structure and on the spatial conformation of the variable regions of immunoglobulin (Ig) and TCR molecules. Both Ig and TCR harbor homology units, each of approximately 110 amino acids, folded into a typical Ig V-like domain that can pair with another related domain to form a functional unit. The modular properties of Ig and TCR enable the construction of functionally active, chimeric Ig-TCR molecules.

Modification of the TCR itself includes grafting of the VH and VL regions of an antibody to the TCR α- and β-chains, respectively, resulting in functional expression of chimeric TCRs with MHC-unrestricted target cell recognition (Goverman et al. 1990). This strategy, however, requires grafting of T cells with two modified TCR chains. To overcome this limitation, Eshhar et al. (1993) made use of the single-chain fragment of variable regions (scFv) to create an antigen-binding domain consisting of one polypeptide chain. The scFv is derived from an antibody molecule by genetically joining the VH and VL Ig regions via a flexible peptide linker, resulting in a continuous polypeptide chain of the VH-linker-VL or VL-linker-VH type. The antigen-binding domain constitutes the extracellular moiety of the chimeric receptor, which is combined with the transmembrane and intracellular moieties within one receptor molecule. The intracellular moiety harbors a signaling domain preferentially derived from the CD3 ζ-chain of the TCR/CD3 complex or, alternatively, derived from the highly homologous γ-chain of the high affinity IgE Fc receptor (FcεRI; Fig. 2). Taken together, at least three prerequisites enable the design of chimeric receptors that exhibit both antibody-like specificity and cellular activation capacity:

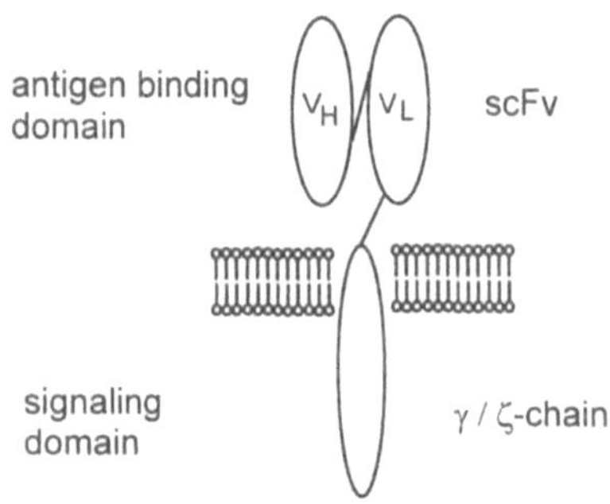

Fig. 2. Design of the chimeric T cell receptor. The chimeric receptor is composed of an extracellular moiety that harbors the antigen-binding domain and an intracellular moiety with the signaling domain. The antigen-binding domain consists of a single-chain fragment of variable regions (*scFv*) derived from an immunoglobulin (*Ig*) by joining the variable region of the Ig heavy chain (*VH*) to the variable region of the Ig light chain (*VL*) via a short flexible linker. The scFv domain is grafted to a transmembrane and cytoplasmic unit with signaling properties, e.g., the γ-chain of the FcεRI receptor or the ζ-chain of the TCR/CD3 complex

1. An antigen binding domain with specificity for a membrane-bound antigen
2. Antigen-driven, receptor-mediated cellular activation
3. Stable expression of the receptor on the surface of immunological competent effector cells.

More recently, a panel of chimeric receptors has been constructed with binding domains recognizing human TAAs. They include ErbB2 (Stancovski et al. 1993; Moritz et al. 1994), 38-kDa-folate-binding protein (Hwu et al. 1993), G250 (Weijtens et al. 1996), CD30 (Hombach et al. 1998a), TAG72 (Hombach et al. 1997), membrane-bound CEA (Hombach et al. 1999), and CD44v6 splice variants (Hekele et al. 1996). Effector cells transfected with the respective chimeric receptor have been shown to acquire the ability to lyse TAA-positive tumor cells in a MHC-unrestricted fashion (review: Abken et al. 1998). Recently, an anti-melanoma chimeric receptor was constructed in our laboratory and shown to be effective in mediating cytolysis melanoma cells in vitro (Reinhold et al. 1999).

The Anti-Melanoma Chimeric T Cell Receptor

We constructed a recombinant TCR displaying both binding specificity for the high-molecular-weight-melanoma-associated antigen (HMW-MAA) and cellular activation after receptor cross-linking (Reinhold et al. 1999). The extracellular antigen-binding domain consists of a scFv derived from an HMW-MAA-specific monoclonal antibody, 763.74. The scFv was generated and enriched by phage display techniques. To facilitate enrichment by panning of recombinant phages that express scFv with specificity to membrane-bound antigens, we used anti-idiotypic monoclonal antibodies instead of isolated antigen (Hombach et al. 1998b). By this procedure, we derived a scFv from the parental monoclonal antibody (mAb) 763.74 with specificity to the HMW-MAA (Reinhold et al. 1999). The scFv 763.74 has retained binding specificity, as it displays specific reactivity in ELISA with a protein extract from HMW-MAA-positive melanoma cells, stains specifically antigen-positive melanoma cells, and is competed by the parental mAb in binding to melanoma cells.

The HMW-MAA-specific binding domain scFv 763.74 was fused to the transmembrane and signaling domains of the FcεRI γ-chain (Fig. 2), resulting in a membrane molecule with an extracellular HMW-MAA binding domain and a intracellular γ-chain signaling domain. MD45 T cells were grafted with the receptor molecule by transfection of the DNA expression construct coding for the receptor. To monitor expression of the chimeric receptor early after transduction, we made use of anti-idiotypic antibodies directed to the antigen-binding domain of the receptor. Furthermore, anti-idiotypic antibodies are found to be suitable for enrichment of receptor-expressing cells after DNA transfection by cell-sorting procedures, particularly magnetic cell sorting. This methodology, however, is limited to a small number of scFv fragments for which an anti-idiotypic antibody or recombinant antigen is available. To make the procedure applicable to a variety of chimeric receptors with different binding domains, we developed a more versatile receptor design by inserting the immunoglobulin IgG1 CH2CH3 domains into the extracellular moiety, between the scFv and the transmembrane domain, of the receptor (Hombach et al. 1999).

Melanoma-Specific T Cell Activation

The anti-HMW-MAA-γ chain receptor grafted on T cells specifically mediates cellular activation, indicated by increased IL-2 secretion, after receptor cross-linking by binding to immobilized or membrane-bound antigen. This was shown by incubation of MD45 T cells grafted with the chimeric receptor (a) on indirectly immobilized HMW-MAA antigen, (b) on immobilized anti-idiotypic antibody directed to the antigen-binding domain of the receptor, and (c) co-incubation with HMW-MAA-positive melanoma cells. It is noteworthy that soluble anti-idiotypic mAb did not stimulate IL-2 secretion by transfected MD45 cells.

Anti-HMW-MAA-receptor-grafted MD45 cells lyse HMW-MAA-positive SK-Mel-5 melanoma cells (Fig. 3), whereas parental MD45 cells do not. Cytolysis is specific because HMW-MAA-negative A375 melanoma cells are not lysed by receptor-grafted MD45 cells. The extent of lysis of HMW-MAA-positive melanoma cells by receptor-grafted MD45 cells is at most 10%. Pre-activation of receptor-grafted MD45 cells by incubation on immobilized anti-idiotypic antibody, however, displayed a marked increase in their ability to lyse SK-Mel-5 cells. The specific cytotoxicity increased up to 25% by increasing the concentration of the anti-idiotypic mAb used for prestimulation. The enhancing effect is specific, as pre-incubation of receptor-grafted cells with an unrelated idiotypic mAb was ineffective in increasing their cytolytic activ-

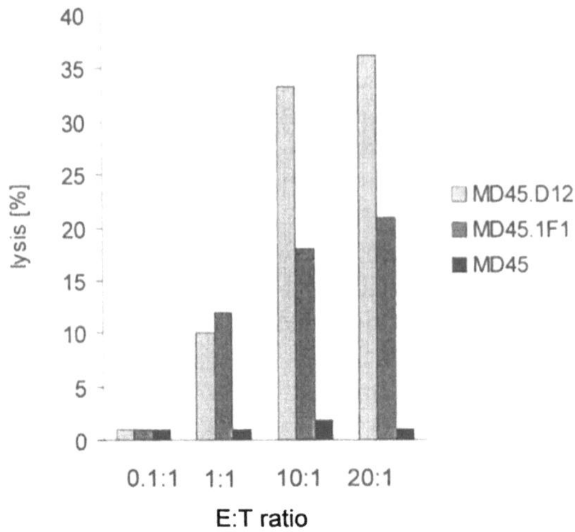

Fig. 3. Specific lysis of melanoma cells by MD45 T cells grafted with the anti-HMW-MAA chimeric receptor. MD45 T cells were transfected with the expression cassette coding for the anti-HMW-MAA-γ chain receptor. Two cell clones with stable expression of nearly similar amounts of receptor molecules on the cell surface were isolated (clone D12, clone 1F1). Receptor-grafted MD45 cells and, as control untransfected MD45 cells, were incubated on immobilized anti-idiotypic monoclonal antibody (mAb) MK2-23 for 48 h, harvested, and cocultured for 16 h with ^{51}Cr-labeled HMW-MAA^{+}Sk-Mel-5 melanoma cells (5×10^{3} cells per well) at the indicated effector:target (*E:T*) cell ratios. Lysis of melanoma cells was determined by standard ^{51}Cr release assay. Data represent the mean specific cytotoxicity of the transfected D12 and 1F1 cell clones and of the parental MD45 cells towards Sk-Mel-5 cells. HMW-MAA-negative A375 melanoma cells are not lysed by receptor-grafted MD45 cells, not even at E:T ratios of 20:1 (not shown)

ity. Untransfected, parental MD45 cells did not acquire the ability to lyse melanoma cells after pre-incubation with the anti-idiotypic mAb. According to the observation that cross-linking of the Fc receptor subunit is required to trigger its signaling pathway (Wirthmüller et al. 1992), enhancing the specific cytolytic activity of receptor-grafted MD45 cells requires immobilization of anti-idiotypic mAb, whereas soluble anti-idiotypic mAb has no effect. The enhancing effect of immobilized anti-idiotypic mAb is nearly similar to that of immobilized HMW-MAA. The use of immobilized anti-idiotypic mAb to enhance the cytotoxic activity of grafted CTLs appears to be preferable to that of immobilized antigen, as monoclonal antibodies can be well standardized and easily prepared in large amounts. An additional advantage of anti-idiotypic mAbs is their potential use in combination with a cross-linking agent for in vitro stimulation of transfected CTLs.

Prestimulation of receptor-grafted cells is dependent on the degree of receptor cross-linking, as the enhancement of cytotoxicity by anti-idiotypic mAb is concentration-dependent, and incubation with Colo38 melanoma cells that express HMW-MAA in low amounts had no detectable effect on increasing the cytolytic activity of receptor-grafted cells. Obviously, the level of HMW-MAA expression on Colo38 cells does not reach the minimum required to trigger significant activation of the receptor signaling pathway.

The analysis points out that the cytolytic activity of receptor-grafted MD45 T cells can markedly be increased following in vitro incubation with immobilized HMW-MAA antigen or an anti-idiotypic antibody which recognizes the idiotope expressed on the HMW-MAA-binding scFv domain of the chimeric receptor.

Residual Disseminated Melanoma Cells: A Chance for T-Cell-Based Immunotherapy?

Immunotherapeutic strategies for the elimination of disseminated melanoma have to take into account the biological characteristics of micrometastases, i.e., dormant melanoma cells that can be reactivated to initiate aggressive metastases and clinical relapse even after long periods of time, poorly or not vascularized micrometastases and the low but balanced rate of cellular proliferation and programmed death.

The attractiveness of the recently developed approach for targeted immunotherapy is based on permanently endowing immunocompetent effector cells with chimeric receptors for specific targeting and activation, thus combining the antigen-binding specificity and MHC independence of an antibody with the cytolytic activity of activated effector cells. In vitro results obtained with established melanoma cells indicate the effectiveness of the strategy. The in vivo application of the treatment of melanoma micrometastases takes advantage of effector cells that are expected to have the potential to penetrate tissues beyond the blood stream, thereby targeting micrometastases that are not vascularized. It remains unresolved, however, whether transduced, receptor-grafted effector cells still have retained their homing capabilities after genetic manipulation and propagation in vitro. The crucial question in the treatment of micrometastasis is whether receptor-grafted effector cells indeed accumulate and penetrate micrometastasis of melanoma after systemic administration. Specific penetration of receptor-grafted cells to the tumor, however, is basically fulfilled by the strategy, because, in the case of ovarian carcinoma, tumor-specific chimeric receptors were shown to drive T cells to accumulate at the tumor site in vivo (Hwu et al. 1995).

The chimeric receptor strategy, moreover, makes use of effector cells that are able to recycle lytic capacity, to expand by cell division after activation, and to enter apoptosis when no sufficient restimulation by antigen has occurred, thus limiting the immune response. Even if the cytolytic capacity of grafted T cells may still be low, this potential limitation in the application of chimeric TCRs may be overcome by taking advantage of the marked enhancement of the cytotoxic activity of grafted CTLs by cross-linked anti-idiotypic antibodies. Most importantly, receptor-grafted CTL can recycle their receptor-triggered lytic acticity, namely one CTL enters into multiple lytic cycles with the target cells as assessed in vitro (Weijtens et al. 1996). Once activated, T cells are expected to induce a second wave of local inflammatory response by secretion of proinflammatory cytokines, potentially resulting in a systemic immune response effective against distant and antigen-negative metastases.

TAA, frequently found in high concentrations in serum of cancer patients, may block the TAA-binding domain of the receptor thus avoiding binding of the receptor-grafted T cell to the tumor cell. In the situation of melanoma, serum concentrations of HMW-MAA are usually low and do not inhibit the localization of radiolabeled anti-HMW-MAA mAb in melanoma lesions (Ferrone et al. 1988). We therefore do not expect efficient blocking of the chimeric receptor by such low concentrations of soluble HMW-MAA present in sera of melanoma patients.

Conclusions and Future Perspectives

Numerous clinical attempts to recruit the cellular arm of the immune system for adoptive anti-tumor immunotherapy have not fulfilled expectations. The question remains whether the chimeric receptor strategy will be effective in vivo in counteracting the mechanisms used by tumor cells to escape from immune destruction.

One of the major hurdles of antibody-directed immunotherapeutic strategies is the heterogeneity of antigen expression within the malignancy, because the antigenic heterogeneity of melanoma cell populations negatively affects the efficacy of the immunotherapeutic approach. HMW-MAA fulfills this criterion with respect to nearly homogeneous expression in the melanoma lesion. Whereas HMW-MAA-positive melanoma cells may be successfully eliminated by specific CTLs, antigen-negative tumor cells, will not be recognized by the grafted receptor. This potential limitation might be overcome by utilizing mixed populations of effector cells transfected with chimeric receptors recognizing different TAAs of the same tumor. On the other hand, activation of immunological effector cells at the tumor site led to the speculation whether IL-2, secreted in high concentrations by grafted, activated T cells into the tumor microenvironment, may be effective in attraction of a second wave of nonspecific inflammatory cells, thus locally enhancing the anti-tumor effect and eradicating antigen-negative tumor cells. Experiments with antibody-cytokine fusion proteins teach us that, in an animal model, antigen-negative melanoma cells are indeed eliminated when co-inoculated with antigen-positive melanoma cells and that the T cell-mediated immune response is followed by a long-lived, transferable protective immunity (Becker et al. 1996b).

A beneficial effector cell:target cell ratio at the tumor site is likely to be required for efficient target cell lysis. As an estimation based on clinical data, however, is not yet available, we assume that systemic application of about 10^8 transduced cells is likely to be necessary for efficient elimination of residual tumor cells in vivo. This situation requires a prolonged lymphocyte expansion in vitro prior to application in vivo, a high proportion of lymphocytes effectively transduced, and stable expression of the receptor on the cell surface.

One of the major potentials of the chimeric receptor strategy lies in the modular composition of the receptor molecule that combines the antigen-binding domain with different signaling domains required for the particular effector cell, e.g., CTLs, NK cells, or basophilic granulocytes. It is still open whether other types of effector cells, e.g., NK cells or macrophages, may be more effective than CTLs or may act synergistically when administered together with receptor grafted CTLs.

Several questions still have to be answered to adopt the strategy for clinical use in elimination of residual tumor cells:

1. How can trafficking and homing of the cells to the tumor site be significantly increased?
2. How can specific activation of the receptor-grafted T cells be modulated?
3. Cells of tumor-bearing patients have been reported to have abnormalities in their TCR signal-transducing machinery (Levey and Srivastava 1996). Although chimeric receptors bypass the endogenous TCR signaling, it is unresolved whether potential downstream defects in the signaling cascade impair signal transduction triggered by the signaling domain of the chimeric receptor.
4. Does cytokine secretion of activated receptor-grafted cells induce an immune response of nontransduced bystander immune cells to those tumor cells that lack the particular target antigen?
5. Is the chimeric receptor molecule immunogenic and how can the risk of immunogenicity be minimized? Is a binding domain with a humanized scFv less immunogenic than a murine scFv?
6. What are the optimal time and dose schedules for administration of transduced T cells? Will large-scale, long-term propagation of transduced cells prior to administration be necessary, or can the propagation period be reduced to a minimal short-term culture? Will their repeated administrations induce anti-idiotypic antibodies to melanoma-associated antigens? If so, will anti-idiotypic antibodies activate CTLs by costimulation or will they inhibit activation and homing of transduced T cells to malignant lesions? In vitro experiments suggest the two conflicting possibilities: addition of anti-idiotypic antibodies to mixtures of grafted CTLs and target cells inhibits lysis of target cells, but cross-linking of the receptor by immobilized anti-idiotypic antibodies enhances their lytic activity (Reinhold et al. 1999).
7. How can blocking of the antigen-binding domain of the receptor by soluble TAA, frequently found in high titers in sera of tumor patients, be avoided? A binding domain of the receptor with improved discrimination between cell-bound and soluble forms of TAA will be required, as recently demonstrated for CEA-positive tumors (Hombach et al. 1999). Because the antigen-binding domain is not limited to antibody-derived domains, other recognition domains, e.g., antigen-ligand domains, might fulfill this requirement more effectively.
8. Upon complete elimination of residual, antigen-positive tumor cells, most of the effector cells will die by apoptosis. Do some effector cells differenti-

ate further into memory cells, allowing surveillance and prevention of relapse of disease?

The T cell-based receptor strategy is not a simple modus operandi, since its application is limited by being individualized and patient-specific. Problems may arise with the clinical situation of the individual patient. Particularly, patients subjected to immunotherapeutic strategies are frequently pretreated by standard chemotherapy protocols that are known to exert immune-suppressive side effects and to adversely affect the T cell-dependent immune system. Consequently, immunotherapeutic approaches that rely exclusively on the induction and/or redirection of cytotoxic T cell responses are of limited value in clinical situations accompanied by immunosuppression.

Taken together, the stable genetic modification of immunocompetent effector cells harbors the potential to extend the current scope of adoptive cellular immunotherapy of minimal residual disease by combining MHC-independent tumor cell recognition with the cytolytic activity of effector cells. Although questions remain, clinical trials likely to be implemented in the near future will determine the feasibility of the strategy in counteracting the escape of tumor cells from immune surveillance.

ACKNOWLEDGEMENTS. We are grateful to Drs. Z. Eshhar (Weizman Institute of Science, Rehovot), S. Ferrone (Roswell Park Cancer Institute, Buffalo), R.L. Bolhuis (Daniel den Hoed Cancer Center, Rotterdam) for stimulating discussions and sharing materials. Work in the author's (H.A.) laboratories is supported by grants from the Deutsche Krebshilfe, the Deutsche Forschungsgemeinschaft through SFB502, and the Fortune Program of the University of Cologne.

References

Abken H, Hombach A, Reinhold U, Ferrone S (1998) Can combined T-cell- and antibody-based immunotherapy outsmart tumor cells? Immunol Today 19: 2–5

Bajorin DF, Chapman PB, Wong G, Coit DG, Kunicka J, Dimaggio J, Cordon-Cardo C, Urmacher C, Dantes L, Templeton MA, Liu J, Oettgen HF, Houghton AN (1990) Phase I evaluation of a combination of monoclonal antibody R24 and interleukin-2 in patients with metastatic melanoma. Cancer Res 50: 7490–7495

Barnhill RL, Piepkorn MW, Alistair JC, Flynn E, Karaoli T, Folkman J (1998) Tumor vascularity, proliferation, and apoptosis in human melanoma micrometastases and macrometastases. Arch Dermatol 134: 991–994

Becker JC, Pancook JD, Gillies SD, Furukawa K, Reisfeld RA (1996a) T-cell-mediated eradication of murine metastatic melanoma induced by targeted interleukin-2 therapy. J Exp Med 183: 2361–2366

Becker JC, Varki NM, Gillies SD, Furukawa K, Reisfeld RA (1996b) An antibody-interleukin-2 fusion protein overcomes tumor heterogeneity by induction of a cellular immune response. Proc Natl Acad Sci USA 93: 7826–7831

Boon T, Cerottini J-C, Van den Eynde B, van der Bruggen P, Van Pel A (1994) Tumor antigens recognized by T lymphocytes. Ann Rev Immunol 12: 337–365

Coulie PG, Ikeda H, Baurain J-F, Chiari R (1999) Antitumor immunity at work in a melanoma patient. Adv Cancer Res 76: 213–242

Crowley N, Seigler H (1992) Relationship between disease-free interval and survival in patients with recurrent melanoma. Arch Surg 127: 1303–1308

Eshhar Z, Waks T, Gross G, Schindler DG (1993) Specific activation and targeting of cytotoxic lymphocytes through chimeric single chains consisting of antibody-binding domains and the γ or ζ subunits of the immunoglobulin and T-cell receptors. Proc Natl Acad Sci USA 90: 720–724

Ferrone S, Marincola FM (1995) Loss of HLA class I antigens by melanoma cells: molecular mechanisms, functional significance and clinical relevance. Immunol Today 16: 487–494

Ferrone S, Temponi M, Gargiulo D, Scasselat GA, Cavaliere R, Ratali PG (1988) Selection and utilization of monoclonal antibody defined melanoma associated antigens of immunoscintigraphy in patients with melanoma. In: Srivastava SC (ed), Radiolabeled Monoclonal Antibodies for Imaging and Therapy. Plenum Press, New York, London

Goverman J., Gomez SM, Segesman KD, Hunkapiller T, Lang WE, Hood L (1990) Chimeric immunoglobulin-T-cell receptor complex formation and activation. Cell 60: 929–939

Guerry DP, Schuchter LM (1992) Disseminated melanoma – is there a new standard therapy? N Engl J Med 327: 560–561

Hekele A, Dall P, Moritz D (1996) Growth retardation of tumors by adoptive transfer of cytotoxic T lymphocytes reprogrammed by CD44v6-specific scFv:zeta-chimera. Int J Cancer 68: 232–238

Hombach A, Heuser C, Sircar R, Tillmann T, Diehl V, Kruis W, Pohl C, Abken H (1997) Specific T cell targeting of TAG72+ gastrointestinal tumor cells by a chimeric receptor with antibody-like specificity. Gastroentereology 113: 1163–1170

Hombach A, Heuser C, Sircar T, Tillmann T, Diehl V, Pohl C, Abken H (1998a) An anti-CD30 chimeric receptor that mediates CD3-zeta independent T-cell activation against Hodgkin's lymphoma cells in presence of soluble CD30. Cancer Res 58: 1116–1119

Hombach A, Koch D, Sircar R, Heuser C, Diehl V, Kruis W, Pohl C, Abken H (1999) A chimeric receptor that selectively targets membrane-bound carcinoembryonic antigen (mCEA) in presence of soluble CEA. Gene Ther 6: 300–304

Hombach A, Pohl C, Heuser C, Sircar R, Diehl V, Abken H (1998b) Isolation of single chain antibody fragments with specificity for cell surface antigens by phage display utilizing internal image anti-idiotypic antibodies. J Immunol Meth 218: 53–61

Hwu P, Shafer GE, Treisman J, Schindler DG, Gross G, Cowherd R, Rosenberg SA, Eshhar Z (1993) Lysis of ovarian cancer cells by human lymphocytes redirected with a chimeric gene composed of an antibody variable region and the Fc receptor γ chain. J Exp Med 178: 361–366

Hwu P, Yang JC, Cowherd R, Treisman J, Shafer GE, Eshhar Z, Rosenberg SA (1995) In vivo antitumor activity of T cells redirected with chimeric antibody/T cell receptor genes. Cancer Res 55, 3369–3373

Irie RF, Morton DL (1986) Regression of cutaneous metastatic melanoma was observed by intralesional injection with human monoclonal antibody to ganglioside GD2. Proc Natl Acad Sci USA 83: 8694–8698

Joshi SS, Kessinger A, Mann SL, Stevenson M, Weisenburger DD, Vaughan WP, Armitage JO, Sharp JG (1987) Detection of malignant cells in histologically normal bone marrow using culture techniques. Bone Marrow Transplant 1: 311–315

Lee PP, Yee C, Savage PA, Fong L, Brockstedt D, Weber JS, Johnson D, Swetter S, Thompson J, Greenberg PD, Roederer M, Davis MM (1999) Characterization of circulating T cells specific for tumor-associated antigens in melanoma patients. Nature Med 5: 677–685

Levey DL, Srivastava PK (1996) Alterations in T cells of cancer-bearers: whence specificity? Immunol Today 17: 365–368

Maeurer MJ, Gollin SM, Martin D, Swaney W, Bryant J, Castelli C, Robbins R, Parmiani G, Storkus WJ, Lotze MT (1996)) Tumor escape from immune recognition: lethal recurrent melanoma in a patient associated with downregulation of the peptide transporter protein TAP-1 and loss of expression of the immunodominant MART-1/Melan-A antigen. J Clin Invest 98: 1633–1641

Maeurer MJ, Storkus WJ, Krikwood JM, Lotze MT (1996) New treatment options for patients with melanoma: review of melanoma-derived T cell epitope-based peptide vaccines. Melanoma Res 6: 11–24

Maio M, Parmiani G (1996) Melanoma immunotherapy: new dreams or solid hopes? Immunol Today 17: 405–407

Moritz D, Wels W, Mattern J, Groner B (1994) Cytotoxic T lymphocytes with a grafted recognition specificcity for ErbB2-expressing tumor cells. Proc Natl Acad Sci USA 91: 4318–4322

Nguyen TD, Smith MJ, Hersey P (1997) Contrasting effects of T cell growth factors on T cell responses to melanoma in vitro. Cancer Immunol Immunother 43: 345–354

Piepkorn M, Barnhill RL (1996) A factual, not arbitrary, basis for choice of resection margins in melanoma. Arch Dermatol 132: 811–814

Piepkorn M, Weinstock MA, Barnhill RL (1997) Theoretical and empirical arguments in relation to elective lymph node dissection for melanoma. Arch Dermatol 133: 995–1002

Reinhold U, Liu L, Lüdtke-Handjery H-C, Heuser C, Hombach A, Wang X, Tilgen W, Ferrone S, Abken H (1999) Specific lysis of melanoma cells by receptor grafted T cells is enhanced by anti-idiotypic monoclonal antibodies directed to the scFv domain of the receptor. J Invest Dermatol 112: 744–750

Reinhold U, Lüdtke-Handjery H-C, Schnautz S, Kreysel H-W, Abken H (1997) The analysis of tyrosinase-specific mRNA in blood samples of melanoma patients by RT-PCR is not a useful test for metastatic tumor progression. J Invest Dermatol 108: 166–169

Rosenberg SA, Packard BS, Aebersold PM, Soloman D, Topalian SL, Toy ST, Simon P, Lotze MT, Yong JC, Seipp CA, Simpson C, Carter C, Bock S, Schwartzentruber D, Wie JP, White DE (1988) Use of tumor-infiltrating lymphocytes and interleukin-2 in the immunotherapy of patients with metastatic melanoma. A preliminary report. N Engl J Med 319: 1676–1680

Rosenberg SA, Yannelli JR; Yang JC, Topalian SL, Schwartzentruber DJ, Weber JS, Parkinson DR, Seipp CA, Einhorn JH, White DE (1994) Treatment of patients with metastatic melanoma with autologous tumor-infiltrating lymphocytes and interleukin-2. J Natl Cancer Inst 86: 1159–1166

Schadendorf D, Worm M, Algermissen B, Kohlmus CM, Czarnetzki BM (1994) Chemosensitivity testing of human melanoma cells: retrospective analysis of clinical response and in vitro drug sensitivity. Cancer 73: 103–108

Seliger B, Maeurer MJ, Ferrone S (1997) TAP off–tumors on. Immunol Today 18: 292 –299

Serrone L, Hersey P (1999) The chemoresistance of human malignant melanoma: an update. Melanoma Res 9: 51–58

Stancovski I, Schindler DG, Waks T, Yarden Y, Sela M, Eshhar Z (1993) Targeting of T lymphocytes to Neu/HER2-expressing cells using chimeric single chain Fv receptors. J Immunol 151: 6577–6582

Weijtens MEM, Willemsen RA, Valerio D, Stam K, Bolhuis RLH (1996) Single chain Ig/g gene-redirected human T lympocytes produce cytokines, specifically lyse tumour cells, and recycle lytic capacity. J Immunol 157: 836–843

Wirthmüller U, Kurosaki T, Murakami MS, Ravetch JV (1992) Signal transduction by Fc gamma RIII (CD16) is mediated through the gamma chain. J Exp Med 175: 1381–1390

Yee C, Riddell SR, Greenberg PD (1996) Prospects for adoptive T cell therapy. Curr Opin Immunol 9: 702–708

Subject Index